THE HOSTAGE BRAIN

BRUCE S. MCEWEN
HAROLD M. SCHMECK, JR.

THE ROCKEFELLER UNIVERSITY PRESS
NEW YORK

Copyright © 1994 by The Rockefeller University Press
All rights reserved
Library of Congress Catalog Card Number 94-67849
ISBN Number 0-87470-054-X
Printed in Japan

Medical Illustrator: Lydia Kibiuk
Graphic Designer: Heather Leahy
Editor: Dianne Mitchell
Cover art: Heather Leahy

CONTENTS

ACKNOWLEDGMENTS

I n this final decade of the twentieth century science is seldom an entirely solo undertaking. So it is with the writing of a book on as broad a subject as the brain. Authors need the counsel of other knowledgeable people to help keep the facts accurate and the concepts in reasonable perspective. In that sense, the authors of this volume are indebted to many men and women engaged in studies of the brain and the human mind and to others active in a broad range of additional fields, because the brain, after all, influences everything in the body and is influenced by everything. This field is so vast that many whose ideas and findings were valuable to this book must remain unnamed. Many others are cited in our section on "Sources and Suggested Further Reading." In addition, we would like to extend our specific thanks to the following people for taking the time and effort to help us get started or stay on track.

Nancy Adler, Becky Alhadeff, W. French Anderson, Paul Brown, Karen Bulloch, Grace Castellazzo, Joe Carey, Carl W. Cotman, Richard Harlan, Mony DeLeon, Wayne Drevets, James German, Roger A. Gorski, Terry Keane, Al Kildow, Doreen Kimura, William L. Nyhan, Eugene Redmond, Robert M. Sapolsky, Larry R. Squire, David Thaler, Annemarie Walsh-Mullen, Daniel Weinberger, Torsten Wiesel, and Stuart Zola-Morgan.

In addition to those who gave direct help on *The Hostage Brain*, each of us would also like to thank some others who contributed ideas and, in some cases, guidance and inspiration over the years, all of which have contributed to the knowledge, concepts, and fascination with biological science that have coalesced into this book.

In this category BSM would like to thank, among many other people who deserve mention as well, Roberta Brinton, Mary Dallman, Howard Fillit, Elizabeth Gould, Seymour Levine, Victoria Luine, Michael Meaney, Fernando Nottebohm, Donald Pfaff, Judith Rodin, Robert Rose, Robert Sapolsky, Catherine Woolley and Richard Zigmond, and especially, the late Eliot Stellar. More than sixty-five present and former laboratory colleagues, postdoctoral fellows and Ph.D. students have made innumerable contributions over twenty-eight years. BSM would also like to thank The Rockefeller University, which has been his scientific home for more than twenty-eight years and has provided the rich intellectual environment and freedom to explore many areas of science whether or not they were fashionable at the time. In particular, BSM acknowledges with warm appreciation his teachers, Vincent Allfrey and the late Alfred Ezra Mirsky, for having made him aware of the complex interactions between genes and the environment, and to Holger Hyden and Neal Miller for having first introduced him to the wonders of the brain and behavior.

HMS owes similar debts of aid and insight to Katherine L. Bick, Floyd Bloom, Robert N. Butler, Theodore Friedmann, Clarence J. Gibbs, Jr., Murray Goldstein, Frederick K. Goodwin, J. Allan Hobson, Paul D. MacLean, Michael Merzenich, Neal Miller, William E. Paul, Nathan Shock, Solomon Snyder, Novera Herbert Spector, Richard J. Wurtman, and, especially, the late James A. Shannon and DeWitt Stetten, Jr. HMS would also like to thank *The New York Times* for encouraging him to explore the rapidly expanding frontiers of science for nearly thirty-three years, for insisting always that he set down the results accurately in language anyone could understand and get it all done in time for first edition deadline.

A special note of thanks from both of us goes to Heather Leahy and Dianne Mitchell of The Rockefeller University Press for their conscientious and highly professional design and editorial efforts, respectively.

After these expressions of sincere thanks, however, both authors must assure the reader emphatically that any errors or other shortcomings in this book are ours alone.

THE HOSTAGE BRAIN

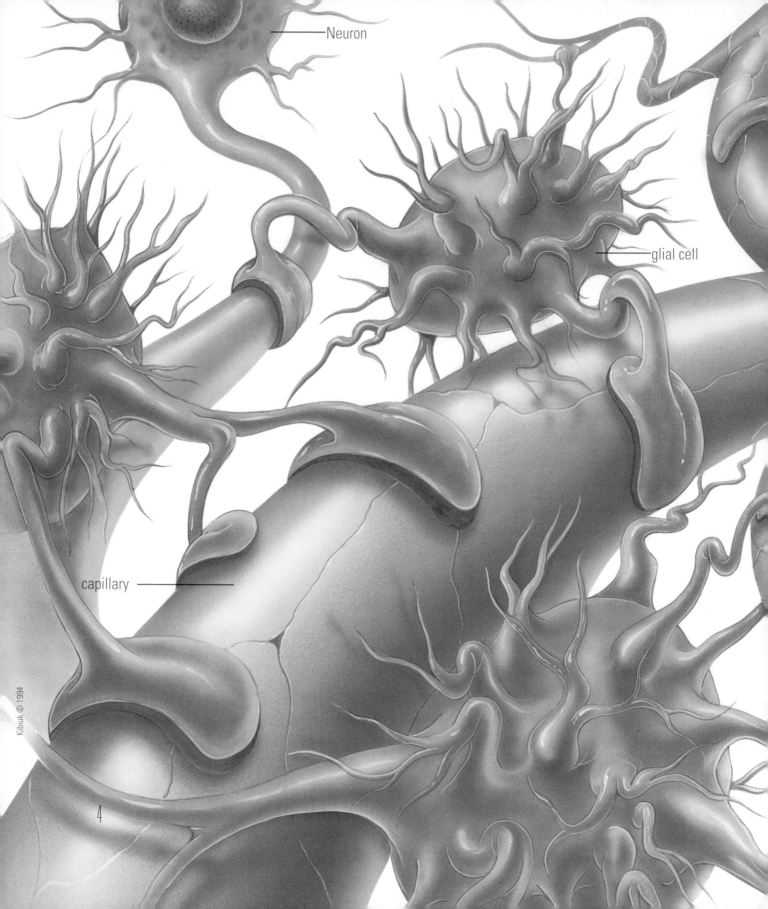

Neuron

glial cell

capillary

Kibiuk © 1994

4

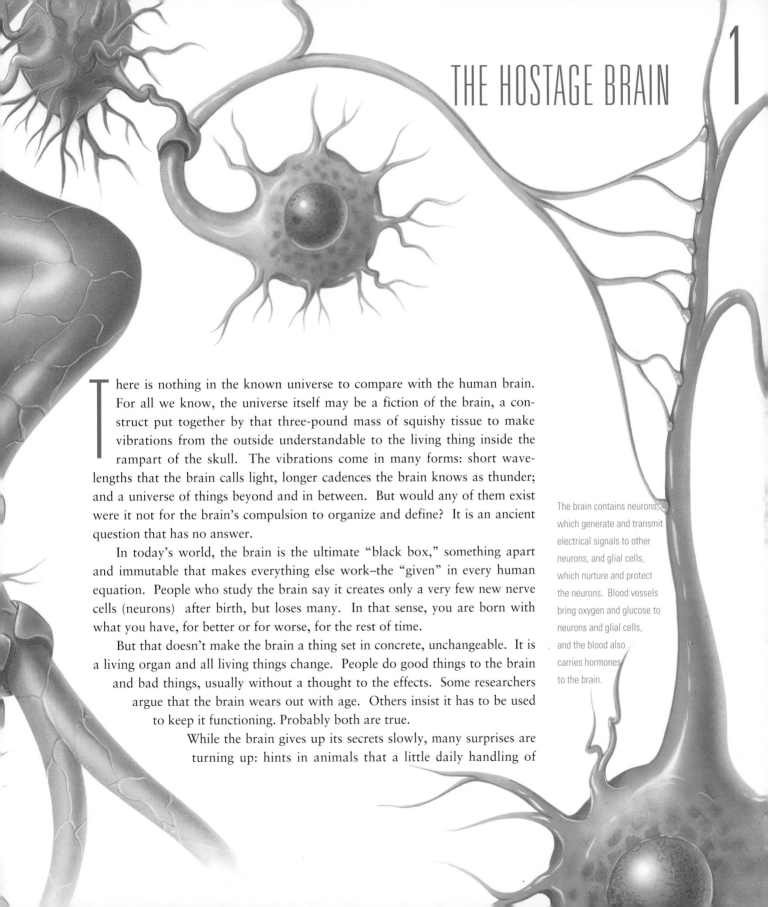

There is nothing in the known universe to compare with the human brain. For all we know, the universe itself may be a fiction of the brain, a construct put together by that three-pound mass of squishy tissue to make vibrations from the outside understandable to the living thing inside the rampart of the skull. The vibrations come in many forms: short wavelengths that the brain calls light, longer cadences the brain knows as thunder; and a universe of things beyond and in between. But would any of them exist were it not for the brain's compulsion to organize and define? It is an ancient question that has no answer.

In today's world, the brain is the ultimate "black box," something apart and immutable that makes everything else work—the "given" in every human equation. People who study the brain say it creates only a very few new nerve cells (neurons) after birth, but loses many. In that sense, you are born with what you have, for better or for worse, for the rest of time.

But that doesn't make the brain a thing set in concrete, unchangeable. It is a living organ and all living things change. People do good things to the brain and bad things, usually without a thought to the effects. Some researchers argue that the brain wears out with age. Others insist it has to be used to keep it functioning. Probably both are true.

While the brain gives up its secrets slowly, many surprises are turning up: hints in animals that a little daily handling of

The brain contains neurons, which generate and transmit electrical signals to other neurons, and glial cells, which nurture and protect the neurons. Blood vessels bring oxygen and glucose to neurons and glial cells, and the blood also carries hormones to the brain.

newborn pups may affect their brains in ways that actually delay the aging process; in humans, suggestions that there may be a good time of day and a bad time for breast cancer surgery in women or a best time of year for men to take college examinations, all because of the rhythmical ebb and flow of hormones controlled, ultimately, by the brain. There are even hints that a too avid reduction of cholesterol or other fatty materials in the blood may raise the toll of violent deaths including murders.

The human brain has an agenda of its own as it confronts and adapts to a changing world. It changes in chemistry and even in architecture day by day, possibly even minute by minute, reshaping itself continually to cope with experience. It is obvious that the brain must change if it is to perform in the incredible fashion we take so much for granted, but the changes go deeper and are more pervasive than scientists had realized until now. Brain cells take on new duties when needs or opportunities arise. Just how they do this is still a mystery.

The brain also produces hormones that used to be considered the sole property of the body's endocrine glands. What does the brain do with those hormones? That too is still a mystery. On another front, scientists have discovered much that is new about the plasticity and everchanging nature of the brain. It may produce few more neurons, but the vital connections, the synapses, and the connecting links called dendrites, do change and reorganize parts of the brain continually. It is those billions of synapses and dendrites that link the vast throng of brain cells into a complex and everchanging skein. Without these changes there would be no habits, no thoughts, no consciousness, no memories, in fact, no mind. There would be nothing human at all.

Infection and physical injury can also buffet the brain from the outside. The brain is shaped by quirks of its own experience and, even more strange, it can become the creature of its own thoughts. For millennia humans have grown accustomed to some of these effects. The ancient Norse berserkers were known to work themselves into combat frenzy to achieve prodigious feats of strength oblivious to pain. The legendary Assassins wrought the same kind of changes with the drug hashish. In both, the performance was really the brain's influence on the body. It has even been argued that the first use of cereal grains may not have been porridge but beer—"Drink this and gods will enter your soul!" In today's world, everyone knows of the man who gets "fighting drunk" or the person who claims to become poetic or musical "under the influence." Many brains fall hostage to alcohol and other chemicals. That has always been one of the greatest human tragedies.

There are many ways the human brain can be taken hostage and there are ransoms to be paid. We humans need to know the price our brains pay for all the things we do and leave undone. All vertebrate animals have brains, but only among some of the more complex creatures is the brain conscious of its own existence. This self-conscious state is the strangest and most important sense in which the human brain has become a hostage. It has become hostage to its own great power and its own knowledge. The ransom is responsibility. Whether, and how long, the species survives will depend on how well we pay that ransom. That fact is the most compelling reason for studying the brain. We need greater understanding of its nature, its possibilities, and its limits to help it cope with life. The brain changes continually to confront reality. The question is whether or not it can change well enough to survive the changes it is making in the rest of the world.

The everchanging brain seems a farfetched concept only to people who persist in thinking the "mind" is somehow distinct from the brain and that the brain just sits there, running the whole show, aloof and inviolate on top of the backbone. In fact the brain is the whole show. The heart may be the symbol of St. Valentine's Day, but it is the human brain that falls in love, gets angry, goes mad, explores the core of the atom and the farthest reaches of the universe. The brain, sculptured by the whole gamut of experiences from birth onward, is the mind and the whole personality. All this is what makes one person a poet, another a rock star, a third a traffic cop or a sheep herder. The brain is a dynamic, living organ affected by body chemistry and every nuance of life. In turn, the brain affects everything else: the individual's body, the community of humans and other animals, even world climate, as students of the greenhouse effect are learning today.

As a personal matter, thoughts influence hormone flow, the action of sweat glands, the pulse, and the heart, as everyone knows full well who has ever been frightened, angry, or in love. And thoughts, essentially, are the everchanging electricity and chemistry of the brain, perhaps even its physical architecture.

At the heart of all this is the brain's enormous population of neurons. They send and receive the signals through which the brain governs the body and responds to its needs. There are billions of neurons in the human brain, and a hint of awe creeps into the voice of the scientist who tries to explain them to a layman. The cliché is that neurons are the fundamental units, the building blocks, of the nervous system. But "building block" is far too simple a label. Neurons are alive, sophisticated, and semiautonomous. They perform a multitude of tasks. They generate and react to both electrical and chemical signals in the brain. They shape our hates, fears, and joys, our every strategy for coping with the universe.

Neurons come in a bewildering array of different sizes and shapes. No other species of cell has such variety. Some neurons appear small and simple. Others look like tall trees in silhouette. Still others resemble garden shrubs that have grown luxuriantly unpruned. But there is little or nothing random in these brain cells. The extensions that look like twigs and branches connect one neuron to a myriad of others in a supremely purposeful, yet mysterious, network of cells. Working together through their billions upon billions of connections, the neurons orchestrate all the signals through which the brain functions. In this labyrinth of connections, the nerve cells are the embodiments of the human mind.

The neuron has three fundamental parts: the cell body, which includes its nucleus and cytoplasm, the many extending branches called dendrites, and the single main extension called the axon. The classically simple definition was that the axon transmits a nerve signal through a combination of electricity and chemistry. In turn, it is influenced by signals received from the thicket of dendrites from other cells. As neuroscientists piece together the details of this process, they find the classic definition far too simple. The interconnected neurons influence each other in many unexpected ways. No one claims to understand the entire process.

The most intricate part of the system is the chemistry. It used to be thought that each neuron used only a single neurotransmitter, a chemical that sends or relays nerve signals. The identity of the neurotransmitter in any circuit depended on the type of nerve cell and its location in the structure of the brain. Now it is known that one neuron may use several signaling chemicals and that they can restrain or augment each other in a multitude of ways. Some neurotransmitters even switch on or off the functions of genes, adding another level of complexity to the brain's controlling influence. Several dozen such signal chemicals are known and the number is still rising. But the chemicals themselves are only half of their own story. To deliver its message, every neurotransmitter must home in on a matching structure, called a receptor, on or inside the destined target cell. The receptor catches the message from the signal chemical and translates it into action.

Working closely with the neurons is another class of brain cells called glia, from a Greek word meaning glue. The glial cells provide structural support for the forest of neurons.

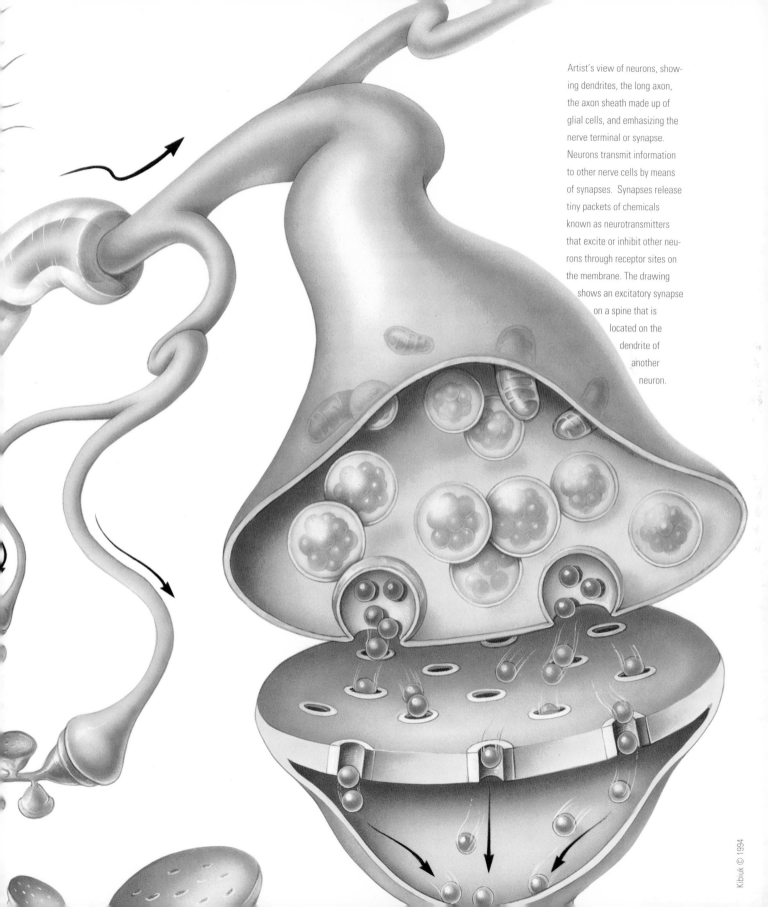

Artist's view of neurons, showing dendrites, the long axon, the axon sheath made up of glial cells, and emhasizing the nerve terminal or synapse. Neurons transmit information to other nerve cells by means of synapses. Synapses release tiny packets of chemicals known as neurotransmitters that excite or inhibit other neurons through receptor sites on the membrane. The drawing shows an excitatory synapse on a spine that is located on the dendrite of another neuron.

Kibiuk © 1994

They soak up and screen out chemicals the brain doesn't need and feed the neurons with other substances for energy and nutrition. They produce an insulating chemical called myelin to sheath some nerve fibers. In many respects, the neurons, glial cells, and other elements of the brain are shielded from the rest of the body by a chemical fence called the blood-brain barrier. But that doesn't mean the brain is a thing apart and aloof. It affects everything in the body and is affected by all the body's ups and downs, demands and quirks.

Your brain is affected by what you eat and even more powerfully by what you drink. It responds to light and darkness, time of year. It can be damaged by heat or a sudden blow, even by invading bacteria and viruses, including the AIDS virus. The brain stores an immense library of memories and can call up concepts with speed, precision, and flexibility that amaze computer scientists. The intimate relationship between the human brain and the rest of the world appears more and more wonderful as scientists explore brain function, using sophisticated tools that, of course, the brain has invented. For many years, philosophers debated the proposition that the mind is an entity somehow apart from the brain. Some still believe it, but nobody has real evidence for that view. In the tangible world of reality, the mind is the orchestration of the brain's functions as it confronts experience. During human life, the mind does not exist without the brain. Whether the human brain will ever fully understand itself no one can guess. There is something mystical in the very question.

But important advances are percolating today. Effects of the brain's experience on its own performance continue to amaze. Unexpected links between cause and effect abound. Take, for example, a subject that seems to have nothing at all to do with the brain: new medicines that reduce the amount of fatty materials in the human bloodstream to protect against heart disease. These anticholesterol drugs have helped lower the number of heart attacks and the deaths these attacks cause in many Americans. So, the drugs must reduce the overall death rate, right?

Well, no, not exactly. Among those who use the drugs, the death rate from heart attack has plummeted, but the total death rate has changed hardly at all.

At first, that seems to defy logic. The drugs do save lives. Specialists convened by the National Institutes of Health recommended: "All Americans (except children younger than two years of age) should be advised to adopt a diet that reduces total dietary fat intake." Experts of the European Atherosclerosis Society gave essentially the same opinion.

But these expert conclusions were not quite the whole story. Several major studies showed that lowering cholesterol still left the overall death rate unimproved. That same point came up time after time, like the loser's three lemons in an old-fashioned slot machine. Some people who might have died from heart disease must be dying of something else. Cancer seemed a logical answer. It is the other great killer of Americans. Faced with the puzzling data from much research, a University of Pittsburgh team took a hard look at the evidence. They analyzed studies that had covered nearly twenty-five thousand male patients many of whom took the anticholesterol drugs. The life stories were followed for years. During that time more than eleven hundred of the men died. A painstaking review produced some clear conclusions: lowering patients' cholesterol levels did reduce the toll of heart attack deaths. Furthermore, the Pittsburgh team found "no consistent link between reduction of cholesterol concentrations and mortality from cancer." Instead, they found that the deaths did not come from disease at all. They came from violence: auto accidents, mishaps in sports or in the home, drownings, suicides, and even murders. The cause seemed not to be the anticholesterol drugs themselves, but the very act of lowering the blood fats. Unexpectedly, this abrupt lowering seemed to affect the chemistry of the brain. Some studies showed that aggressive behavior often went with low blood cholesterol in violent psychiatric patients, criminals, and people who habitually fight when drunk. Large human populations whose customary diets are low in cholesterol don't seem to be affected, but in rats and monkeys, experimental diets that reduced cholesterol unnaturally produced exactly the kinds of behavior likely to raise the risk of violent death. Almost inadvertently, the numerous study results stumbled into territory that had been little explored: the effects of the blood serum's cargo of fatty materials on brain and behavior.

Scientists at Bowman Gray School of Medicine in North Carolina put groups of adult male monkeys on two different diets to study the effects of too much fatty food. For almost two years one group ate a fat-rich "luxury diet." The others were on a "prudent" low fat diet. At the study's end it was obvious that the luxury diet was bad for hearts and arteries, but even earlier something else became obvious. The dominant monkeys on the prudent diet were more aggressive on the average than those in the other group. It wasn't because those on the rich diet grew fat and lazy. They didn't. Perhaps the luxury diet somehow had a pacifying effect, but there wasn't much evidence of it. On balance, it appeared that animals on the prudent diet were more violent than the others.

Writing in the journal *Psychosomatic Medicine*, the authors said their results did fit well with studies in humans suggesting that "relatively low serum cholesterol concentrations are prevalent among persons who characteristically engage in violent behavior."

Maybe Shakespeare, as usual, had it all figured out 300 years ago. Consider the famous words he put in Julius Caesar's mouth:

"Yond' Cassius has a lean and hungry look. He thinks too much: such men are dangerous."

The team at Bowman Gray didn't say the prudent diet made people think too much. They did suggest a clue to the violence: lack of the important brain chemical serotonin. The scientists said they observed that monkeys fed a low cholesterol diet also had low serotonin activity in their brains when compared with animals that consumed a relatively high fat diet. Some violent criminals also showed a similar pattern of blood chemistry. Serotonin is one of the brain's main neurotransmitters. Like many important brain chemicals, it was first discovered in the intestine and the bloodstream and was later found to function in widespread portions of the brain. There is also evidence that poor function of nerve circuits that use serotonin occurs in severe depression and suicidal behavior. Some of the most effective antidepressant drugs act by increasing the effectiveness of nerve signal transmission via serotonin.

Predictably, not all the evidence on blood fats is on one side. A small study done recently in the Midwest showed that symptoms of depression improved in patients who were treated to reduce their severely high levels of blood fats. The authors of the study cited other research tending toward the same conclusion. This kind of divergence in results is common, even typical, in good biomedical research. There is great variation among human beings. We are individuals and we do differ from one another in a multitude of ways, including responses to drugs.

Where does all this leave the anticholesterol crusade? Certainly, it doesn't cloud the value of reducing cholesterol and other fats in individuals whose blood is seriously overloaded. These people need to lower blood fats to survive and their sense of personal well-being may improve with the treatment. But much research does suggest that sharp dietary reduction in cholesterol is not a harmless panacea or even necessarily a prudent diet for the entire population. The brain has its own special needs. People ignore these at their peril.

The cholesterol conundrum may be only the latest episode in humans' failure to pay enough attention to their own behavior that might make hostages of their brains. No one can guarantee that a course of action will leave the brain alone, just because the intentions were not directed at the brain.

There have been many other examples, including the use of alcohol and the so-called recreational drugs. The cholesterol-lowering drugs are at least used under medical supervision with doses that have been established after thorough study. Most drug use is much more haphazard and more dangerous. The sorry example of steroid drug use by muscle builders is just such a case. These drugs have important medical uses, but no one ever asserted they are totally risk free. The wholesale use adopted by some athletes takes the question of ill-effects into frighteningly uncharted territory. As usual, the last thing any user of such drugs considers is that this effort at muscle building might also affect the brain. Part of the reason is tragically obvious. Often the drug user starts the habit at the age of fifteen or even younger when life seems limitless and nobody worries about abstractions like bad drug reactions. A study in 1988 estimated that more than 6% of all male high school seniors under the age of eighteen were using, or had used, anabolic steroids, the kind that help build muscle. That, according to one authority in sports medicine, means something between 250,000 and 500,000 young adult males. When asked, teenagers and young athletes give several reasons for taking the drugs. One survey put them in this order: first, to improve athletic ability; next, to improve appearance; and also for "social reasons," for injury prevention, and injury treatment. Worries about the mind at that age? Who needs it?

Yet for more than fifty years, doctors have known that these drugs can have powerful mental effects. So obvious were these effects that at least one steroid drug—testosterone, the male sex hormone—was used deliberately as an alternative to electroshock treatment for severe mental illness. Early reports said the drug treatment seemed to be as effective as the shocks.

One of the earliest studies of the psychiatric uses of steroid hormones, published in 1938, involved six mental patients who were described at the start as "disturbed, anxious, and broken in spirit." Two of the six men had earlier been castrated for reasons that were not specified; two were cases described as "psychic impotence," and two "hypogonadal," a term that means abnormally low function of sex glands. All of the patients suffered from depression and emotional instability, as well as chronic mental and physical fatigue. They took a testosterone preparation three times a week and their mental attitudes bloomed. Depression changed to elation and, interestingly, to a state their doctors described as "rational aggressiveness."

In another case, doctors tried two drugs simultaneously, methyltestosterone and imipramine, in two severely depressed patients. The depression vanished to be replaced by what the doctors described as "a paranoid reaction." The drug treatment was halted. That effect of the combination of two different drug types is interesting in the light of what muscle builders often do to themselves today.

Unlike medical patients, who will usually take one specific steroid for a limited time, some athletes gobble them as though they were jelly beans. The amounts and combinations some men take are far greater than anything ever prescribed for any medical treatment. Athletes refer to this steroid gorging as stacking. Typically, several different steroids are taken in gradually increasing dosages, some daily and some at intervals of one or two weeks. This is likely to be followed by a period of several weeks without the drugs and then the cycle is repeated.

The steroids do seem to accomplish some of the users' objectives, including the building of muscle tissue, production of more energy, and a decreased need for sleep. They also show effects that can be good or bad depending on the degree and the circumstances. Some users say they get elevated mood, faster speech, quicker mental function, sharper eyesight and hearing, and heightened sexuality. One expert said they also tend to develop "very aggressive personalities that allow more intense training." It all sounds good, but these effects can shade into makings of tragedy: irritability, heightened impulsiveness, grandiose delusions, and a broad range of psychiatric problems, including paranoia, mania, and hallucinations. Reports of such bad reactions began to appear in the medical literature in the early 1980s, but it is seldom clear whether the drugs are entirely to blame or whether these are stories of people who were on the borderline before they took the drugs and might have tipped over the edge with them or without. Many people apparently can take steroids without disastrous effects.

A team of sports medicine specialists, in a letter to the *New England Journal of Medicine*, said they gave psychological tests to more than fifty athletes who used the drugs at the time or had done so in the past, and compared these people with athletes who did not use steroids. The research turned up no significant differences at all between the two groups in aggression, hostility, or tension and anxiety. The only behavioral difference the doctors found was that the men who were taking the steroids had more feelings of guilt than the others. They went beyond the nonusers in feelings of "being bad, having done wrong, or suffering pangs of conscience." Were these direct psychological effects of the drugs or were they just evidence of the "bad press" those drugs have received in recent years? For the athlete, however, there is another problem. The gains in muscle size and strength disappear rapidly as soon as drug use stops. This could lead to continued use just to maintain the hard-won gains of training.

If the medical issue is still clouded, steroids seem to be making an impact on the American legal system. In today's blame-anything-but-me atmosphere, defendants and their lawyers find it tempting to blame violence and antisocial acts on steroids much as earlier generations might have claimed "the Devil made me do it." Another condition sometimes blamed for strange or socially unacceptable behavior is premenstrual syndrome in women, known in today's popular jargon as PMS. The condition occurs in some women a week to ten days before menstruation and usually ends quickly after menstrual flow begins. It is thought to be related to fluctuations in the hormones estrogen and progesterone. A wide range of symptoms has been attributed to the syndrome, including nervousness, agitation, anger, lack of self control, and difficulty in concentrating. Both PMS in women and excessive steroid use, usually in male athletes, have been used in court cases to explain abnormal behavior. How often these explanations are justified can be debated, but PMS is a real biological phenomenon and not the result of any voluntary personal action. In contrast, abuse of steroid drugs is something the athlete does deliberately to himself. So well-publicized has the blaming of steroids become that reporters covering legal cases have called it "the dumbbell defense."

Whether the drugs be the cause or just a weight that tips the scales, some users of the hormones for bodybuilding have suffered major episodes of depression when withdrawing from the drugs and some have claimed the steroids are seriously addictive. The case histories are often compelling.

A young man took large doses of several steroids for bodybuilding over a period of months and went to a doctor because he found it impossible to stop taking the drugs without becoming depressed and fatigued. He developed an intense craving for them and feared he was becoming addicted.

The physician gave him a drug used for opiate addiction and the patient promptly went into the typical set of withdrawal symptoms: his hair stood on end; his pulse rate and blood pressure went up. He vomited, suffered chills, headache, and profuse sweating. The doctor gave him clonidine to cope with the withdrawal symptoms. A week after this "fight fire with fire" attempt to use other drugs to cope with damage from the first batch, the man telephoned to say that he couldn't stand it any longer. He was going back to the steroids.

Another case involved a seventeen-year-old athlete who was diagnosed as schizophrenic and who improved markedly during treatment with the widely used antipsychotic drug haloperidol. After about a year, he stopped the treatment and his symptoms returned. At this point he confided to his doctor that he had been weight lifting during the six months before his first diagnosis and had been taking large quantities of steroids. Had the drugs contributed to his mental illness? Perhaps yes, perhaps no, but the case alerted doctors to the possibility. Several other reports have appeared in medical and psychiatric journals since then, but, of course, large numbers of young men and women are taking these drugs for muscle building yet the tales of disaster are relatively rare.

One extensive study involved interviews with thirty-nine men and two women who took steroid hormones in the course of weight lifting and body building. These athletes took the drugs by themselves and in many cases used amounts that were 10 to 100 times the doses ordinarily prescribed in medical studies. None of the drug-takers had any evidence of mental illness before their self-initiated medical experiments. Most of them continued to appear essentially normal while they were taking the drugs, but five reported hallucinations or delusions during the drug-taking periods and an additional four reported what their doctors called "mild or equivocal psychotic symptoms."

Said Drs. Richard E. Harlan and Meredith M. Garcia, of Tulane University School of Medicine, in discussing such effects: "Despite the limitations of this kind of retrospective study, these results, combined with several case studies, clearly suggest adverse changes in mental status during exposure to large doses of androgenic-anabolic steroids."

These are the types of steroid drugs most often used in bodybuilding. The scientists noted with particular interest that of the athletes most seriously affected all used not just one type of steroid, but several drugs embracing both of the major categories.

The authors, studying the chemistry as well as the psychology of these effects, have a hypothesis to explain the effects. While evidence compiled by others points suspicion at reduction of serotonin activity as a clue to violence, Drs. Harlan and Garcia propose that steroids lead to an increase in dopamine, another of the brain's major neurotransmitters, and that this increase perturbs networks in the brain

Neurons have many shapes and forms.

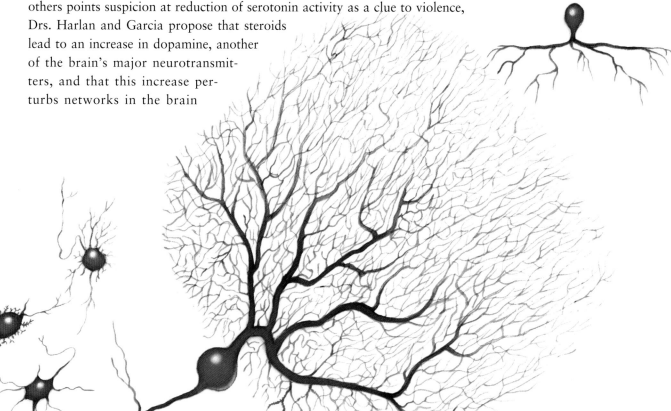

that are intimately concerned with emotional outlook and goal-directed behavior. The two ideas—serotonin down and dopamine up, to oversimplify them drastically—need not be altogether in conflict and neither idea has yet been proved. The chemistry by which networks of neurons communicate in the brain is extraordinarily complex and far from totally understood. Dopamine and serotonin are each vital to that chemistry and there is evidence linking each to brain functions that are intimately related to emotion and reaction to danger.

Furthermore, the mystery is not all chemistry. The brain is also an organ that uses electrical signaling in the transmission of nerve signals. The electricity and chemistry work closely together. As long ago as the early 1960s, Dr. José M.R. Delgado of Yale University startled the world by showing that he could stop a bull in midcharge by electrical stimulation to the animal's brain. He set up the experiment by putting hair-fine electrodes into carefully chosen parts of the animal's brain and linking them to a small radio receiver strapped to the animal's head. With this equipment, he could deliver electricity at long range by pressing a button on a transmitter. He also demonstrated that he could convert a dominant monkey in a social group to a subservient one by the same long-range electrical brain stimulation. Several years after those experiments in animals, Drs. Vernon H. Mark and Frank R. Ervin, working at Harvard, reported success in halting violence in a few epileptic patients by the same means, using equipment developed by Dr. Delgado. These experiments highlight the complexities of the hostage brain concept. The brain of Dr. Delgado's bull seemed to be captured by the radio signal. But the patients of Drs. Ervin and Mark are more complicated examples. Were they hostage to the electrical signals that were intended to rescue them from violence, or to the epileptic attacks that produced the violence?

Neither the animal nor the human experiments seem to have been pursued in recent years. The attempts by Mark and Ervin got a lot of adverse publicity and charges that they were attempting brain control and were seeking to shift the blame for human violence from social injustice to brain defects. Also the internal complexities of the brain raised some questions on what the animal and human experiments actually proved. Dr. Delgado himself noted that the individual neurons that he stimulated were parts of intricate systems in which signals passed continually to and from widely separated parts of the brain. His electrical signals did hit their targets precisely, but the effects must have reverberated widely through the brain. How does one pin down precise causes and effects in that situation? Vital to the story of the hostage brain is heredity because that is where everything in life begins. While each newborn baby has at least the hope of vast opportunities and broad horizons, the genes set the outer limits. It is those 100,000 or so messages written in the language of DNA, that make us human rather than hummingbird or giant octopus. The concept of heredity has been mangled beyond recognition by the racist atrocities and totalitarian idiocies of this century, but the basic truths remain. We are, to a major extent, the creatures of our genes.

Yet even the functioning of the genes isn't totally impervious to harm. That seems particularly true of the developing brain although many details are still murky. The brain of the unborn child can be taken hostage by the deprivations, infections, and other wounds inflicted on the mother, as later chapters will show.

Like every good romance, our story of the hostage brain begins with sex because there is nothing more important to any mammal. The true compulsion of the genes is to get themselves reproduced in the next generation. To the DNA, each bride and groom are simply the vehicles. After discussing the little fragment of DNA that decides which wears the bridal veil and which the striped tie, the story will proceed to the genetic system itself: how it carries out the orders of the great blueprint and how errors and accidents can capture the brain early in life.

No forces set to work by the genes are more powerful or more crucial than the hormones. They affect almost every function of the brain, not the least its conscious thoughts. The fact that the mind can be captured by its hormones is one of mankind's oldest stories, and one of the newest. Stress, which can also capture and distort the brain, is largely a matter of hormones. This subject is so important that it deserves two chapters with topics that range from the stresses that keep us alive and vibrant to the shock of armed combat and even the stress of hopelessness. Science today is coming to grips with the anatomy of fear. Specialists have traced the brain circuits by which terror echoes through the mind. They have probed the small, deep-set center where fear begins. These stories are followed by the saga of that other great language, the language of immunity. This is the great biological system that keeps us healthy long enough to pass on our genes. In the later decades of life, more and more mistakes creep in, allowing infections and other more complicated diseases. Could it be that the genes lose interest in the body after the reproductive years?

There are strange ways in which the immune system too can take the brain hostage—and vice versa, as a little tale of witchcraft will make clear.

Although many of us ignore the primeval facts of our solar system, time of day and season of year can also warp the brain's perceptions. Here our story will tie together the birds, the bees, and breakfast time to show why humans should not forget their biological clocks.

For all of its wonders and mysteries that we can only dimly glimpse, the brain is a physical organ. It weighs only a few pounds and occupies no more volume than a half gallon of milk. What is this object that has invented music, truth, and justice, and may have invented the universe? For that matter, is it more the product of its "nature" or its "nurture" and what is the good news and the bad news of what we can and cannot do to help the brain?

Among the most tragic items of the bad news are dementias that steal the mind from itself. Some of these thefts that take the brain hostage are infections and some, like that great mind plague of our era, Alzheimer's disease, are of unknown cause. Finally, the story will touch on questions that call for the highest wisdom to reach the bottom line. Why should we want to learn about the brain at all? Has the human brain finally become hostage to its own consciousness; its own powers of reason and judgment? Is our ransom the debt of responsibility not only to our families and our species, but to all life on Earth? If so, what should we do to improve the human brain? What should we avoid doing?

Research on the everchanging brain has never been a single clear voyage forward. It is a series of quests launched from many ports into a vast unknown. As we will see, many of those ventures set out through seaways defined by disease and injury to the brain. Science does not always steer straight toward its predetermined goals. It goes where opportunity beckons.

Today, the quest for knowledge seems to beckon more enticingly than ever before. In July 1990, President George Bush proclaimed the 1990s the Decade of the Brain. The proclamation said in part:

"Over the years, our understanding of the brain—how it works, what goes wrong when it is injured or diseased—has increased dramatically. However we still have much more to learn. The need for continued study of the brain is compelling: millions of Americans are affected each year by disorders of the brain ranging from neurogenetic diseases to degenerative disorders such as Alzheimer's, as well as stroke, schizophrenia, autism, and impairments of speech, language, and hearing.

Today, these individuals and their families are justifiably hopeful, for a new era of discovery is dawning in brain research..."

Some scientists look at the brains of people who have died in extreme old age for clues to the nature of aging and to the tragic parody of that process that erases the mind in Alzheimer's disease. At the other end of the spectrum, researchers study the burgeoning of the human brain in embryo and fetus. The organ takes shape from a tiny cluster of neurons-to-be in the ball of new cells that are growing, multiplying, and evolving to become a human being. Even this seemingly esoteric frontier of embryology and fetal research is producing some bitter controversies today. It all starts during the embryo's twelfth week of life in the womb.

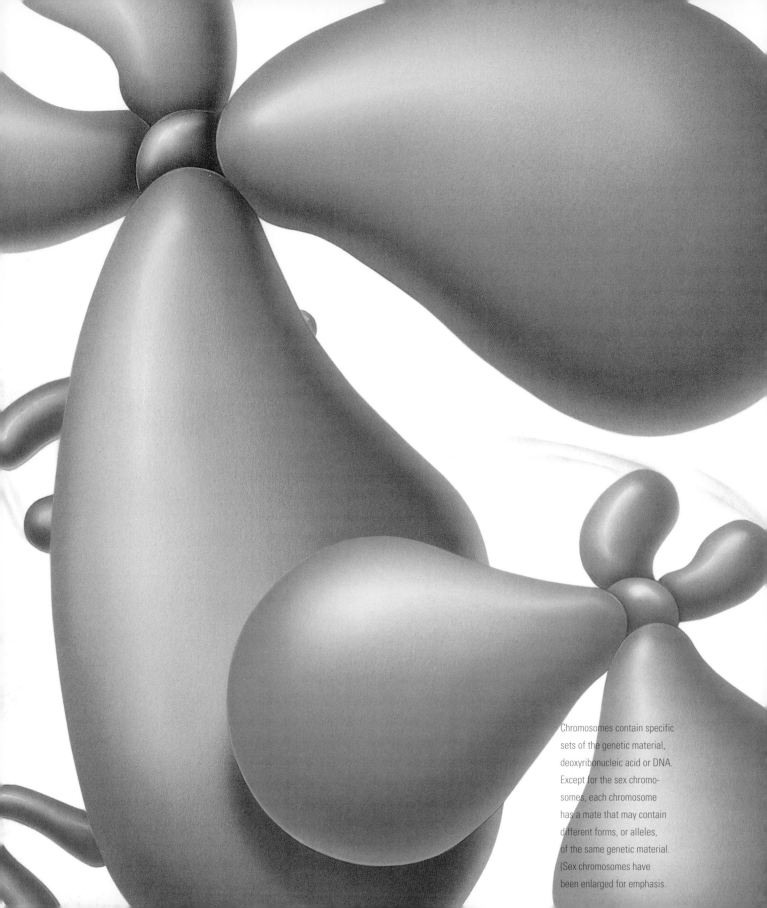

Chromosomes contain specific
sets of the genetic material,
deoxyribonucleic acid or DNA.
Except for the sex chromosomes, each chromosome
has a mate that may contain
different forms, or alleles,
of the same genetic material.
(Sex chromosomes have
been enlarged for emphasis.

SEX AND THE SINGLE GENE

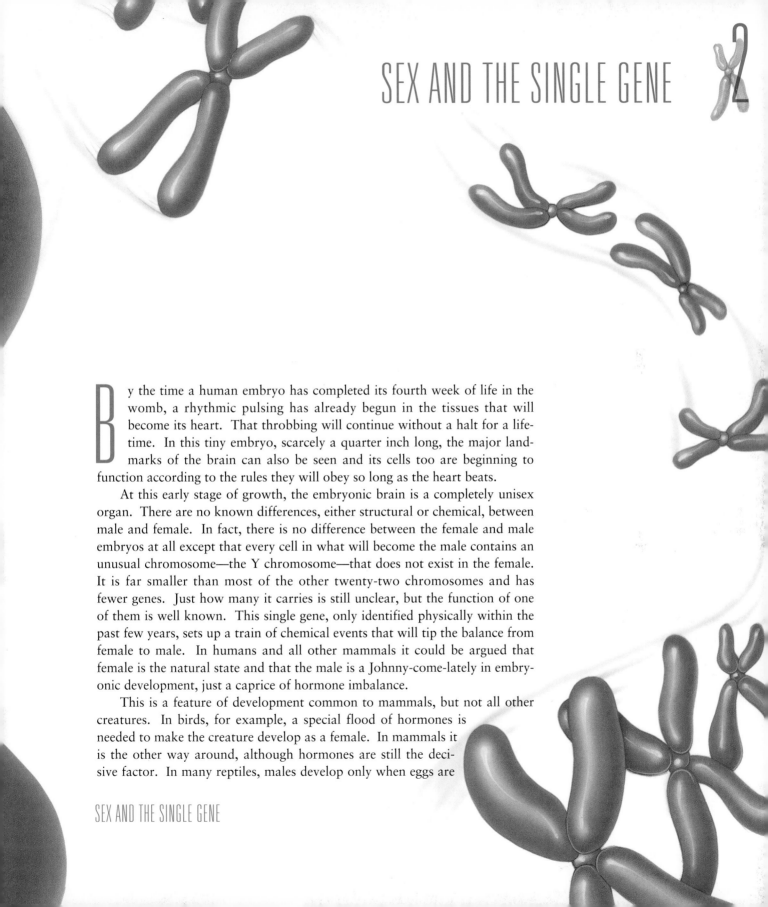

By the time a human embryo has completed its fourth week of life in the womb, a rhythmic pulsing has already begun in the tissues that will become its heart. That throbbing will continue without a halt for a lifetime. In this tiny embryo, scarcely a quarter inch long, the major landmarks of the brain can also be seen and its cells too are beginning to function according to the rules they will obey so long as the heart beats.

At this early stage of growth, the embryonic brain is a completely unisex organ. There are no known differences, either structural or chemical, between male and female. In fact, there is no difference between the female and male embryos at all except that every cell in what will become the male contains an unusual chromosome—the Y chromosome—that does not exist in the female. It is far smaller than most of the other twenty-two chromosomes and has fewer genes. Just how many it carries is still unclear, but the function of one of them is well known. This single gene, only identified physically within the past few years, sets up a train of chemical events that will tip the balance from female to male. In humans and all other mammals it could be argued that female is the natural state and that the male is a Johnny-come-lately in embryonic development, just a caprice of hormone imbalance.

This is a feature of development common to mammals, but not all other creatures. In birds, for example, a special flood of hormones is needed to make the creature develop as a female. In mammals it is the other way around, although hormones are still the decisive factor. In many reptiles, males develop only when eggs are

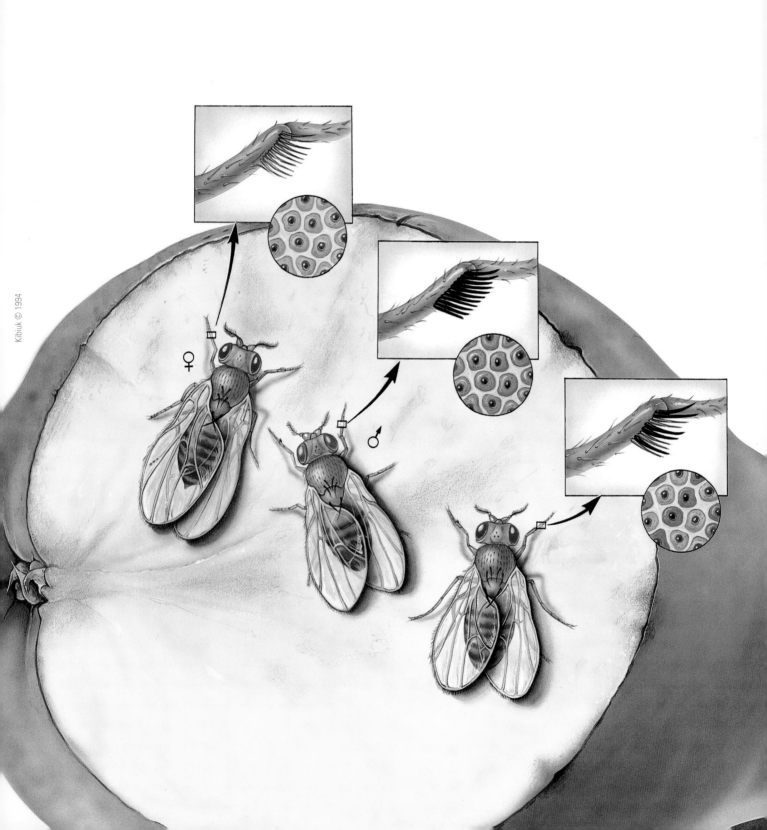

incubated at a critical temperature. Above or below that temperature the eggs hatch females. In insects such as the much-studied fruit flies, *Drosophila*, individual cells have a large measure of autonomy. Laboratory workers can construct strange male-female mosaics by transplanting cells in an embryo. As one example, a typically male antenna can be made to grow on a fly that is otherwise female.

Particularly among Americans, it sometimes seems that the discussion of sex is only safe when it doesn't seem to matter; when it is something long ago or in a far distant species. Current biology hasn't bowed to those prim restraints. Are males and females different in their mental abilities? Are the brains of men different from those of women? For that matter, are the brains of homosexuals different from those of heterosexuals and is there a homosexuality gene variant? Recent research has raised each of these questions and each issue has been denounced by one or another fiery advocate of sameness. Nevertheless, sex is biological reality. It has much to teach about the brain, and the brain reveals much about sex. For one thing, sex starts early and exerts a multitude of effects throughout the life span.

In humans, the process of sexual differentiation begins at about the twelfth week of embryonic development and lasts for eight weeks. During this crucial period of a little less than two months, hormones generate a cascade of changes in the developing male with each new phase multiplying the effects that have gone before. The first step, under the guidance of that single gene on the Y chromosome, is to prepare a welcome for testosterone, the male sex hormone on which much of the process will depend. To make the hormone's actions possible, the gene triggers action by other genes in many cells so that they are able to respond to the chemical message the hormone brings. To be more specific, receptors appear inside the cells destined to become targets for testosterone. These receptors serve as bull's-eyes that the hormone molecules seek and occupy. All of the myriad events that follow stem from that initial flow of hormone and the presence of receptors that give the testosterone places to act.

In the female embryo, development is more a strengthening of the status quo, but here too the embryo takes steps to prepare for its own torrent of hormones.

Hormones are messengers produced in special tissues. They flow with the bloodstream to distant target cells where their messages are delivered and put into action. Those messages can only be acted on by cells already prepared to do so. Through the flow of genetic instructions, genes in the potential target cells become active, causing the cells to produce proteins that serve as receptors for the particular hor-

Sex characteristics in the fruit fly are not dependent on circulating hormones but rather on messages emanating from sex chromosomes in individual cells. Thus a mosaic fly, made up of male and female cells, shows coexisting male and female characteristics.

mones those cells will use to start new processes valuable to the cell and the body in general.

The hormone is like the ignition key for a car. The receptor is the ignition switch turned on by that key to start the complicated engine of the cell. In reality the system is much more complicated than that. Every cell has many different receptors–inside, or protruding from the surface. Cellular receptors are among the vital elements in the body's, and the brain's, grand design for using chemistry to communicate and execute orders. Cells react to many substances, each of which fits one particular type of receptor. There are many copies of each type and the numbers of receptors rise and fall with changing needs and conditions in the body. In the process of determining sex, hormones have a crucial advantage. As they flow through the body, they can coordinate the development of many diverse tissues along paths to the same sexual identity.

The steroid hormones that figure so importantly in human development are only one broad class of messenger molecules. But the production of steroid receptors inside cells is a potent event that shapes the anatomical, chemical, and mental future of the person. Only with those receptors in place can the whole torrent of changes proceed by which the embryo that has no Y chromosome will develop as a female while the embryo equipped with the Y will change to become a male. Recent studies of the brain show that neurons have receptors for all of the six classes of steroid hormones and the brain actually manufactures hormones itself. No one has yet figured out completely how these so-called neurosteroids are used.

Among the steroid hormones, testosterone is particularly crucial to sexual differentiation. Produced by the embryonic tissue that will grow into the testes, it has many familiar effects on the male body, including development of the male sex organs and the fading away of some female features such as the Müllerian duct that would otherwise become the fallopian tubes and uterus. The process of differentiation actually unfolds in two parts that are quite distinct from each other in developmental terms. These are masculinization and defeminization. The sensitive periods for inducing them do not necessarily coincide, nor are the processes equal in degree in all species. In animals, such as rats and monkeys, that have been most studied in embryology, masculinization includes such behavioral results as rough and tumble play in the young and male sexual and aggressive behavior later. Defeminization is the suppression of feminine sexual behavior, maternal behavior, and ovulation. But are these changes in behavior foreshadowed by physical modifications of the brain? Are the brains of males and females physically different from each other? It was long assumed that they were not.

While the main physical differences between human males and females have been obvious to every human since the species began, the fact that sexual differentiation shapes the brain itself has only gradually become accepted. Perhaps that is a mental legacy of the bias that sees the brain as a black box too mysterious and powerful to be subject to change.

One startling glimmer of truth came with the discovery that chemistry can change the attributes of sex itself. This can occur only during the sensitive period of sexual development. In rats this period stretches from a few days before birth to a few days after. Females given heavy doses of testosterone during this period develop physical traits and behavior like those of normal males. Male rats castrated during this sensitive period, to deprive them of the male sex hormone, develop as though they were females. Genetically, the sexes were not altered. The males still have the male chromosome while the females do not, but the functional and behavioral attributes of sex are switched. Timing of the experiments is crucial. No hormone bombardment in adulthood will produce the change. It can only be done during the sensitive period near birth.

The comparable period of sensitivity in humans is the twelfth to twentieth week of embryonic life. An obvious question is whether or not a similar hormone disruption would have a like effect on a human embryo. It is a plausible guess, but difficult to prove and it is not easy to imagine how the hormonal accident could happen. In any case, the special capacity to change an animal's functional sex was not direct evidence that sexual differentiation affected the brain. It simply showed the powerful effects of hormones on development in general.

Do hormones actually alter the physical architecture of the embryonic human brain? Many people prefer to dodge the question. Sex differences in the brain go beyond science and become an incendiary social issue. The reasons aren't hard to guess. Not too long ago, it was "common knowledge" in many societies that men and women were different in the way their minds worked. Their thought processes were simply not the same. People who believed this saw ample evidence and it was seldom convenient to ask whether the differences were strictly hormonal or the sum results of upbringing, much less whether they really existed beyond the prejudices of the observer. The bottom line was usually that women should stay meek and not be troubled with such things as having careers outside the home, or the vote, or even personal freedom. Over several generations, American women have fought free of those shackles. Even today, some don't believe the battle has been won. Many are suspicious of anything that seems like a counterattack under the camouflage of science.

In short, some people don't like the new biological evidence. It is dangerous and therefore not to be believed. But one ingrained form of prejudice does not justify another. Scientists are studying the black box of the brain with a sophistication never achieved before. The results are seldom palatable to dogma on either side of the sex issue.

Thus, in the 1960s, research workers took further steps into the unknown and discovered that cells in the brain do have receptors for sex hormones and are therefore almost certainly targets for those hormones. The details of the evidence gave strong hints that the hormones act to influence, even to turn on, behavior. Men and women differ in the ebb and flow of sex hormones, but still the new data did not budge the politically charged dogma that the brains of men and women must be identical.

Then, a direct hit on the dogma was made by Donald Pfaff, then at Massachusetts Institute of Technology, now at The Rockefeller University. He turned an inquiring eye on the hypothalamus of the rat's brain.

The hypothalamus is a small region deep in the brain that is the focus of much research. It is part of the "old" brain, the portion that goes farther back in evolution than even the common ancestor of man, mouse, and rat. In humans, as in all other mammals, it has many vital functions. Among these are the regulation of hormone production in the pituitary gland; the maintenance of proper water balance in the body; and the regulation of the autonomic nervous system–the system that controls such largely involuntary functions as the beating of the heart, the movements of the intestines, and the functioning of the glands.

The hypothalamus is also crucial to feeding and drinking behavior and to sexual reproduction. All of these are functions on which survival of the individual and the species depend. They arose long before the brain of act-and-react, fight-or-flight evolved into the thinking human brain that clothes all of those ancient imperatives in a cloud of new concepts–"should," "shouldn't," "maybe" and "shame!"

Analyzing the structure of rat brains, Dr. Pfaff found significant differences between males and females in the size of nerve cell bodies in the hypothalamus. But, again, there was the old chicken-or-the-egg problem. Did these differences arise from hormone effects in the adult or were they the results of sexual differentiation "hard-wired" in the brain during development? The research could not answer the question.

Then came a discovery in 1971 by two scientists at Oxford University. It is now considered a landmark in the study of sexual dimorphisms–differences between male and female. When they did the work, the two scientists were not concerned with differences between male and female brains. They were look-

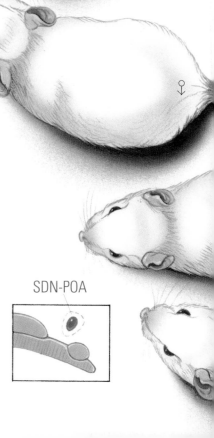

SDN-POA

SDN-POA

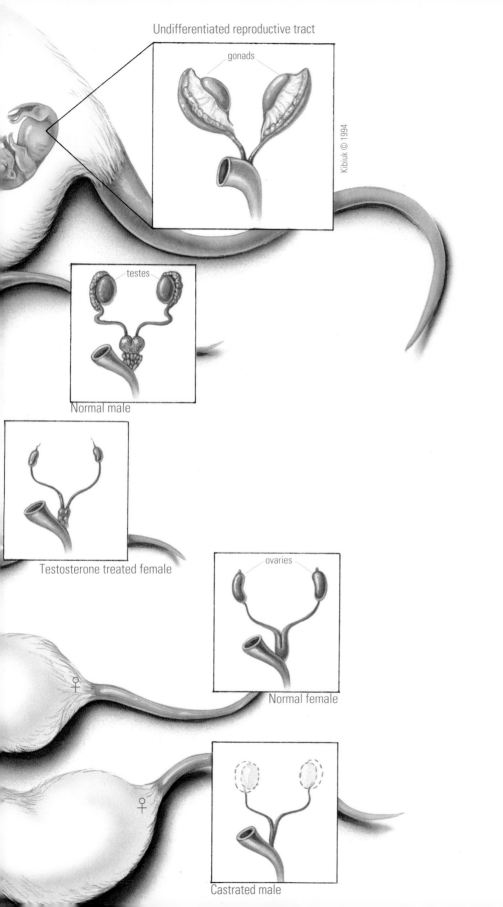

Undifferentiated reproductive tract

gonads

Kibiuk © 1994

testes

Normal male

Testosterone treated female

ovaries

Normal female

Castrated male

For mammals, like the rat, sex is determined for the whole organism by the presence or absence of testosterone during early development. Brain structures like the SDN-POA (sexually dimorphic nucleus of the preoptic area) become larger as a result of early exposure to testosterone and are therefore larger in males than in females; other brain structures are larger or of different shape in the female compared to the male brain, presumably because testosterone was not present during an early stage of their development.

ing for new ways of treating nerve disorders in patients.

"I wasn't looking for sexual dimorphism in the brain originally," Dr. Geoffrey Raisman recalled twenty years after the event. "I was looking at the ability of the brain to form new connections after injury and during development and learning."

He and his co-worker, Pauline M. Field, were searching through the animal brain with the electron microscope, studying minute slices of tissue at high magnification to find synapses, the connections between one brain cell and another. Each neuron and each of its projecting tendrils (called dendrites) establish thousands of connections and make the whole brain an almost infinitely interconnected skein of cells. It is the evolution of this complex web that gives the human brain its marvelous flexibility and power to think, remember, and react. All mammalian brains share a measure of that sophistication.

Dr. Raisman said their study marked the first time he and his colleague, Dr. Field, were able to use the electron microscope to see the synaptic connections in the brain. They were looking for new synapses that the rat's brain made after injury, but they found something much more important.

In an interview with the *Journal of NIH Research*, Dr. Raisman explained: "The head of my department, Geoffrey Harris, was interested in the way the brain controlled sexual function, particularly, in controlling female egg production. This is a function that depends on the release of hormones and is controlled by the brain."

It was obvious that only the females would ever produce eggs. Males were not equipped to do it. This clear difference would give a promising way to study changes in the brain and match them with specific causes related to the animals' sex. There was evidence from other studies that the hypothalamus was a key to the process and would be the place to look. But, even though the hypothalamus is a relatively small part of the total brain, it is still a continent-sized hunting ground to anyone searching through it with the electron microscope. The scientists picked a particular brain region of the hypothalamus, called the preoptic area because there was evidence that a lot of hormone action involved that region and it might be easiest there to find the new synapses the two scientists were seeking.

Drs. Raisman and Field knew the history of earlier research on sex differentiation in the brain: that the process depends on the flow of hormones to the embryonic brain tissues and that the wrong hormone would upset the pattern and change the functional sex of the animals. So they waded into the laborious task of counting and classifying thousands of synapses in their chosen area of the rat brain. Each of the two researchers counted about a half million synapses by Dr. Raisman's estimate. It was a huge task that took them four months.

They did the research in a way that is called a blind experiment. While they were counting and analyzing the brain slices of rat after rat, they kept themselves deliberately ignorant of the sex of the animals from which the specimens came. Each brain slice was identified by a code number and the sex of each coded specimen was kept in a sealed envelope. All of this crucial material was held by another member of the department who was not involved in the actual research. The counting and analysis of synapses is tedious and repetitive. It is the kind of work that threatens to numb the most alert mind, yet it requires skill and continuously sharp judgement. In such a situation, a blind experiment is a necessary safeguard. It insures that the resulting data are objective and not distorted by any unconscious bias that might make the researcher see what he or she had expected to see under the electron microscope instead of what was actually there.

At the end of the process, the scientists made a ceremony of opening the sealed envelopes. As they opened one after another, the team's delight increased. The data fell beautifully into groupings by sex. The synapses in the male brains were structurally different from those of the female brain and the numbers of new synapses were different too. New brain connections were lacking in the males and present in the females in just the pattern the scientists had hypothesized. In the areas of the hypothalamus that they studied, Drs. Raisman and Field showed clearly that the brains of male and female rats were physically different. These and later research results showed unmistakably that the differences in hormonal secretions of males and females produced differences in the anatomy and wiring pattern of the brain. The circuits were not hard-wired from earliest embryonic development, but had changed in the course of sexual differentiation. The ebb and flow of hormones had done it. Next, the team repeated the research strategy that had given early hints of male–female differences. The team castrated newborn male rats to reduce

corpus callosum

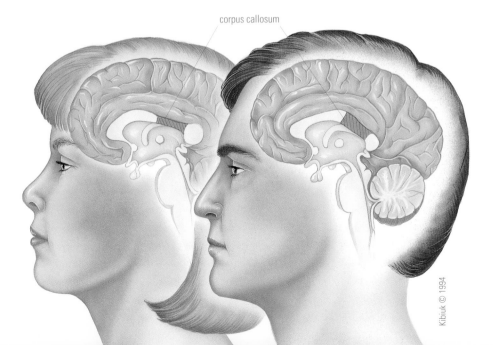

The corpus callosum, the bundle of nerve fibers that connects the two hemispheres of the brain, differs in shape and in size between left and right handers and between men and women.

Kibiuk © 1994

male sex hormone production and gave testosterone to females to raise the dose. From the early work, the scientists knew that these treatments had effects on the animals' sex characteristics and behavior. But what would actually happen in the brain regions they were exploring? They found that the large number of synapses that normal females developed were also present in the castrated males. The testosterone-treated females had the low number characteristic of normal males. There was no longer any reasonable doubt that sex differences did exist in the brain.

This early research focused on just two areas of the rat brain that are involved in the control of reproduction: the preoptic and the ventromedial areas of the hypothalamus. Throughout the 1970s and 1980s, brain researchers expanded the landmark discovery to other areas of the brain and to other species including humans.

Today, the catalogue of known differences between the brains of males and females is impressive and extends well beyond aspects that are directly related to reproduction. Experts on the brain have known for a long time that the cerebral hemispheres—the two sides of the "thinking brain"—are almost symmetrical, but not quite. It is also known today that the asymmetry is different between men and women. That may account for the observation in medical studies that injury, such as stroke, affecting only one part of the cerebral hemisphere on one side of the brain results in different losses of function in men and women. Some complex functions, such as organizing words into speech, depend on the front of the left hemisphere in women and on the posterior left hemisphere in men. Moreover, in assessing the meaning of words, women use the two hemispheres more equally than men. Thus, the geography of basic speech mechanisms in the brain is known now to be somewhat different in men than in women although the differences are neither large enough nor sufficiently clear-cut to be described simply. There are differences also in one of the great trunk nerve cables of the human brain: the corpus callosum that connects the right and left cerebral hemispheres. Some of the major tracts of the corpus callosum are larger in women than in men, while other tracts are larger in men. Why this is true and what effect the differences have on brain function is still a mystery.

Beyond the ancient prejudices concerning men's and women's roles, there is also some modern evidence for differences between the sexes in certain mental abilities. On the average, women appear to be more skilled in verbal tasks and fine motor coordination, while men are better in perceiving spatial relationships and in physical skills like throwing a ball or kicking a football. Men, on the average, are more adept in certain realms of mathematics and logic.

The reports of mental differences between men and women have had some incendiary social effects: charges of bias, insensitivity, and worse. Is it discrimination against women in general to discover such differences? Some people assert that it is. Much of the smoke and fire of controversy has been fanned by debaters who seem intent on ignoring most of the facts and the simple word "average." There is ample evidence that differences among individuals in almost any skill will be far greater than the average differences between the sexes. To reduce the argument to familiar territory only partly related to brain function: men, on the average, are taller and stronger than women and no one would expect the world's top woman tennis player to beat the first-ranked man. But any ordinary male player who parlayed that proposition into the hope that he could beat Steffi Graf or Monica Seles would be in for a rude six-love, six-love, six-love shock. Indeed, Billie Jean King proved the same point decisively many years ago against the overoptimistic Bobby Riggs.

An entirely different kind of controversy erupted in August 1991 via another study published virtually on the twentieth anniversary of the report by Raisman and Field. Early brain studies in animals had demonstrated that it was possible to produce permanent changes in sexual behavior by aberrant internal chemistry during a critical period of embryonic development. There is no real animal model of homosexuality, but the evidence from hormone studies hinted that some feature of chemistry might produce that condition in humans. It was by no means clear how such abnormal hormone exposure could come about, but the question lurked in the air: were the brains of homosexual humans different in any way from the brains of heterosexuals of the same genetic sex? To brain specialists and biologists in general, the concept is no great surprise. The brain, after all, is the organ that controls behavior and also is an organ that changes with behavior. Homosexuality is behavior and it should not seem amazing to find traces of either its causes or its effects in the brain. But such brain effects are exceedingly difficult to study in humans and there has been an almost total lack of data on the subject. A report in the journal *Science* on August 30, 1991, gave one of the early pieces of solid evidence on where in the brain the differences may lie. The report was published under the headline "A Difference in Hypothalamic Structure between Heterosexual and Homosexual Men."

The research that found this difference was another tedious, but illuminating, search through microscope slides of the brain, not in rats or monkeys but in forty-one humans on whom routine autopsies had been done. Dr. Simon LeVay, then of the Salk Institute for Biological Studies in San Diego, explored small hypothalamic structures in postmortem studies of sixteen men who were presumed to be heterosexual even though six had AIDS, eighteen homosexual men all of whom had AIDS, and one bisexual man. The postmortem examinations also included six women one of whom had AIDS. Dr. LeVay explained that a study like this had not been possible before the AIDS epidemic made autopsy material available from large numbers of humans who were known to be homosexual. In the past, he noted, sexual behavior toward members of one's own or the opposite sex has been studied mainly in psychology, anthropology, or ethics. There has not been much opportunity for studies correlating the biology or anatomy of the brain with sexual preferences.

Given the new autopsy material made available by the AIDS epidemic, Dr. LeVay focused on four minute clusters of cells in the front portion of the hypothalamus known to pathologists as interstitial nuclei of the anterior hypothalamus. They were discovered and named in the late 1980s by Dr. Roger A. Gorski and Laura Allen of University of California at Los Angeles who also showed that there were differences between men and women in the sizes of these nuclei. In the shorthand jargon of the field the nuclei are known as INAH 1, 2, 3, and 4. Each of these nuclei is spherical or ellipsoidal in shape. In volume they are only about as big as medium-sized grains of sand. Dr. Gorski's team found that INAH 2 was twice as large in males as it was in females and that the male INAH 3 was nearly three times larger than the female. Monkeys in which tissue in this part of the hypothalamus was cut surgically showed derangements in heterosexual behavior even though their sexual drive was not eliminated. That and evidence from other animal species raised the possibility that at least two of the nuclei are involved in regulating human sex behavior.

"These two nuclei could be involved in the generation of male-typical sexual behavior," Dr. LeVay said, so he decided to test the proposition that they might differ in size depending not on biological sex itself, but on sexual preference. It was an ingenious idea that brought the anatomy of the human brain into studies of sexual behavior. It may have been only the second scientific report to do so. A few years previously, D. F. Swaab and M. A. Hofman of Amsterdam reported finding size differences between heterosexual and homosexual men in another portion of the hypothalamus, the suprachiasmatic nucleus. This nucleus is of particular interest to brain scientists because it is a pacemaker that governs the body's natural day-and-night rhythms. Yet another structural difference between brains of heterosexual and homosexual males has been found by Drs. Allen and Gorski: a difference in a strand of nerve fibers called the anterior commissure.

In Dr. LeVay's recent work, his hypothesis was that the nuclei INAH 2 or 3, or both, would be large in men and women who were sexually attracted to women and that the nuclei would be small in men and women who were oriented toward men. It wasn't likely that the other two nuclei, INAH 1 and 4, would reflect these preferences, but they were useful as study controls.

Among his forty-one autopsied brains, none of the six women who died of AIDS had been known to be lesbians. That part of the hypothesis could not be tested. But Dr. LeVay did have enough male brains to test. As was expected there were no significant clues in either nucleus 1 or 4. It turned out that there were no marked differences in nucleus 2 either. But in INAH 3 there

The human brain has structures which differ in size, on the average, between men and women. Groups of nerve cells, known to neuroanatomists as "nuclei," are larger in the male hypothalamus, whereas the average size of the anterior commissure (c) and massa intermedia (b) tends to be larger in women than in men. The corpus callosum (a), connecting the two hemispheres of the brain, differs in size and shape between men and women.

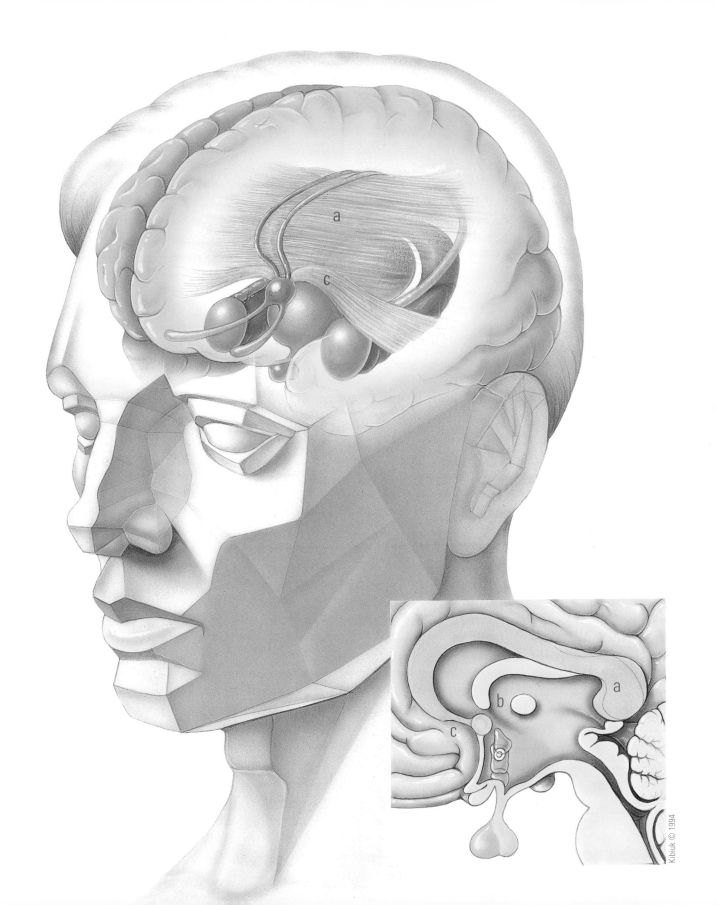

were. This nucleus solidly confirmed Dr. LeVay's theory. In heterosexual men, INAH 3 was more than twice as large, by volume, as it was in the homosexuals. Something linked, not to genetic sex, but to a behavioral trait—sexual preference—was mirrored unmistakably by an anatomical feature of the human brain.

Dr. LeVay, known as a meticulous research worker, did not make any extravagant claims. His report noted that the evidence was an association, not a proof of cause or effect, and that the findings might well have uncovered a factor in a larger biological process that produces sexual preferences in humans. His report warned that "further interpretation of the results of this study must be considered speculative." But he also noted that his discovery shows that sexual orientation in humans, a behavioral trait, may now be open to objective biological study. He suggested that it might be possible now to find neurotransmitters or receptors that help regulate this aspect of human personality. Information of this kind would be a major advance in understanding the brain and the way it organizes behavior.

Sexual preference is a touchy subject, and suggestions that it may be a question of biology rather than either morals or free choice is touchier still, even though biologists and students of the brain know that it is certainly biology. What else is the human brain if not a biological organ?

Dr. Thomas A. Schoenfeld, of Clark University, put it succinctly in a letter in *Science* commenting favorably on Dr. LeVay's report. After noting that the biological basis of behavior is a premise for psychobiology, he wrote, "...it is still all too common to see early experience, social learning, or choice pitted against biology, but these are false dichotomies. This is because the brain has been shown or is assumed to be the underlying mechanism in these processes. Several decades of empirical work have shown that the brain is a product of early experience, social environment, and genetic instructions. So, it manifests the workings of both nurture and nature. Moreover, while the effects of both nurture and nature on the brain and behavior can be enduring and resistant to change, they need not be inexorable... Choice may be a forceful biological process in its own right."

About two years after Dr. LeVay's report, another study was published in *Science* that seemed to take the issue even farther toward nature and away from nurture in its broad sense of total life experience. Dr. Dean H. Hamer, of the National Cancer Institute, was the leader of the new research effort. His team was trying to determine whether or not male sexual orientation is influenced by heredity. Some family studies and other evidence indicated that this might be true.

Through a detailed study of 114 families, Dr. Hamer's team discovered a small piece of genetic material near one tip of the X chromosome that seemed to be strongly associated with male homosexuality. Starting with a panel of seventy-six homosexual men, the research team compiled family histories of all the 114 families that included homosexual members. This was followed by detailed studies of the DNA. The gene that determines male biology is on the Y chromosome, but the focus of the new research was on the X. The family studies by Dr. Hamer's group showed that inheritance of the homosexuality trait seemed often to come through the mother. That route ordinarily means that the X chromosome is involved. The work brought the scientists to a small stretch of genetic material that, statistically, was strongly linked to male homosexual preference and behavior. There was no immediate clue to a specific gene that might be responsible, nor what the biological function of that gene might be. Dr. Hamer's report estimated there is room in that stretch of the X chromosome for several hundred genes.

"Once a specific gene has been identified, we can find out where and when it is expressed and how it ultimately contributes to the development of both homosexual and heterosexual orientation," the report said. The study also made it clear that the segment of DNA is, at most, a clue to one source of homosexuality in men. From the study results, it appeared that there must be other factors too. The findings offered little information on women. But the research team suggested that the evidence should be useful "for identifying additional genes or environmental, experiential, or cultural factors (or some combination of these) that influence the development of male sexual orientation."

Specialists, including Dr. Hamer, emphasized that the research at the National Cancer Institute must be repeated and confirmed by others before it can be taken as fact. Modern genetics research is strewn with reports of strong associations between genes and behavior, genes and disease, that have had to be discarded. Confirmation of research results by other groups working in the same field is a crucial requirement in all scientific work. This is particularly true of studies on a subject as complex, variable, and socially volatile as the contributions of nature and nurture in human sexual behavior.

By the usual definition, nature is genetics and nurture is everything else. All of these issues, including nature, nurture, choice and the limits of choice, will arise again as later chapters deal with many disparate forces that threaten to take the human brain hostage.

But, first, all the issues, including many aspects of behavior, do ultimately go back to the genetic archive of DNA. The puzzles in that realm are as intriguing as any other component of the human brain's great quest to understand itself. Just such a case was the search for the elusive but powerful sex gene on the Y chromosome.

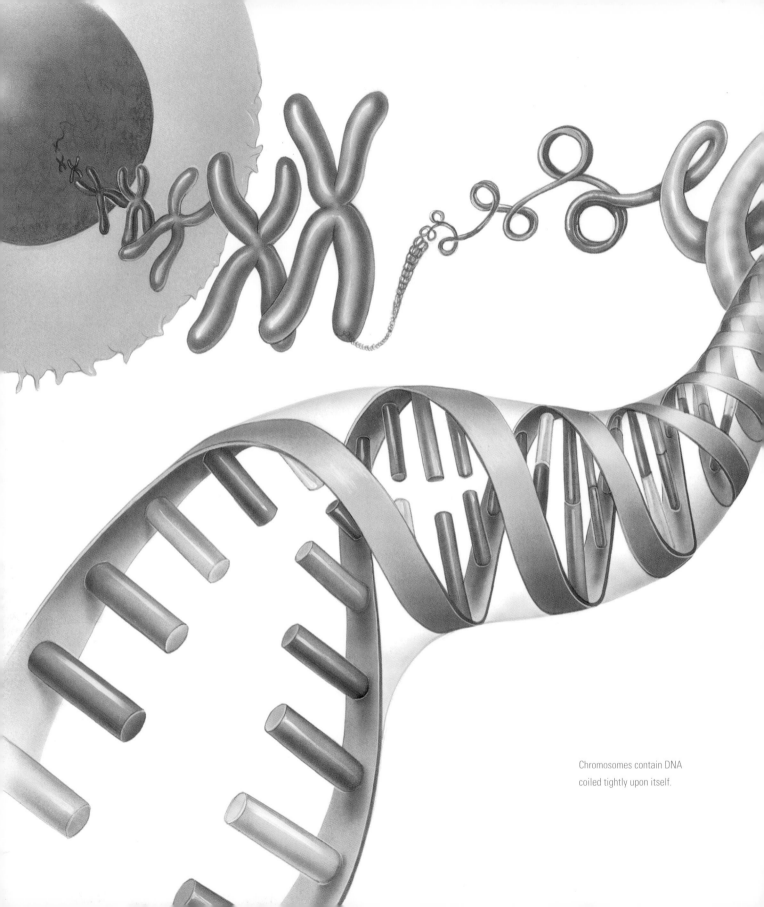

Chromosomes contain DNA
coiled tightly upon itself.

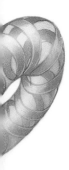

Genes are the common currency of heredity. Every trait and every chemical process in the body is controlled by a gene or a constellation of genes. Consider that singular gene on the human Y chromosome. For more than thirty years geneticists have tried to find it. There must be a switch to turn on the complicated process of male development, so a gene to play that role must exist. It must be on the Y chromosome, because that tiny thread is the only piece of genetic apparatus that distinguishes the male from the female human. The long-sought gene must take the first step: triggering a speck of embryonic tissue to develop into the male testes rather than the female ovaries. Thus begins a cascade of events, rousing a host of other genes into action and quieting still others. It starts the dance of hormones that makes hair sprout on the male chin, the voice change in the adolescent boy, and all the other developments that spark the male's compulsion to find a companionate set of chromosomes that have no Y. The gene had to be discovered if scientists were ever to understand sex. It was crucial to brain research because sex has powerful effects on the brain and the brain governs virtually every aspect of sex. In fact, sex is probably the most compelling case for the entire concept of the everchanging brain. But where in the Y was that gene?

Today the question seems an obvious one to ask. Research teams are hard at work trying to find and map every single gene in the whole human genome–the total archive of human heredity. In recent years, molecular biologists have learned how to read the messages of the genes. Now they thirst to open up the whole encyclopedia of genetic information. Not only can educated biologists read the messages of the genes, they can even write messages of their own and have those messages understood and obeyed by living cells. We are becoming literate at last in the oldest language on earth, the language that spells out the form and functions of all creatures and has always done so since life began.

The messages are coded in the chemical structure of deoxyribonucleic acid, familiar to the world as DNA. The discovery of that code and molecular biologists' rapidly growing ability to read and write in that most ancient language has been one of the greatest triumphs of the human imagination. It is already affecting our lives, our health and wealth, and our whole conception of the place of humans in the world of life. It has all happened within the last half century and most of it within the past thirty years. The genes of spiders, blue whales, bacteria, giant sequoia trees, and human beings all use the same language of DNA. All life on Earth has probably always done so. Recently, scientists found a twenty-million-year-old magnolia leaf that, through some incredible series of accidents, had evidently escaped destruction since the earliest days of the mammals. To no one's surprise, its DNA is about the same as that of modern plants and animals.

So, the search for the gene that triggers sexual differentiation in humans was an obvious as well as an important quest. Even today the total number of human genes is still only a rough guess; 50,000 was the accepted estimate in recent decades, later revised to 50,000–100,000 and now often put at 100,000 or more. Most of the human genes are located in the cell nucleus on twenty-three pairs of chromosomes, joined threads of genetic material that look like wiggly Xs when the microscope makes them visible. On the average, a chromosome holds several thousand genes. Most of them are still to be identified, although gene mapping, an important specialty of the new biology, has come into being in the effort to find genes and establish their locations on charts of the chromosomes. The Y chromosome is peculiar in many respects. It is among the smallest of the forty-six human chromosomes and its cargo of genes is divided into two domains. One of these is much like the X; in fact, the two have many genes in common. The other portion of the Y chromosome is different and evidently is devoted exclusively to developing the state of being a male. It is on that portion of the Y chromosome that the gene for starting the process of male development must exist. The search for it has involved an ingenious strategy: searching for the gene in patients who didn't

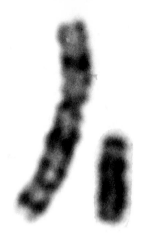

Human chromosome set was provided by Dr. Becky Alhadeff and Dr. James German of the New York Blood Center.

40

have it. Among those who followed that scheme was an international team led by Dr. David C. Page of the Whitehead Institute in Cambridge, Massachusetts. Their strategy went this way: while females have two X chromosomes and males have one X and one Y, there are a few rare people in whom this tidy arrangement fails. A few individuals have two X chromosomes and should be female, but actually turn out to be males. A few others have most of the normal Y, but nevertheless develop as females. Why? To people who follow this subject, the conclusion was that the XX males must actually have a small fragment of the Y chromosome while the XY females lack that same tiny piece. Dr. Page and his colleagues saw this strange fall of the genetic dice as a chance to find the elusive gene because it must lie somewhere on this tiny fragment of the Y chromosome. Even such a region, small in terms of a whole chromosome, is a big territory for gene hunters. Genes are far too small to be measured in inches or fractions of an inch. Instead they are usually measured by numbers of the chemical subunits that make up the long strand of DNA. These units of gene function and measurement are called bases or base pairs. In painstaking studies, the research team narrowed down the field of search to a region of 140,000 base pairs on the Y chromosome. There was room here for a fair number of genes, but close study of the DNA indicated that it probably contained only one. That was a strong hint that the scientists had in their grasp the crucial switch that turns on testes development. The scientists' translation of the genetic message of this gene showed it to be a likely candidate. It would be the kind of structure likely to serve as the switching gene. The evidence was strengthened when they found that closely similar passages in the genetic script existed on the chromosomes of other mammals far removed in evolution from humans. Rabbits and cattle have it. Something similar even appears to exist in chickens. Just before Christmas in 1987, the research team published a report in the journal *Cell* saying their candidate gene was probably it.

But it wasn't quite. As so often happens in science, strong circumstantial evidence was not proof. Attempts by other research teams to confirm the finding were stubbornly unsuccessful. Scientists in Britain found patients who had two X chromosomes, lacked the gene identified by Dr. Page's group, but still were males. Studies of mice gave further evidence that the search was not yet over. In mice, the gene was active at the right time in embryonic development, but not in the right type of cell. It couldn't be the right gene.

The British finally solved the puzzle. The team that did so was led jointly by Dr. Robin Lovell-Badge of the National Institute for Medical Research and Dr. Peter Goodfellow of the Imperial Cancer Research Fund in London. They discovered that the Page hypothesis was correct, but that he and his co-workers had not snared the right fragment of the Y chromosome. The British scientists found another fragment geographically close to the first, but distinct from it. This too was sometimes inherited in people who should have been female, but turned out male. The new fragment had a region of thirty-five thousand base pairs. That piece of chromosome was big enough for several small to middle-sized genes, but it too seemed to contain just one. The scenario was the same as in the earlier search. In their reports, the British group labeled their candidate gene SRY, for sex-determining region Y. Was it the right genetic switch at last? The scientists put it to the final test in a way that is not possible in humans, but today is relatively easy to do in mice.

Using the mouse chromosomes comparable to the human X and Y, the research workers developed transgenic mice that carried the suspect fragment. Research with transgenic animals is one of the strangest and most potent skills of modern molecular genetics. Scientists grow animals which are actually chimeras, to use the ancient Greek term. These modern animals are not quite so fanciful as the monster the Greeks imagined to have a lion's head and a goat's body, but are much more important and, if anything, more bizarre: goats that give human blood substances in their milk, mice that carry human cancer genes, chickens that carry a genetic antidote to a common disease of fowl, and many other strange combinations. This kind of gene transplantation has become a potent tool for research. The foreign genetic material is implanted in the female's fertilized egg even before it has had enough time to become an embryo. As the embryo does develop, it replicates the foreign gene as though it was part of its own normal complement. In successful cases, the animals born from these experiments have the foreign genes and put them to work in the normal fashion. In the search for the male testes-producing gene, female mice were grown that carried the normal genes for female development, but also had the crucial fragment of the Y chromosome. These transgenic "female" mice nailed down the discovery because they developed testes and were functionally male even though all the rest of their genetic inheritance was female. The difference was just the fragment of the Y chromosome and the single gene that it contained. Beyond argument it was the long-sought switch that turned on the process of becoming a male. One of these historic mice, who probably didn't care, had its picture immortalized against an

42

appropriately blue background on the May 9, 1991 issue of *Nature*. It was the journal in which the British scientists reported their discovery.

The single sex gene on the Y chromosome has profound effects on the brain as well as large effects on many of the body's other organs and tissues. It also appears to be the first mammalian gene to be identified that clearly acts as an on–off switch to begin the development of an entire organ system. Inevitably, the story does not end here. In science, the stories never really end. They are all parts of the evercontinuing saga: a series of approximations that should come ever closer to truth. The newfound gene is not by any means the only gene on the Y chromosome. The latest catalogue of known and provisional genes has several pages devoted to the Y. Now scientists want to know what else is percolating on that chromosome. When the switch for maleness is thrown, what are the precise next steps in the rush of genetic events that follow? In the process, scientists will come closer and closer to understanding the development and the genetics of sex.

This, of course, is only one of the many issues in modern brain research, but much of the current excitement is centered on genetics. All cells in the body have the same complement of genes, but only express a very few of them in any tissue. The word "express," in this usage, means turn on for action. One can imagine a geneticist deciding to express a light bulb when he flips the switch to turn on the light. In any case, a skin cell has the full complement of three billion base pairs of DNA, totaling the entire 50,000 to perhaps more than 100,000 genes, yet the cell's destiny in the body calls only a handful of those genes into action during the cell's entire life. In contrast, specialists who study the brain say that organ uses as many as 30,000 active genes and many of them go to work after the individual's birth. This is no cause for surprise, but further testimony that the human brain is the most complex and intricate assembly of living cells yet produced in the four billion years of life on Earth. It is because of that huge assembly of active genes within the human skull that the powerful new tools of molecular genetics have offered so much information on the functions of the brain. Today the genes are providing clues to an incredible array of questions: why do people age? Why do a few develop schizophrenia and many fall prey to Alzheimer's disease or alcoholism? What do people have in common who think best in terms of shapes and spaces? What is the common denominator of the talent for using numbers? It would

Kibiuk © 1994

When the piece of DNA containing the testicular-determining factor is transferred from a Y to an X chromosome, the female mouse containing this X chromosome develops testes.

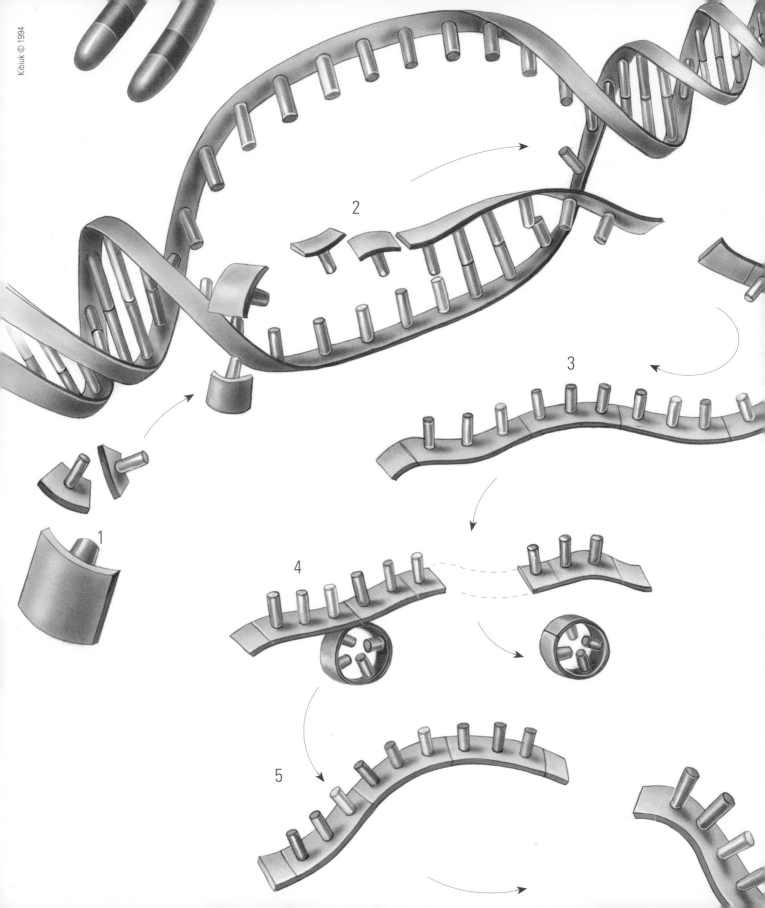

be naive to say that it is all in the genes . . . or would it? The genes are at least a happy hunting ground for clues in what has always been an impenetrable jungle of reverberating chemical effects. Until the past few decades, genetics used to be nine-tenths observation and one-tenth philosophy, guesswork, and dogma. Today it is mostly the chemistry of the DNA molecule and the other nucleic acid—RNA or ribonucleic acid. DNA and RNA work together. DNA is the substance of the genes, the genetic blueprints. Multiple forms of RNA turn the instructions of the genes into action within the living cell, seeing to it that the instructions of the DNA are carried out in the manufacture of all the proteins that give the cell its life and functions.

DNA is a long, twisted, double-stranded molecule: the famous "double helix," a spiral staircase of life in which the treads of the staircase—the links that join the two long strands of the helix—are the letters in the code. There are four letters, the chemical bases adenine, thymine, cytosine, and guanine; known in the geneticists' shorthand as A, T, C, and G. In forming the rungs of the twisted ladder, or steps in the stairway, A is always paired with T and C with G. That system of base pairs was nature's ingenious device, discovered by James D. Watson and Francis F. C. Crick in 1953, by which genes replicate to pass on their messages of heredity to future generations. When the two strands of the helix split apart during the process of cell division, a new strand is formed on each of the old ones, each producing a new double helix identical to the original. The new ones have to be identical to the originals because the base called A will seek out and join to every exposed T while every C will find its companion G. In that way the messages of the genes are perpetuated from generation to generation. It is because genes are strings of the pairs of those four bases that the size of genes is commonly measured in bases or base pairs. A gene may be a message as short as about 800 base pairs, as in the gene for alpha globin, a blood substance, or as many as two million as in the muscle fiber gene that is defective in the disease Duchenne's muscular dystrophy. Until 1953, the gene itself, the basic unit of heredity, was little more than the useful intellectual concept it had been since the rediscovery of Gregor Mendel's research. Now the genes are recognized as messages coded in the chemistry of the DNA.

After the discovery of DNA structure, the next crucial step in the modern chemistry of genetics was the achievement of Marshall Nirenberg and Herbert Matthei of the

Separation of the two strands of the DNA double helix allows enzymes to produce complementary copies of one strand in the form of a messenger RNA (mRNA). At step 1, building blocks, called ribonucleotides, are mobilized and activated; and at step 2 they are assembled along the template on one strand of DNA. At step 3, the messenger RNA leaves the DNA template and at step 4 it is spliced, removing extraneous pieces called introns, in order to put together the exons into a finished messenger RNA that codes the information for the formation of proteins.

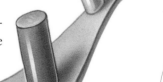

mRNA
tRNA
rRNA

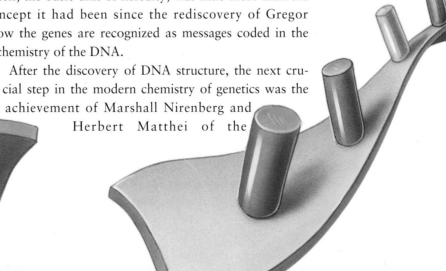

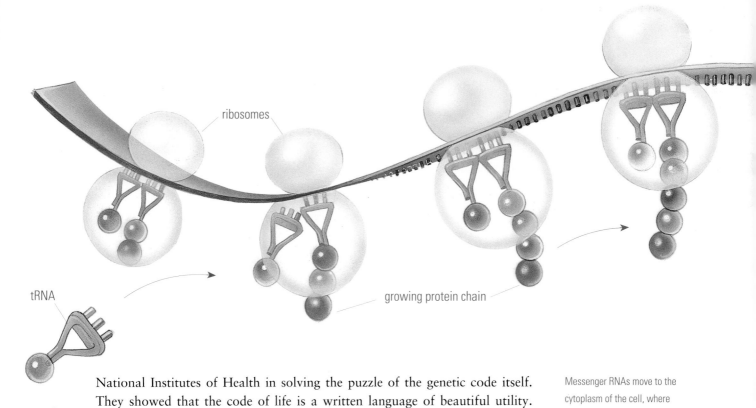

ribosomes

tRNA

growing protein chain

National Institutes of Health in solving the puzzle of the genetic code itself. They showed that the code of life is a written language of beautiful utility. Each sequence of three bases, called a triplet, is a "word" that identifies one of the twenty-odd amino acids that are the building blocks of all the proteins in living things: plants, animals, and microbes. The proteins are the "sentences" in every story of biology. In this somewhat crude analogy, a "chapter" might be a kidney or a pituitary gland, and a whole human being is the "book" called *Homo sapiens*. The entire alphabet of this code has been translated, together with its start and stop signals. For example, the triplet G-G-A is a code message telling the cell to assemble the amino acid glycine into the protein under construction. The sequence A-G-A calls for arginine, but the sequence T-G-A is one of the stop signals. These examples show also how some of the devastating genetic diseases can arise from chance minor errors in spelling in the language of life. When a spelling mistake puts a stop signal in a place where it shouldn't be, the assembly stops and the protein is ruined. Some spelling errors are harmless because the code has a substantial amount of redundancy. For example, not only A-G-A, but also A-G-G, C-G-C, and some other combinations are code words for the same amino acid—arginine. But some spelling errors create the disasters of genetic disease. More than three thousand of these so-called single gene disorders are known. Perhaps the

Messenger RNAs move to the cytoplasm of the cell, where they attach to ribosomes upon which the assembly of proteins takes place. Transfer RNAs have amino acids attached to one end and a coding region at the other end that binds to the messenger RNA. When the transfer RNAs attach to the messenger RNA, the amino acids are coupled to other amino acids to form the growing protein chain. The diagram shows the step-by-step addition of new amino acids to growing protein chains.

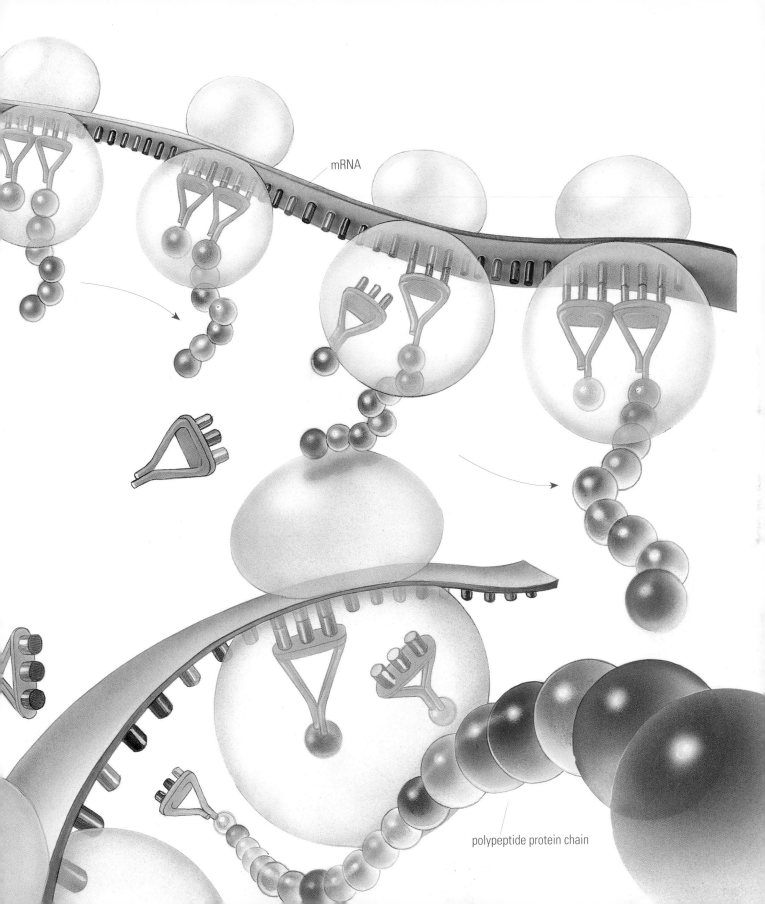

mRNA

polypeptide protein chain

wonder is that they are all so rare. Many genetic disorders affect the brain and nowhere has the great flux of scientific progress been more illuminating than in brain research.

Only portions of the DNA in any gene are actually coding regions, called exons, that serve as the genetic blueprints. The other portions, called introns, are still mysterious in purpose. They may be just the genetic debris of evolution, but probably they do have functions yet to be discovered. Meanwhile, these introns are spliced out of the genetic message by one kind of RNA before the working gene is shipped from the nucleus to the cytoplasm—the main body of the cell—so it can be put to work as the blueprint for making something the cell needs.

Altogether, the several decades of discoveries in human genetics have opened a new universe of biological knowledge: how genes are spelled out in the genetic book of specifications that exists in every cell; how genes are controlled and how they control other genes; how proteins, the building blocks of all tissues, are strung together in response to the genes' coded instructions. There are few realms of science in which this has been more important than in study of the brain. Indeed much of modern brain research depends on the new talents of molecular genetics. These new tools and concepts show promise of revealing much of what one neuroscientist has called "the molecular hardware of the brain." Of the roughly estimated thirty thousand active genetic messages that are found in the brain, more than half have not been found elsewhere in the body.

Some genes bring other genes into action by causing the cell to make proteins that tell the DNA to start or stop action at particular points. They are called DNA-binding proteins because they work by binding themselves to the DNA at critical points in the strands of that immense molecule. The estimate that thirty thousand human genes function in the brain is based on a variety of clues. Probably the strongest evidence is provided by "sequencing" the DNA of those genes. The term sequencing means that scientists work out the identity and exact order of each DNA base as it occurs in the long strand of genetic material.

Relatively few genes have been sequenced entirely, but a scientific team led by Dr. J. Craig Venter, then at the National Institutes of Health, developed a technique that makes it possible to identify genes rapidly by using partial sequences as identifying tags. Using the new tools of DNA analysis with this technique, the scientists identified for the first time 2,375 genes that function in the human brain, most of them never detected before. The team made two reports in the crucial stages of this research, the second published in the

48

February 13, 1992 issue of *Nature*. Together with their earlier gene identifications, the scientists added a total of more than twenty-five hundred genes active in the brain to those already known. They said the new data doubled the number of human genes identified up to that point by DNA sequencing and that their harvest of genes active in the brain may represent as much as one-twentieth of all the genes in the entire human genome–the complete galaxy of human genes. Most of the newly identified genes appear to be distinct from any that have been identified in the past. Their functions are unknown at present, but the process of discovery makes it clear that they are genes that the brain actually uses, at least for a time and at least in certain of its tissues.

Some 217 of the newly identified genes do bear close similarities to known genes in humans and other species. Several genes that govern the growth processes of *Drosophila* have counterparts among those found in the human brain. Newly identified members of known gene families in humans include genes for many different enzyme systems, blueprints for structural components of cells and growth-promoting substances, which scientists call growth factors, or their receptors.

In the early 1990s Dr. Venter's method for identifying genes led to a controversy over patenting genetic material. Scientists, lawyers, and others interested in the practical applications of molecular biology argued heatedly over the question of whether or not genes should be patented. Most controversial was the question of patenting DNA sequences that identified genes whose codes had not yet been totally spelled out and whose functions were still unknown. The debate probably still has a long life ahead.

One of the strange quirks of the DNA story is that all of evolution—all of progress, if one chooses to call it progress—comes from error. If there had never been any mistake in the copying of DNA from one cell to the next and one generation to the next we would all still be single-cell organisms swimming brainlessly in the pre-Cambrian seas. Emergence of the world's incredible panoply of different life forms, and the evolution of the human brain, all seem to have depended on mutations, rare mistakes such as spelling errors in the DNA or rearrangements in the genetic material of chromosomes. They were all changes that were not supposed to happen. Most such errors were fatal, but a rare few gave the mutated cell some advantage in surviving. With the help of such happy accidents, the descendants of primordial cells learned to live together in peace and profit, and multicelled organisms arose. More errors helped some creatures and plants leave the pools and oceans to find niches on land. It all took several billion years, but this unimaginably long

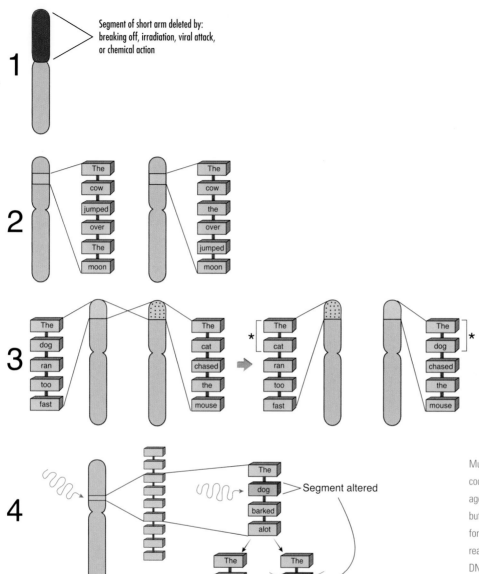

1 Segment of short arm deleted by: breaking off, irradiation, viral attack, or chemical action

2

| The |
| cow |
| jumped |
| over |
| The |
| moon |

| The |
| cow |
| the |
| over |
| jumped |
| moon |

3

| The |
| dog |
| ran |
| too |
| fast |

| The |
| cat |
| chased |
| the |
| mouse |

| The |
| cat |
| ran |
| too |
| fast |

*

| The |
| dog |
| chased |
| the |
| mouse |

*

4

| The |
| dog |
| barked |
| alot |

Segment altered

| The |
| dog |
| barked |
| alot |

Normal replication

| The |
| fish |
| barked |
| alot |

Abnormal replication

Mutations change the genetic code. Radiation and chemical agents directly damage DNA but these are not as important for genetic change as rearrangements of pieces of DNA between chromosomes, and within chromosomes, which may occur during cell division. These rearrangements change the sequence of information in the genetic code. While most mutations are harmful, a few may be beneficial and form the basis for evolutionary change.

50

process gave birth to beetles, dinosaurs, mastodons, Marie Curie, Ludwig van Beethoven, and all the rest of us.

The process is still going on in subtle and imperceptible ways. It is not always a climb to higher horizons. As in any other language, spelling errors are usually bad: many are disastrous, most are fatal. Cancer is a complex and many-faceted process. It may be caused by chemicals, such as those in tobacco smoke, by a virus, by radiation, or any of a host of other insults to the body. But the actual process of malignancy always starts with one or another copying mistake in a chromosome or a simple spelling error in a cell's DNA. The several thousand genetic diseases, and scores of other maladies that are only partly genetic, also begin with harmful variants in the DNA. Such variations can change the brain and, through processes such as prolonged stress, the brain can affect crucial activities and even the performance of genes themselves.

Many of the known human genes were discovered because of the disastrous effects that mistakes in those genes produced in human health. Often, the ill effects involve the brain although there is sometimes no obvious clue to the reason the brain should be affected. Two of the most puzzling among many such tragic "single-gene" disorders are Lesch-Nyhan syndrome and Huntington's chorea. The faulty gene in Lesch-Nyhan disease has been known for many years. The one responsible for Huntington's chorea was only identified in 1993. In each disease, the single gene error produces a whole nightmare of tragic effects on mind and brain. For Lesch-Nyhan patients, the tragedies are apparent from infancy onwards. Nobody knows why the failure of one gene that is the blueprint for one enzyme does so much damage or why it erupts so soon. Huntington's disease is as great a puzzle, but its timing is far different. There is no warning of disaster until early adulthood or middle age when the victim's mind begins a slow and terrifying deterioration that ends years later in physical and mental helplessness and, finally, death. Like most other single-gene disorders, these two diseases are mercifully rare.

A common affliction that also has profound effects on the mind is Alzheimer's disease. It too is mysterious. The disease usually manifests itself late in life and gradually produces a mind-robbing dementia for which there is no present cure, treatment, or even coherent explanation. In a few cases it seems to run in families, a strong hint that some genetic flaw is involved. This is particularly true of cases in which the symptoms begin relatively early in middle age. In a few of these familial cases, as they are called, the tragedy has been pinpointed, not only to a particular gene, but to a particular place in a particular exon, one coding region, of that gene. This is the kind of dazzling precision that has only become possible because of recent strides in the techniques of molecular biology.

One genetic defect associated with these familial cases is a mutation in a gene on chromosome 21, one of the smallest of the human chromosomes. It is only about as large as the Y chromosome, although easily distinguished from that sex chromosome by any competent observer. The gene on chromosome 21 that is altered in some Alzheimer's patients is the code of instructions for making a protein called the amyloid precursor. Specialists in Alzheimer's disease think this is significant because the material called amyloid becomes the core of ball-shaped deposits that clog the brain tissues of Alzheimer's patients. The plaques disrupt the architecture of the brain and may interfere with communications between nerve cells. Some amyloid can also be found in the brains of extremely old people who are free of the devastating symptoms of Alzheimer's disease. The amyloid deposits appear to be important in the disease process, but whether they are part of the ultimate cause or one of the effects is still unknown. Dr. Kenneth S. Kosik of the Harvard Medical School and Brigham and Women's Hospital, Boston, reviewed the biology of Alzheimer's disease in the journal *Science*. In the cases that appear early and often in members of certain families, the gene defect is a tragically small spelling error in a gene for making amyloid. Dr. Kosik says it has been pinned down to the change of a single base in a sequence of over twenty-one hundred of these subunits. In one case, this minute spelling error changed a C to a T at the 2,149th base pair in one of the coding regions of the gene. This change in spelling altered the identity of just one of the 717 amino acids in a protein molecule. The error changed a valine to an isoleucine. The two are among the twenty amino acids that make up all the proteins of humans. In another Alzheimer's disease case, there was a change from a valine to either an isoleucine or a glycine.

Just what these highly specific and circumscribed errors do in biological terms is not known, but patients who had them did develop Alzheimer's disease and postmortem studies of their brains showed that they had the typical Alzheimer's disease senile plaques of amyloid and the tangles of tissue called neurofibrillary tangles in their brains.

This and other research shows the importance of studying the human genes in the search for clues to such puzzling disorders as Alzheimer's disease. One research team has recently found a patient suffering from chronic schizophrenia, an entirely different mental disorder, who also has a single base mutation in a gene on chromosome 21.

But provocative as the changes in chromosome 21 may be in some Alzheimer's patients, these cases are rarities. In the majority of Alzheimer's cases—those that don't run so closely in families—no one has been able to demonstrate any clear and consistent genetic flaw. The symptoms of familial Alzheimer's and the much more common sporadic cases are essentially the same although the familial cases develop earlier in life. Perhaps there are somewhat different causes that lead to common effects.

At the opposite end of the age spectrum is another relatively common brain disorder that has some features in common with Alzheimer's disease, but is known without question to involve a quite specific disorder of the genetic apparatus. This is Down's syndrome, the most common cause of mental retardation in the United States, affecting an estimated one baby in every 700 born alive. The disease has apparently been present in the human race for many centuries, perhaps far longer. An English physician, Dr. John Langdon Haydon Down, who cared for patients at an asylum in Surrey, gave the first thorough description of the disorder in 1866.

Almost a hundred years passed after his painstaking catalogue of signs, symptoms, and consequences before doctors found any clue at all to the cause, although there were many wrong guesses. Today, Down's syndrome is known to result from a disorder of chromosome 21, although a much more obvious one than in the case of familial Alzheimer's disease.

While a normal person has two copies of chromosome 21, a Down's syndrome patient has three, or at least two and a portion of a third. The abnormality is called a trisomy, meaning three where there ought to be two. It took a long time for the medical profession to recognize this rather gross departure from the normal. The current explosion of knowledge of the human genes and chromosomes is remarkably recent. Chromosomes are easy to see under a microscope, but they tend to look like a plate of spaghetti. Not until the 1950s was there any reliable way of spreading them apart to look at them individually. Indeed, so confusing was the tangle, that geneticists even had the number of human chromosomes wrong. Today everyone knows that normal humans have forty-six chromosomes in twenty-three pairs, one set from each parent. Twenty-two of the pairs are called autosomes. The twenty-third pair consists of the sex chromosomes: two Xs in the female and an X and a Y in the male. This is such fundamental knowledge that it is hard to remember how recently that fact was discovered. It was not known until the 1950s after Dr. Joe Hin Tjio and Dr. Albert Levan of the Institute of Genetics in Lund, Sweden, developed a new and simple way of spreading chromosomes apart to look at them. With their technique, the chromosomes could at last be counted accurately. So poor were the previous methods of chromosome analysis that the conventional wisdom of science had the human number fixed at forty-eight. With the new technique it became obvious that forty-eight was wrong and that forty-six was the correct number. Now the two nonexistent human chromosomes have vanished into the mists of ignorance.

No doubt the nineteenth century Dr. Down would be gratified by the new discovery about chromosome 21, but how does the trisomy really explain the cause of the syndrome? It doesn't. No human embryo that lacks chromosome 21 altogether will ever survive. Why does too much of a necessary thing create another kind of disaster? No one knows precisely, but the chromosome 21 connection is helping scientists close in on that mystery, because now they have something specific to dissect and the tools to do it. To date no known case of Down's syndrome has ever occurred without some excess material from chromosome 21 and no person who has trisomy 21 seems ever to have escaped the disorder. The next set of questions is obvious: what genes are located on those extra portions of the chromosome and what functions do those genes serve? Alternatively, what normal genetic arrangement does the excess material disrupt?

That is where the evidence from Alzheimer's disease becomes most interesting. Down's syndrome patients who live to adulthood all develop the amyloid deposits, neuritic plaques, and neurofibrillary tangles that are the physical hallmarks of Alzheimer's disease. They also develop the same degeneration of the mind. It would seem that something related to amyloid must be a key to the puzzle.

But the puzzle is still unsolved. The meaning of the common findings in Down's syndrome and Alzheimer's disease is much disputed among brain specialists. There must be individual genes and individual proteins that offer clues to solve the disputes, but these needles in the great haystack of the brain have yet to be found.

Meanwhile, the techniques of molecular biology are so powerful and so new that it is a temptation to think they are the answer to everything. In fact there is still ample room for some of the old tools. Consider, for example, one of the hot new research tools of 120 years ago. It was developed by a man whose name is famous in brain research—Camillo Golgi—who first learned to use silver nitrate to stain nerve tissue so that the nerves in the brain could be seen clearly enough for close study. Even today, his nineteenth century technique can bring new truths into focus from the depths of the brain. And that brings the story back from the intricacies of the molecules and the genes to some of the most important products of those genes, hormones in particular.

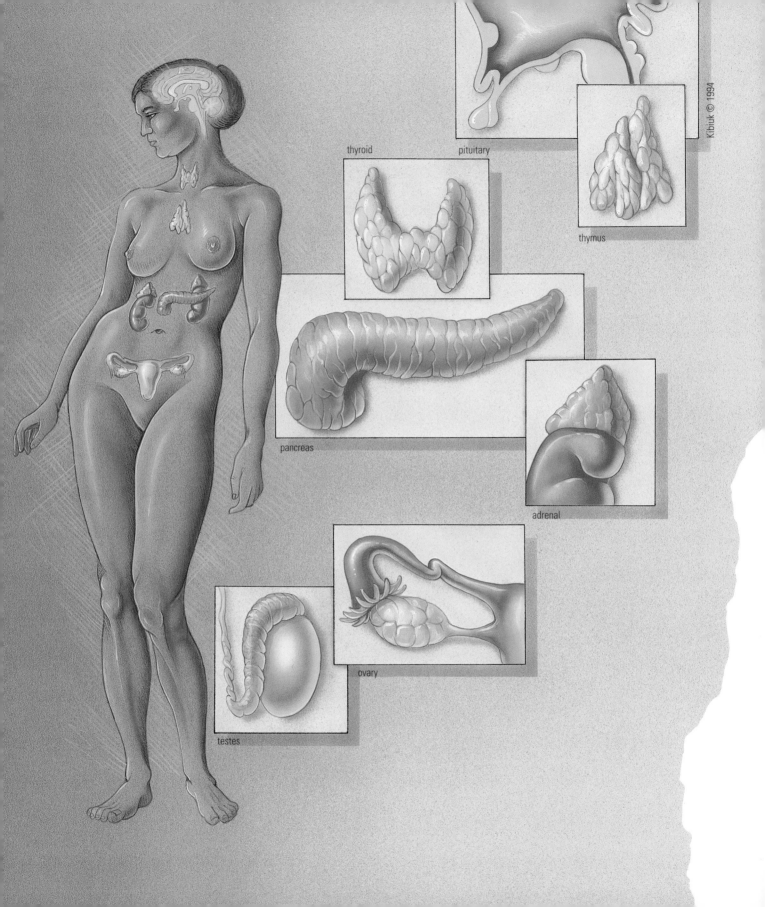

thyroid

pituitary

thymus

Kibiuk © 1994

pancreas

adrenal

ovary

testes

Nobody ever accused Camillo Golgi of being the shy, self-effacing kind of scientist. He worked hard to develop a brain research method that few people thought was plausible before he perfected it. Yet that method of staining nerve tissue with a concoction of silver nitrate and other substances opened scientists' eyes to the true complexity of the human brain.

Golgi, an Italian physician, was also a man of strong opinions that were hard to dislodge. He saw the brain as a network of connected cells, but he backed the wrong horse, so to speak, in guessing what kind of a network it really is and how the cells are connected.

In the late nineteenth century, he was a leader among those who espoused the so-called reticulum theory. The idea was that the brain was a web of cells directly fused (anastomosed) to each other to form a close network or reticulum. The concept was persuasive. Under the microscope, brain tissue did look that way. Furthermore, the idea possessed what scientists like to call elegant simplicity. It was like a painting in which a few deft brush strokes evoke a whole complex scene. The reticulum idea explained a lot about the brain with a minimum of footnotes and caveats. Golgi also liked the concept because it seemed to drive the final stake through the heart of the old idea that the brain functioned through a quasi-miraculous "vital force" that could never yield to scientific analysis.

By the time he was awarded the Nobel Prize for medicine/physiology in 1906, the truth was solidly on the side of another concept of the brain, called

The endocrine system produces hormones and releases them in response to signals from the brain, either nerve signals or hormones released from the pituitary. The pituitary is the master gland of the body, and its hormones control the thymus, the thyroid, the pancreas, the adrenals, and the ovaries and testes. The pancreas produces important hormones that affect metabolism, such as insulin. The thymus gland (over the heart) is a producer of hormones that affect both the immune and endocrine systems, as well as being a master organ of the immune system (see Chapter 7).

the neuron theory. It was far less simple than the reticulum idea and promised to be much more difficult to prove. It required some special kind of connection between separate nerve cells. The details of how those connections might work was a mystery. Today they are called synapses. Nerve signals are transmitted across them with a combination of chemistry and electrical activity that has taken most of the present century to understand. These connections, billions of them, link the separate neurons and the many dendrites that grow from each neuron like the tendrils of climbing vines. The man who was most responsible for the neuron theory, although he didn't coin the word, was the Spanish anatomist, Santiago Ramon y Cajal. He had used Golgi's own staining technique brilliantly to advance the neuron theory and he shared the 1906 Nobel Prize with Golgi. But his co-winner devoted his Nobel lecture to a passionate last defense of the reticulum theory. His lecture created something of a storm. By that time most students of the brain considered the theory outdated and using the Nobel lecture to push it was considered insulting to Cajal.

The whole issue seems a trifle quaint today. Scientists have been using Golgi's technique and Cajal's concept of the brain with immense profit ever since. Nearly a century after the confrontation at the Nobel ceremonies, scientists of the Laboratory of Neuroendocrinology of The Rockefeller University used the old staining technique to settle an issue that might well have amazed the two men of the nineteenth century. The question: can hormones actually bring about physical changes in the adult brain? It is an issue that has all manner of ramifications today and it brings up some possibilities that are downright frightening.

To the experimenters at Rockefeller it was obvious that hormones could influence the adult brain chemically. Everyone has felt the adrenalin rush of focused attention and emotion that comes with sudden crisis. That experience is clear evidence of hormones at work in the brain. But many scientists thought the effects came from the hormone's effects on nerve signaling chemicals–the neurotransmitters, perhaps even by influencing the number and activity of the action sites called receptors on nerve cells. Studies of tissues other than those of the brain had shown this kind of effect to be possible. But actual physical change in the brain, perhaps even alterations of its wiring? That was something else entirely. Few believed it was likely.

The question the research team addressed was quite specific and potentially illuminating. They wanted to know if the cyclic hormone changes that go with the female's ovulatory cycle produce physical changes in the brain. If so it would mean that the female brain would actually change month by month in its physical organization. This was an intriguing possibility because it went beyond such relatively obvious concepts as a brain that might change gradually with age or with chronic disease. The new issue was whether or not the mammalian brain was plastic enough to change and rechange in response to the monthly cycle of the sex hormones. Looked at more broadly, it is an issue that has social and political implications too. Can the adult brain be taken hostage by physical changes caused by the body's own hormones? The answer to this question also solves another: whether or not premenstrual tension in women is a real phenomenon. Judges and lawyers are apparently ahead of many scientists in being sure it is. The mental effects of premenstrual tension, a totally taboo subject for centuries, has recently been used by lawyers as a defense of violent behavior in their clients and some judges have ruled in their favor. Menopause in women is clearly a function of changing hormone flow that has major health consequences for a large and increasing part of the population. A typical response from male doctors, who don't experience female menopause, has been to shrug off the effects and tell their patients to stop imagining things and that menopause is just a part of life and they must adjust to it. Until recently, it has been a neglected area of medical research. But the National Institutes of Health began paying serious attention to the subject in the early 1990s under Dr. Bernadine Healy, the first woman to serve as director of the NIH.

Hormones have a multitude of effects on health and they are by no means limited to one sex only. After all, the male brain is presumably no more resistant to hormone effects than the female.

Molecular biology, for all its powers in experiment and analysis, did not offer any good way for the team at The Rockefeller University to grapple with their question concerning changes in the adult brain. Dr. Golgi's ancient staining method did. It allowed the scientists to look for physical changes in the dendrites, the threads of tissue that extend from neurons and hold most of the cell-to-cell connections—the synapses. The studies had to be done in animals, of course, but the point was crucial to understanding the human brain too: just how plastic and changeable was the adult brain?

That question has only begun to have meaning in recent years. Just a few decades ago it was close to heresy to suggest that the brain might change even in the course of sexual differentiation. The charge of heresy was probably more social than scientific. In the era of unisex this and unisex that, the idea that there were actual physical differences between the brains of men and women was seen by some as a declaration of war. How a totally unisex brain could possibly give rise to childbirth and milk production in some people, while others were totally incapable of these feats, was not much addressed.

Belief in the body-as-miracle didn't die altogether with the nineteenth century.

What nobody doubts today is that the human body produces hormones and that hormones have powerful effects. By definition hormones are biological messages produced in one set of cells to be read, marked, and, almost literally, inwardly digested in far distant parts of the body. Scientists often call hormones chemical messengers. In fact, they are both the messenger and the message. There are many kinds of chemical messages that continually flow to and fro in the body and scientists divide them into three categories; autocrine, which are substances that act directly on the very cells that produce them; paracrine, which act on nearby cells; and endocrine, which act at a distance. The endocrine substances are the hormones and the field of their study is endocrinology.

While most of brain research is remarkably new, endocrinology has a history of nearly 150 years. It began in 1849, most experts agree, with a scientist named Arnold A. Berthold at the University of Göttingen in Germany. He devised a clever experiment to find out just what it was that made roosters crow and fight and act like roosters. He started with a commonplace. Everyone knew that a capon, a castrated rooster, will stop fighting, crowing, and showing a normal interest in hens. But what did the castration actually do to achieve this effect? Did it interrupt nerve circuits, upset some mysterious anatomical arrangement, or disrupt the natural scheme of things in some totally unimagined way?

What would happen, Berthold asked himself, if he put some testicular tissue back into the altered rooster? He tried it, transplanting testes into the abdominal cavities of castrated roosters. They quickly regained their entire cock of the walk personalities. With that simple operation they were roosters again. There was no regrowth of nerve tissue from the implants to the birds' brains and the testes certainly hadn't been put back in the anatomically proper place; but blood vessels had soon formed, connecting the transplanted tissue to the rooster's circulation. There was only one logical conclusion. Something from the testes was circulating in the blood and affecting the birds' brains and their personalities. Today those early tissue transplants are regarded as the first experiments in endocrinology. The "something" that flowed in the blood from testes to brain was the male hormone, testosterone.

It was more than 100 years later, 1969 to be precise, that Ronald J. Barfield of Rutgers University put Berthold's discovery to the final test. He implanted minute amounts of testosterone directly into the brains of castrated roosters. He put the hormone into a part of the brain called the preoptic area; a region of nerve cells that has a truly ancient history going back to the days before the ancestors of birds and mammals diverged from those of the reptiles. In humans, as well as other mammals, and in birds, this so-called "primitive" brain is vital to the fundamental acts and decisions on which life depends—including sex. Just as in Berthold's nineteenth century experiments, the castrated birds at Rutgers promptly became roosters again. Of course, the two experiments were not just isolated sparks of light in a vast fog of ignorance. Scientists have been trying to clear away the fog bit by bit at an ever accelerating pace for a century.

The state of knowledge today would be astonishing to anyone of Berthold's era. The brain responds to the endocrine organs' hormones and the brain is itself an endocrine organ. There are more kinds of hormones than anyone had imagined even a few years ago and they have more complicated effects. They are also produced in unexpected places. The classic definition was that hormones are produced by the endocrine glands; testes, ovaries, thyroid, the islet cells of the pancreas, and the adrenal and pituitary glands. Today it is known that even the heart produces hormones although that organ used to be thought of as nothing but life's most important pump. The brain produces hormones too. It is still a mystery why the brain produces some of them and what these locally produced substances, called neurohormones, do for and to the body's master organ. Some brain substances that have nearly hormone-like actions do have known effects. Among these are the enkephalins and endorphins that seem to be the body's natural equivalents of the opiate drugs. They have been found to kill pain and produce mental "highs" of their own. Some students of the brain think they give successful

Chemical messengers can act on the cell that produced them (autocrine effect) as well as on adjacent cells (paracrine effect). Hormones are chemical messengers that are released from one type of cell and act at a distance on receptors expressed by another type of cell (endocrine effect). Sometimes the same chemical messenger can have all three types of actions.

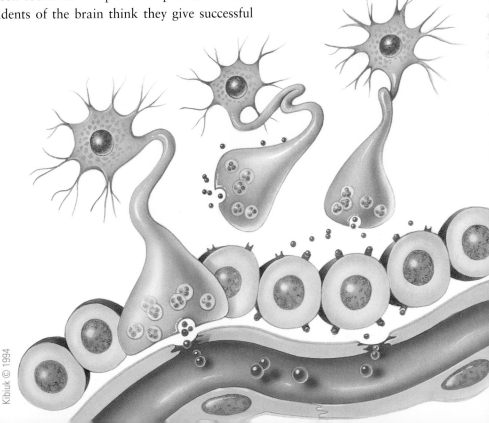

Kibiuk © 1994

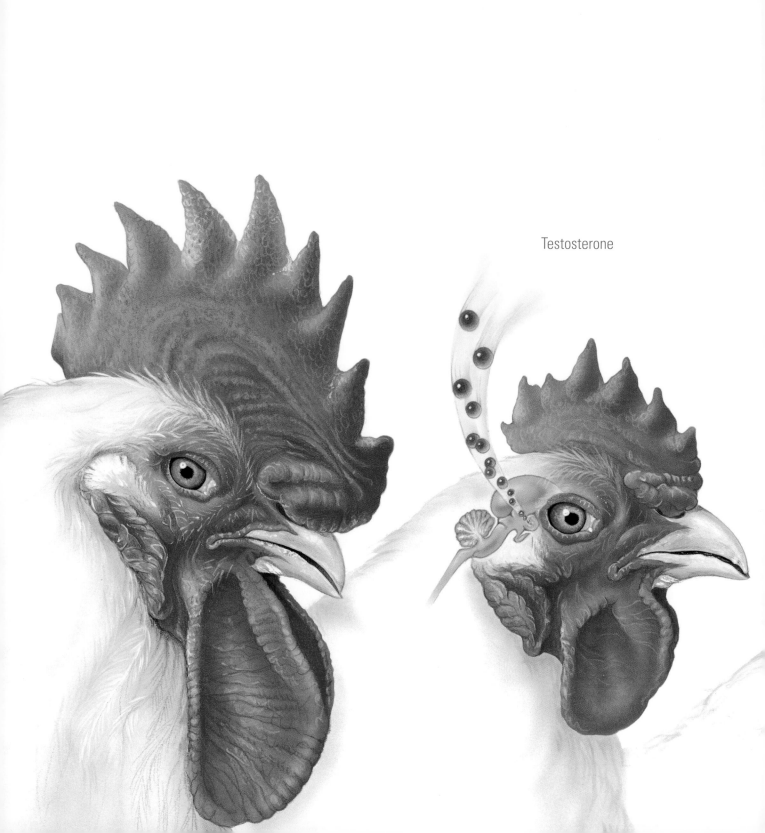

Testosterone

long distance runners the drive and satisfaction that goes with their lonely calling. The existence of endorphins as natural brain chemicals is also thought to explain why such totally foreign substances as opium, which comes from poppy plants, and its man-made variants, have such powerful effects on the human brain. The drugs are acting on chemical pathways already in place for use by the endorphins.

A multitude of growth factors that act more locally than true hormones has also been discovered. Important among them is nerve growth factor which has direct effects in stimulating the growth of nerve cells. In 1986, Dr. Rita Levi-Montalcini, its discoverer, and Dr. Stanley Cohen were awarded a Nobel Prize for years of research with this substance at Washington University in St. Louis.

Scientists' questions about the actions of true hormones on the brain have proliferated and evidence that hormones are important to the brain has been building for years, amid controversy and differences in scientific opinion. How, after all, does the brain influence the hormones everywhere in the body and what is there in the brain itself that lets hormones affect the body's main control center? It has taken decades of research in laboratories all over the world to get just some of the answers.

In 1849, the first experiment in endocrinology, the scientific study of hormones, demonstrated that the sexual, aggressive, and crowing behavior of the rooster depends on hormones secreted by the testes. In this experiment by A. A. Berthold, castration caused male traits of the rooster to regress, including appearance of the comb and wattle, as well as the characteristic crowing and aggressive and sexual behavior. The castrate rooster, or capon, resembles the hen. Testes transplanted into these capons made them look and behave again like normal roosters. More than 100 years later, it was recognized that it is testosterone secreted by the testes that is responsible. Testosterone implants in the hypothalamus of the "capon" restore male-typical behavior.

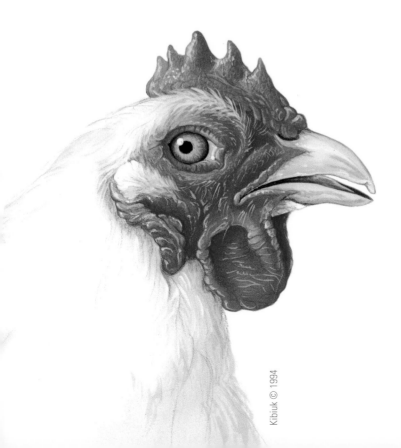

Kibiuk © 1994

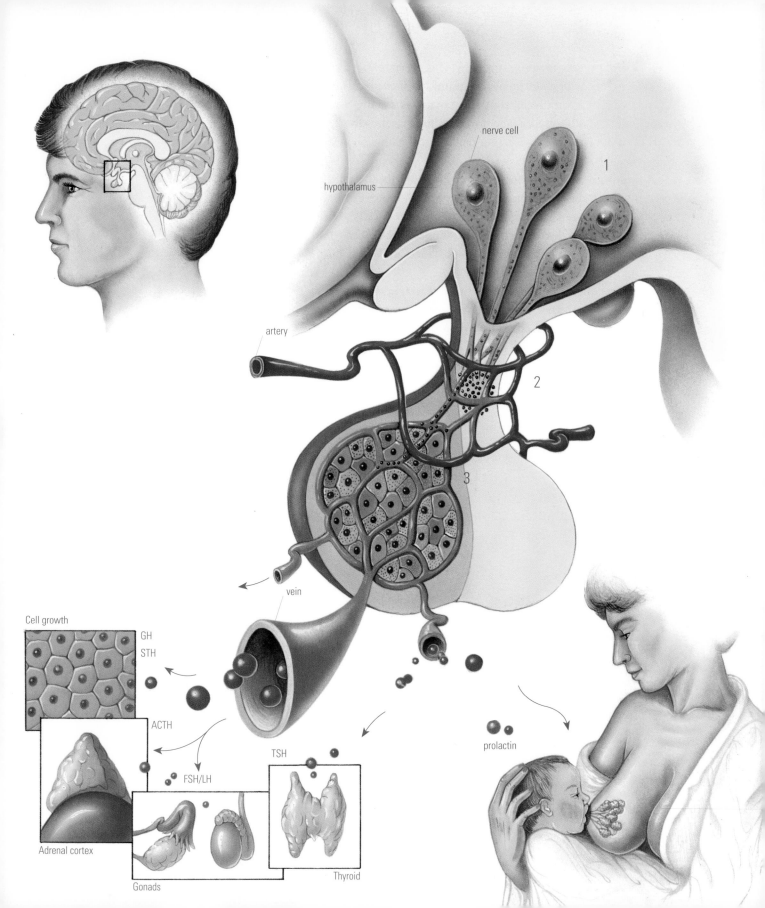

nerve cell

hypothalamus

1

artery

2

3

vein

Cell growth

GH
STH

ACTH

FSH/LH

TSH

Adrenal cortex

Gonads

Thyroid

prolactin

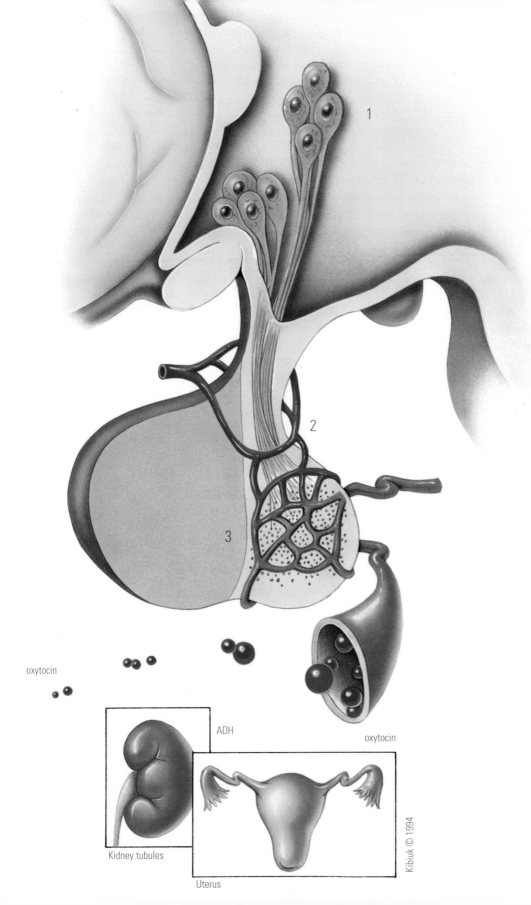

1

2

3

oxytocin

ADH

oxytocin

Kidney tubules

Uterus

Kibiuk © 1994

The pituitary "master gland" consists of anterior and posterior lobes. The anterior lobe (*left*) receives signals from the brain (1) via hormones released into blood vessels from nerve endings at the base of the hypothalamus (2). These blood vessels (3) transport the so-called releasing hormones to cells of the anterior pituitary (4) where they stimulate release of the major hormones into the bloodstream: growth hormone (GH), adrenocorticotrophic hormones (ACTH), follicle-stimulating hormones (FSH) and luteinizing hormone (LH), thyroid-stimulating hormone (TSH), and prolactin. Each of these hormones has specific target cells, containing specific receptors, in various parts of the body.

The posterior lobe (*right*) of the pituitary receives signals from the brain (1) that stimulate the release of hormones from nerve cells in the hypothalamus (2) that have synaptic endings in the posterior lobe of the pituitary. These nerve endings (3) release two hormones into the bloodstream: antidiuretic hormone (ADH) that promotes retention of water by the kidney; and oxytocin, that stimulates milk letdown from the mammary gland and contraction of the uterus.

65

The classical concept, still accepted today, is that the pituitary gland is the master of the endocrine system. It is nestled so close to the base of the brain that a layman might pardonably think it is actually a part of the brain. Like many other parts of the body that exert prodigious effects, it is remarkably small; a little stalk of tissue less than a half inch in diameter and weighing little more than one or two aspirin tablets. But the pituitary influences everything from head to toe. It sends out hormonal signals to control the production of other hormones by all the body's other endocrine glands, the testes, ovaries, pancreas, thyroid, and adrenal glands. In this way, it oversees sex in both men and women and governs the entire gamut of chemistry that keeps the body working. The responses to daytime and darkness, hunger and thirst, fear and elation, and almost everything else are evoked by the intricate rhythms of the rhapsody of hormones. It is hormones from the pituitary gland that send out the orders to control the maternal breast's production of milk, stimulate bone growth, induce the skin to grow darker to protect against sunlight. Through all these actions and signals to the other glands, the pituitary is the general overseer that maintains the vital constancy of the internal environment while it copes with the wild ups and downs of the outside world.

But what tells the pituitary when to send out the orders? The brain, of course.

Within roughly the past twenty-five years, scientists have found a series of "hormone releasing factors" that are produced by the hypothalamus in the brain to give the pituitary gland its orders. Dr. Roger C. L. Guillemin, then of Baylor College of Medicine in Houston, and Dr. Andrew V. Schally, of Tulane University, in New Orleans, shared a Nobel Prize in 1977 for a series of brilliant discoveries made independently in this field. The two scientists had competed bitterly for years to reach the goal of discovering and understanding the hypothalamic hormones. So close was their race that the Nobel committee awarded them the prize jointly.

Through their work, and that of many others, it has become clear that the commerce between hormones of the hypothalamus, pituitary, the endocrine glands, and the rest of the body is certainly not a one-way street. Everything that affects the body registers in the brain and, one way or another, affects the brain. And the brain gives the body new orders on the basis of those new messages. It is a continually reverberating exchange that biologists, as well as engineers, call a feedback loop.

Given that state of affairs, one of the next important questions was how a hormone could actually deliver its message to a nerve cell. Chemicals such as hormones serve as keys that turn on actions by the individual cells that they influence. But keys are only part of the arrangement. A key is no good by itself. There must also be keyholes and locks on which the keys can function.

In the world of biology, the special protein structures called receptors serve as the locks. They often protrude through the cell surface, although sometimes they are completely internal. Receptors for the important class of hormones called the steroid hormones are lodged in the nuclei of cells and are believed to act directly on the DNA to turn genes on and off. This pattern of gene control is itself an incredible testimonial to the everchanging nature of the brain. In any case, receptors give the hormone or other floating message something to grab so that message can be received and delivered. That is why they are called receptors. A multitude of different receptors are a main avenue for the cell's use of hormones as well as the myriad other substances that flow from place to place in the body. Like the key and lock situation in the world of mechanics, each hormone or other message substance is designed to interact with only one type of receptor.

In the early 1960s, biologists everywhere were looking for receptors to all manner of things in all kinds of cells. In 1962 a group led by Elwood Jensen found receptors for the sex hormone estradiol in the rat uterus. Only a few years later, Richard Zigmond, a graduate student at The Rockefeller University, found those same receptors in cells of the rat's brain. From this and other research, it soon became clear that the brain does have receptors for many different hormones. Indeed it is now known that brain cells have receptors to all six of the main classes of steroid hormones: androgens, estrogens, progestins, glucocorticoids, mineralocorticoids, and vitamin D. The steroids, named for a particular feature of their chemistry, are among the most important and widely known groups of hormones. From the fact that brain cells had receptors for all of them scientists could now see how they could work on the brain. The next question was: what did they really do? It soon became clear that they do a lot. Hormones were found to alter the brain structure of songbirds and the spinal cords of rats. Many other effects also came to light.

The process begins with a hormone coupling with a receptor, or having direct effects on a cell membrane. Some receptors are known to be DNA-binding proteins. When the hormone turns on those receptors, they attach to the DNA molecule and either activate or halt the activity of a gene depending on the circumstances. Sometimes hormones act more directly by altering the outer membranes of neurons with the result that the nerve cell's electrical activity is changed. In yet other cases, the hormones do it by increasing or decreasing the number of receptors for another substance on the nerve cells. For example, male sex hormones make receptors for the neurotransmitter serotonin appear in the preoptic area of the rat's brain and this may be a key to male sexual behavior. The female sex hormone, estradiol, calls forth receptors for oxytocin in the female reproductive tract and also in a key area of the brain's hypothalamus. Oxytocin is a hormone known to have important effects on female fertility. It all grows more and more complex the closer one looks, but there is a grand consistency in the design.

To help sort out the details in at least one of the brain's multitude of systems, the team at The Rockefeller University decided to zero in on a particular sex behavior of rats and the precise cluster of cells in the brain that dictates this part of the act of mating. The behavior is something called the lordosis response, the posture the female takes to show the male that his attentions are welcome. So finely have scientists narrowed down their search for causes and matching effects that they know that the lordosis response is dictated in the hypothalamus by little clusters of nerve cells called the ventromedial nuclei. These cells take their cue from the sex hormones estradiol and progesterone. They order additional hormone actions and the specific neuromuscular events that produce the physical response. All of this is well known. Scientists have worked out the entire set of nerve circuits that translate the hormonal urge into the final muscular action. So much for the mystery of romance.

Using both light microscopes and the electron microscope, to get an ultra-high magnification view of the nerve cells involved in this behavior, the team at Rockefeller saw the neurons swell and their nuclei get larger and rounder under the hormonal influence. There was also evidence that the cells' capacity to make new protein was increasing. In short, the hormone action was driving some important activities in those key brain cells and the changes all took place in remarkably short time; only a matter of a few hours. It seemed to be a process that got the nerve circuits ready for mating behavior. But was the brain actually changing physically or was it just flexing its neural muscles so to speak?

Having progressed this far with the sophisticated tools and methods of the twentieth century, the Rockefeller team turned for help finally to Golgi's nineteenth century silver nitrate stain. The stain makes the nerve cell's dendrites stand out sharply against the background of other brain tissue. With the Golgi stain, the research workers could actually see not just the dendrites but the spines that grow on them like the thorns of rose bushes. The dendrite spines are the places were the synaptic connections are made with other dendrites and other nerve cells. If a dendrite grows new spines that means either that new synapses are being formed or that existing synapses are being changed. In other words the actual wiring diagram of the brain is being

Steroid hormones and thyroid hormone activate genes by means of protein receptors inside cells. These hormones diffuse from the bloodstream (1) and pass through the cell membrane (2) and then into the cell nucleus (3) where they bind to the receptor (4) and release another protein, called a "chaperone." The hormone-receptor complex attaches to a specific region on one strand of the DNA double helix (5) and stimulates transcription of an adjacent gene (6) to produce a messenger RNA as shown in Figure 3.2. The messenger RNA leaves the nucleus and travels to the cytoplasm, where it binds to ribosomes and codes for the formation of new proteins, as shown in Figure 3.3.

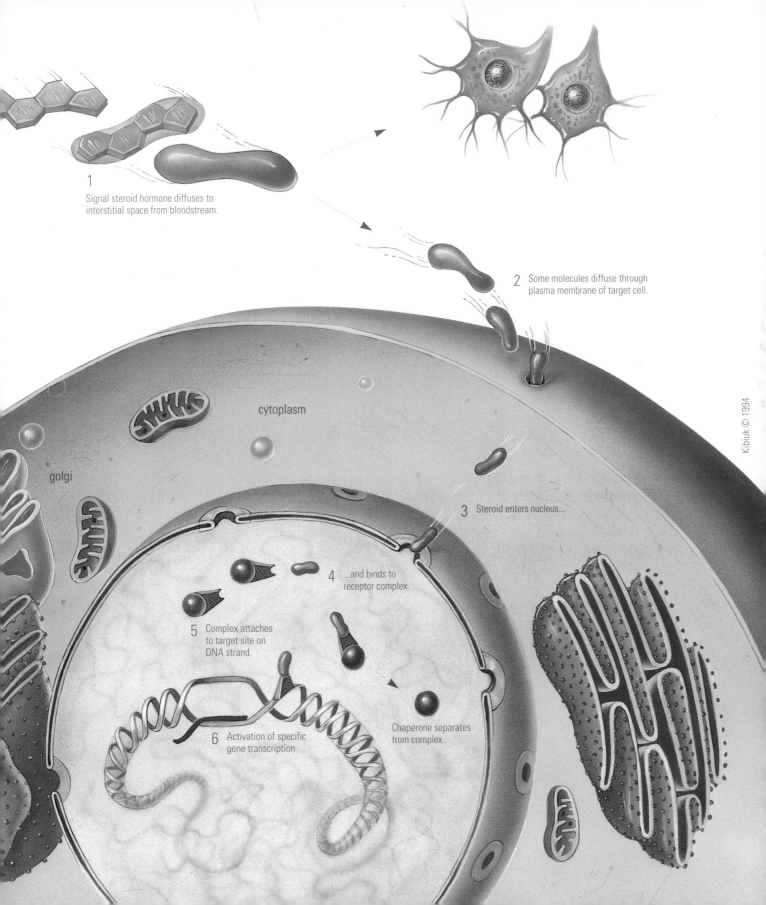

1 Signal steroid hormone diffuses to interstitial space from bloodstream.

2 Some molecules diffuse through plasma membrane of target cell.

cytoplasm

Kibiuk © 1994

golgi

3 Steroid enters nucleus...

4 ...and binds to receptor complex.

5 Complex attaches to target site on DNA strand.

Chaperone separates from complex.

6 Activation of specific gene transcription.

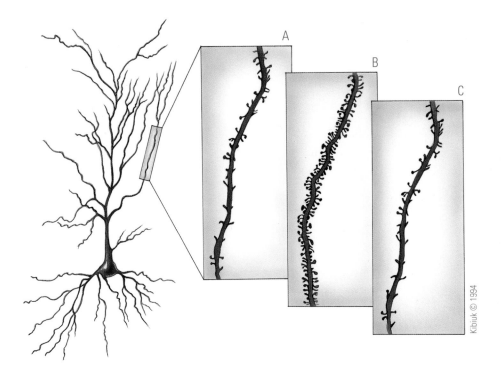

A B C

Kibiuk © 1994

Estradiol causes some neurons in the brain to form more synaptic connections with other nerve cells. This process occurs every four to five days during the reproductive cycle of a female rat and implies that nerve circuits that are needed for reproductive behavior are recreated at the same time of each cycle. Appearance of neurons: early in cycle (A); at the time of ovulation (B); and one day after ovulation (C).

altered. And this wiring diagram and the pattern of synapses are at the heart of all brain function, including thought, memory, and emotion. If the circuitry of the brain was changing under the influence of the sex hormone estradiol, these studies would show it.

When slices of rat hypothalamus were stained with Golgi's method, the answer to the scientists' question came out clearly and unmistakably. The number of dendrite spines did change. That meant synapses changed too. Together with studies by electron microscope, the research showed that the actual number of synapses changed with the progression of the rat's estrous cycle. The adult brain did change in its fine structure with the ebb and flow of hormones.

This was an exciting discovery and further results in several laboratories have amplified it. The brain changes during embryonic and fetal development and it continues to change in adult life. Plasticity, particularly in the synapses and dendrites, is a natural and cyclic feature of life in the adult brain. These natural hormonal rhythms are necessary and life sustaining, but the evidence that hormones are continually at work renewing and revising aspects of the human brain and mind, carries many implications. For one thing, the chemical remodeling of the brain that hormones ceaselessly perform means that transient experiences of life as well as the immutable gifts of heredity play a role in the brain's architecture.

There was evidence to support this idea even before detailed studies of the brain nailed it down. Identical twins start life with the same set of genes. If the endowment of genetics was the whole story, there should never be a case in which one twin develops a serious brain disorder while the other does not. But there are such cases; one twin will develop the mentally crippling disease schizophrenia while the other does not. Something in the life experience of one twin has changed the brain in a way that the other twin has escaped. It is true that the twin of a schizophrenic has a much heightened risk of developing the disorder too, but it is only a risk, not a certainty. Some nongenetic factors must contribute to these tragedies. Many scientists have spent many years trying to learn what the essential differences are. To date it is still an unanswered question, but it is clear that crucial differences must exist. Probably the causes are multiple, but it would be surprising if hormones were not involved in the picture somewhere either among the causes or the damaging effects.

Certainly, hormone effects are known to contribute to serious depression and a recent study by scientists of the National Institutes of Health has even shown hormone deficiencies in the endocrine systems and brains of the puzzling condition called chronic fatigue syndrome. Patients who fit this diagnosis all have debilitating fatigue lasting for many months that cannot be blamed on any detectable disease, yet the typical sufferer from this disorder also has bouts of feverishness, tender lymph glands, muscular aches, sleep disturbances, and depression. The study at the NIH showed that such patients are low, compared with normal people, in the amount of the adrenal hormone cortisol in their blood and urine. Cortisol is an important hormone that has antiinflammatory effects on the body and a calming effect on the brain. The scientists attribute the lack in chronic fatigue patients to a shortage of corticotropin-releasing hormone, one of those many hormones produced by the hypothalamus in the brain to send orders to the pituitary gland. This particular hypothalamic hormone tells the pituitary to make and dispatch adrenocorticotropic hormone, known more widely to the hormone-conscious public as ACTH. It is ACTH that tells the adrenals to produce cortisol to respond to stress.

The chronic fatigue condition appears to be a case in which a hormone deficiency does the harm. That kind of effect is a familiar story in endocrinology. Diabetes is probably the most familiar example. The disease reflects either a shortage of the hormone insulin or an inability to use it properly.

Another well-known disorder is Addison's disease, involving insufficiency of adrenocortical hormones, usually because of atrophy of the cortex of the adrenal glands. Weakness and fatigue are among its early symptoms. There are also many health problems, of course, in which too much hormone, or hormones, is the problem.

All such diseases are reminders that hormones, with the proper timing and amount, are absolutely necessary to human well-being and to life itself. In fact, these substances produced in the endocrine glands are the archetypical two-edged sword. They bring growth and vitality, joy and sex, defense and aggression. They are key factors in giving the brain strong mental and emotional highs. But when the body produces too much or too little at a crucial time, they can damage both the body and the mind. It is hormones that ravage the body when the mind is in the grip of continuing and overwhelming stress. Hormone imbalance is an ingredient in serious bouts of depression. There is growing evidence that hormones can cripple the mind, kill cells, and extinguish life. On the other hand, there would be no human life at all without them.

There are three great fundamentals that underlie virtually all of human biology, including that of the brain. One of these is genetics. The action of the genes sets the ground rules and the limits for everything else. A second is the immune system, which governs the body's ability to defend itself against all foreign invasions, including the viruses and bacteria that cause disease. The immune defenses have many other effects, some of them so subtle that they are only gradually coming to light. The third great force, in some ways the most profound of them all, is in the actions of the endocrine system—the world of hormones. Not surprisingly, these three great categories are all tied together.

Much of the work assigned by the genes is done by hormones. In some cases, hormones decide which genes will become active. Hormones have powerful moderating effects on the immune system. They are crucial to the development and functioning of the brain. They have profound effects on the intellect and the emotions. Rage, love, fear, and exaltation are all a matter of hormones, no matter what the poets say. It is the brain that calls hormones into action, but their effects can alter the brain chemically and, the new research shows, even structurally.

Sometimes the causative effects can be remarkably subtle. It has taken many years and a mountain of work to reveal some of the details. Today, everyone, scientists and laymen alike, appreciate that hormones can affect the mind, behavior, decisions, the flames of anger and affection. It has also been

72

known for decades that hormone aberrations in the body can cause disease while hormones given as drugs can cure disease, raise spirits, build muscles and bones. In recent years, scientists have found that hormones are keys to understanding sexual differentiation, brain development and architecture, and many other fundamentals. Evidence has emerged more and more persuasively to suggest that hormones, acting on the brain or called into action by it, are keys to the destructive power of prolonged stress, to the nature of the aging process, perhaps to some aspects of today's great brain plague, Alzheimer's disease. Such considerations are part of the reason for intense interest in hormone effects. If the normal cycle of hormone flow can cause physical changes in the brain, isn't it possible that the level of hormones over a long period of time might produce physical damage, when the level is wrong, or bolster the defenses of the brain when the level is ideal? One of the most obvious cases on the bad side of the equation is that of the anabolic steroid hormones used in excess by bodybuilders. Whether or not they do cause all the bad mental and emotional effects that have been charged is still open to debate, but showing that hormones can cause physical changes in the brain strengthens the evidence that such changes are possible.

Some of the questions related to hormone effects have come to the fore recently with none too comforting implications. Sudden stress brings hormones into play at higher than normal levels. Can chronic stress cause physical changes in the brain? One scientist who has studied this issue thinks some of the new discoveries are frightening. But there is another side to the equation. Stress is necessary to life. Too much placidity may be more deadly than turmoil. What can be done to help keep the effects of stress within life-sustaining bounds? The search for answers to that question appears to start in infancy. The mild stimulation of a little loving-kindness can last a long time. In laboratory animals it seems to last a lifetime.

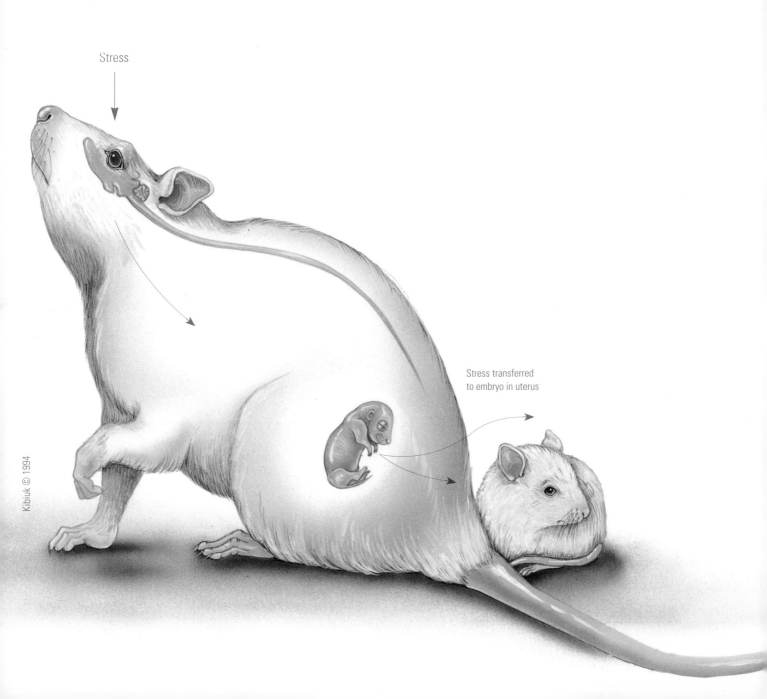

Stress

Stress transferred
to embryo in uterus

Kibiuk © 1994

INSIDE JOB? STRESS, GOOD AND BAD 5

Pregnancy should be a time of hope, calm, and contemplation of the future, but all too often it doesn't work out that way. Take the situation in the Middle East, where the scream of jet fighters, the sudden jolt of explosions, and the unexpected rattle of gunfire often shatter the peace of the expectant mother when she least expects it.

Shakespeare would have called these sudden shocks "alarums." Modern psychologists call them stress. They upset many pregnant women, but do they harm the babies?

Old wives' tales for countless generations have testified that they do. The details of the old folk wisdom are so fanciful that the basic message has usually been ignored. But maybe that's a mark of late twentieth century hubris; a prejudice that there can be no truth without a Ph.D. and a federal grant. Dr. Martha Weinstock, of Hadassah Medical School in Jerusalem, had heard many anecdotes linking wartime stress to babies who were tense, hyperemotional, and colicky. Her city, after all, has not been noted for serenity at any time in this century. Were the frequent eruptions of war and violence reflected in some of the problems of infants whose mothers had been exposed to the noise

Stress to a pregnant rat mother is transmitted to its offspring via nerves and hormones; and the stress causes offspring to become permanently more or less reactive and emotional depending on such early experiences.

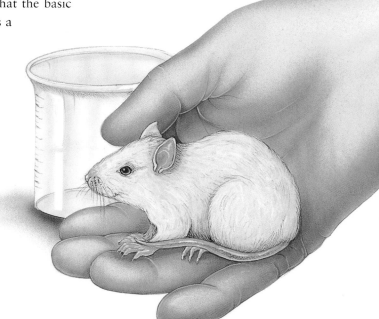

and terror? In humans the issue is probably impossible to prove conclusively, but animal research can be illuminating. What would happen, Dr. Weinstock wondered, if pregnant rats were subjected to the sudden racket of a loud buzzer at irregular and totally unpredictable intervals? These eruptions of noise are not physically damaging in any direct sense, but they do put the expectant mother under stress, which can produce effects on the flow of hormones in her circulation and other things that might affect the fetus. There is little doubt today that psychological stress can produce physical effects, including changes in the brain, but would the effect cross from mother to fetus? The Israeli scientist set up experiments to test the issue by subjecting pregnant rats to sudden noises.

After the rat pups were born, Dr. Weinstock found that the alarmingly loud noises during their mothers' pregnancies had affected a substantial num-

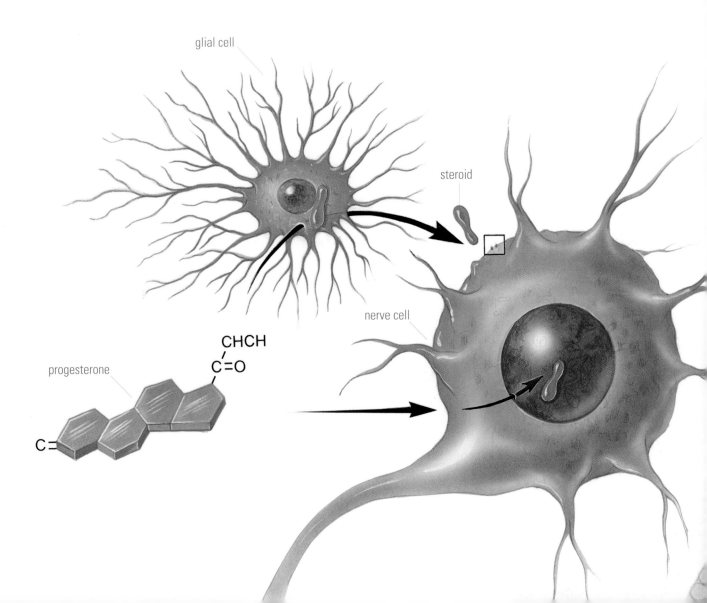

ber of them. They grew up fearful, irritable, and emotionally edgy, much more so than animals that escaped the frightening buzzer. The psychological effects on the mother had physical effects that could be seen in the pups. Their pituitary and adrenal glands were more reactive, producing copious supplies of stress hormones. Since it is the brain that controls those endocrine glands, the prenatal experience must have altered the animals brains too.

The effects on the fetuses seemed to last a long time, well into adulthood, and the scientists did find physical changes in the animals' brains. They had fewer receptors for benzodiazepines than rats whose mothers had not been exposed to the unusual stress. The benzodiazepines are a group of chemicals that calm the brain and promote tranquility. The shortage of receptors meant that the prenatal stress had deprived these rats

Stress frequently activates the secretion of cortisol from the adrenal cortex that is triggered by ACTH from the pituitary. Cortisol secretion is normally "contained" by mechanisms within the brain, but under severe and persistent stress, cortisol secretion can rise above normal and this may cause a variety of damaging effects on the body.

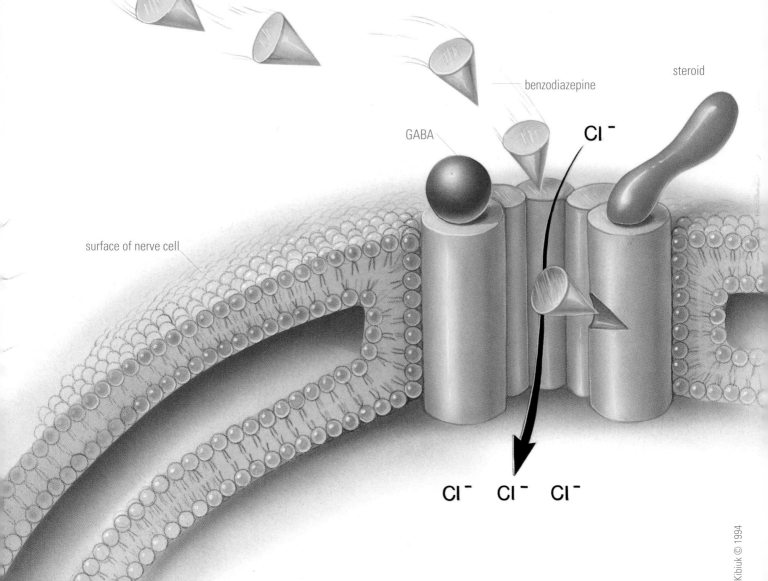

steroid

benzodiazepine

GABA

Cl⁻

surface of nerve cell

Cl⁻ Cl⁻ Cl⁻

Kibiuk © 1994

of a normal mechanism for calming themselves.

Benzodiazepines were originally identified as "tranquilizers" by drug companies, but scientists have discovered that the brain makes equivalents of its own. The homemade variety are called endogenous tranquilizers, meaning that they are produced within the brain itself. The situation is much like that of the endorphins, which are similar to morphine in their painkilling effects. Mammalian brains have been making endorphin receptors for eons; certainly all the way from rodent to human. Brain cells need them to get the painkilling benefit from the endorphins which are also endogenous products of the brain. Indeed, the word endorphin was coined from pieces of the words endogenous, which simply means developing from within, and morphine, the drug.

A similar need for nerve cell action explains the benzodiazepine receptors. They are closely coupled to receptors for the neurotransmitter gamma amino butyric acid, or GABA, which has an inhibitory effect and is therefore important in the brain's natural means of calming itself.

Benzodiazepine receptors were not discovered until 1976. Fortunately, Dr. Weinstock's study was done later than that. Otherwise, she might have missed an important clue to the nature of the effects she saw in the rats whose mothers had been frightened by unexpected noises.

Another surprising discovery emerged from further studies of rats that had been subject to stress while they were still in the womb. It was the effect on these newborn animals of something research workers call handling. Nobody is quite sure why this procedure has the effects it does, but study after study has produced the same results. Handling is a simple matter of taking the newborn rat pups away from their mothers for fifteen minutes or so and then bringing them back. It is done every day for the first two weeks of life. The young animals are treated gently, but they are removed briefly from their mothers' protection and introduced to an alien environment. Intuitively, it would seem to be a stressful experience. In fact, the effects are just the opposite. Unlike the pups whose mothers were exposed to the random noises, the handled pups grew up unmarked by excessive fearfulness and emotion. They seem to have a real advantage in dealing with stress. Biochemical studies showed that the handled animals' hormonal responses to stress were under good control and stayed that way. Moreover, their brains had an excess of the calming benzodiazepine receptors.

Sudden stress in a normal person or animal brings an immediate rise in the "emergency" hormones. But this response to danger is usually brief. Quickly, the brain sends out orders to "cool it." The levels of hormones slide back to normal as soon as the emergency has been confronted. The contrast with the victims of prenatal noise is sharp. In these animals, the stress hormones also rose quickly to face something scary, but their brains' ability to turn off the chemical call-to-arms was impaired. The high levels of stress hormones persisted. This is not only abnormal, but probably damaging. Chronic excess of these steroid hormones can actually kill brain cells. The rats exposed to stress in utero grew up hampered in their ability to take emergencies in their stride. To put their different life styles in human terms, think of the handled animals as "laid back" California rats as contrasted with "uptight" New York rats, the kind whose mothers had experienced the stress of unexpected noise during pregnancy. Not only did the laid back animals cope better with stress in adult life, but studies of their brains showed that the effects of aging develop more slowly in them than in the other group. To cap this line of evidence, however, rat pups born to mothers who were subjected to unexpected noise during pregnancy could escape the ill effects of that experience if they were handled in the first weeks after birth. Not only does the experience of handling rescue the pups from the destructive physical effects, it also seems to give them a better attitude toward life in spite of the early experience. Like other handled pups, these rats also grew up relatively calm and unflappable in the face of stress and these good effects seem to last a lifetime. What the ever-changing brain can take away, it can also give back sometimes.

The sum total of these studies shows how powerfully experience can act on the brain. Stress is a creation of the brain as it interprets sensations and signals from the world at large. Sometimes stress is a figment of the imagination, a danger the brain has concocted within its own circuits. But the consequences are powerful. Stress can cause chemical and even physical changes in the brain; not only the fetal brain and the young brain, but the adult brain as well. Some of these changes tend to protect the brain and help it cope, while others can cause real harm to the brain itself. Meanwhile, of course, the ever-changing brain has physical effects on the body and its health. Discovery of some of those effects many years ago led to the very idea of psychological stress itself.

As a biological concept, stress is little more than fifty years old. The term was borrowed from engineering jargon by the Hungarian-Canadian scientist Hans Selye who noticed, in the 1930s, that laboratory animals suffered serious physical effects, including ulcers and high blood pressure from experiences that were presumably unpleasant, but not physically damaging in themselves. Many scientists since Selye have documented the ill-effects of too much stress in all manner of species, including our own. A particularly important factor is whether or not the individual is prepared and can exercise some control over the outcome. Nearly thirty years ago, Jay M. Weiss, then at The Rockefeller University, and Dr. Martin Seligman of the University of Pennsylvania, did animal experiments that showed this clearly. In the studies, when a rat heard a warning bell and then got a mildly unpleasant electric shock, the animal soon learned to take it without panic. This was especially true if the animal could jump to a safe place where there was no shock. The worst case was when the shocks came frequently with no warning and, particularly, when the animal knew shocks were sure to come but there was nothing that could be done to avoid them. The animals suffered serious physical effects, including ulcers, high blood pressure, and disruptions of the immune defenses. What apparently caused the damage was not the electric shocks at all, but worry and feelings of helplessness.

The total effect was even worse than that, producing an effect that scientists today call learned helplessness. After a certain amount of experience with unavoidable shocks, the animals give up. Even after an avenue of escape is reopened, some animals simply won't take it. Instead, they accept the shocks as inevitable and won't even try to escape.

It is hard to avoid speculating on human equivalents of this phenomenon. Many people in many societies have felt themselves helpless either in the face of human oppressors or the battering of natural disasters. How do these stresses affect the victims' attitudes toward life? How do they affect physical health and even survival? Malnutrition and infectious disease are certainly the major ingredients in shortened life span in these circumstances. But there may be other costs as well. The person who dies in captivity rather than live as a slave is as much a staple of our literature as the person who never gives up.

Recently, psychologists at McLean Hospital in Belmont, Massachusetts, have found evidence that seems to link learned helplessness to some cases of serious depression in humans. In the studies at this major psychiatric research center, the scientists matched the attitudes of severely depressed patients to their bodies' supplies of the substance MHPG, a by-product of the stress hormone norepinephrine. They had noticed that animals suffering from learned helplessness have more MHPG in their brains than do animals still determined to help themselves. In the psychological studies at McLean, gravely depressed patients who were convinced that they were helpless puppets under the control of someone else had unusually high levels of MHPG in their urine. It was a hint at least that more of the substance was being produced in their brains too. Perhaps, in some way yet to be analyzed completely, the chemistry of learned helplessness is acting in these human tragedies. Other studies have shown that

Stress means different things to different people. Whether a situation is perceived to be stressful depends on a person's genetic make-up and prior experiences in early life as well as later on. These combine to sensitize to or protect an individual from particular challenges. How we respond to a threat or challenge plays a big role in how stressful something becomes: that is, behaviors chosen may involve aggression or submission, may result in humiliation or adaptation, and may further increase or decrease vulnerability to subsequent events. There are also individual differences in how much hormone activation results from a stressful event and how long that hormone secretion goes on. Imbalances in hormone secretion accelerate disease processes, and internal imbalances in neurochemical in the brain, such as serotonin (see Chapter 1), have been linked in animals to aggression and in humans to hostility, substance abuse, impulsive behavior and suicide.

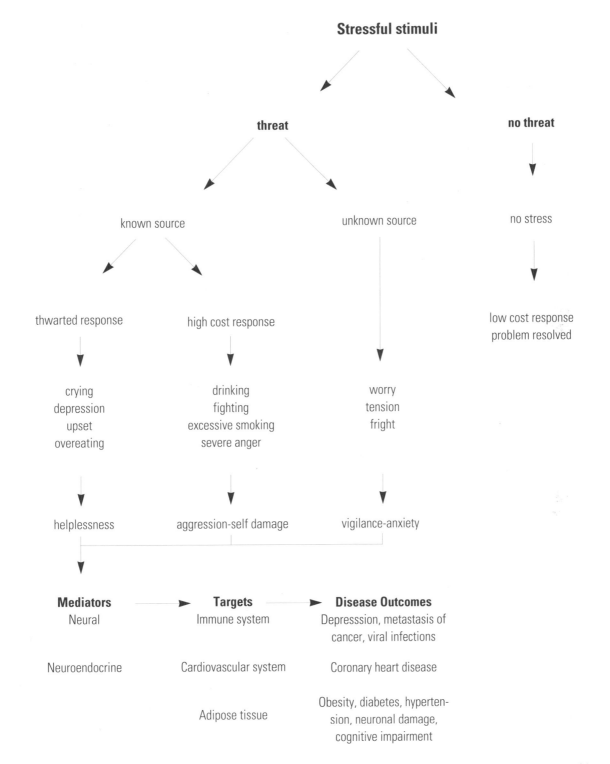

Stressful stimuli

threat → **no threat**

known source   unknown source   no stress

thwarted response   high cost response

crying   drinking   worry   low cost response
depression   fighting   tension   problem resolved
upset   excessive smoking   fright
overeating   severe anger

helplessness   aggression-self damage   vigilance-anxiety

Mediators	→	**Targets**	→	**Disease Outcomes**
Neural		Immune system		Depresssion, metastasis of cancer, viral infections
Neuroendocrine		Cardiovascular system		Coronary heart disease
		Adipose tissue		Obesity, diabetes, hypertension, neuronal damage, cognitive impairment

too much production (hypersecretion) of glucocorticoid hormones is often associated with depressive illness and degenerative brain diseases.

But stress is a universal feature of life, and it hardly requires scientific training to know that stress is both good and bad. No human or any other creature with a nervous system could survive if its natural responses to stress were not jolted into action when sudden emergency erupts. Sounding the call to action in the face of danger is one of the brain's most crucial functions. A tiger bounding down a jungle path and a car swerving suddenly into the wrong lane trigger the same instant responses: a suddenly racing heart and clang of instant attention. This is lifesaving stress. The cliché is "fight or flight." The reaction seems almost instantaneous: the brain sounds the alarm to the muscles and the muscles react so fast that the response may be all over by the time the conscious part of the brain registers the danger.

The first part of the response calls the autonomic nervous system to instant action. The heartbeat and breathing are faster, some arteries relax so blood can flow more readily to the muscles, but vessels supplying the skin constrict so there will be less bleeding if wounded. This is mobilization for war and it blunts or puts on hold any "civilian" concerns that get in the way or can be postponed—sense of pain, digestion, growth, sex, and reproduction. In the emergency they are distractions, expensive in terms of body energy they require and useful only if life is going to continue. Dr. Robert M. Sapolsky, of Stanford University, calls them "optimistic processes."

The second part of the stress response activates the adrenal cortex to produce the hormone cortisol. The brain directs this too by sending signals to the hypothalamus to release a chemical called CRH, for corticotropin-releasing hormone. CRH stimulates the pituitary to release another chemical, ACTH. It is the ACTH which travels in the blood stream all the way to the adrenal glands on top of the kidneys. The adrenal cortex, the outer layer of those glands, produces the cortisol, and releases it into the circulating blood.

Cortisol is a marvelous substance. We put it on skin rashes to sooth the inflammation, and we take it, or synthetic derivatives, for allergies and autoimmune disorders to keep the overzealous immune system from causing us harm. Cortisol also has a calming influence on the brain. It does this through a process called "counterregulation" which prevents many nerve signaling chemicals that respond to stress from reacting too strongly. These include such neurotransmitters as serotonin, norepinephrine, and dopamine. In fact, the disabling symptoms of depressive illness result from an imbalance of these stress-sensitive chemicals in the brain. Normally, cortisol appears to keep them in balance. Evidence from animal experiments suggests that the absence of cortisol makes the brain more susceptible to learned helplessness, that consequence of inescapable stress discovered by Drs. Weiss and Seligman, which may be an animal equivalent of severe depression in humans.

One of the surprising findings of recent research on hormones and stress is that the body also takes one of the adrenal steroids secreted in response to ACTH and converts it to another steroid that acts like a benzodiazepine tranquilizer on what is known as a GABA-benzodiazepine receptor. Thus, the brain has its own means of calming things down in the aftermath of stress, even as it also has the means to increase arousal and anxiety.

Of course, too much placidity can be as deadly as too much excitement. It is the brain, with the help of the adrenal cortex, that defines both states and there is great variation among individuals. Some people are frightened in thunderstorms. Other people ignore the high altitude pyrotechnics. Some like the mild excitement of routine flying, others hate the whole experience from takeoff to landing. The brain decides.

But marvelous as the brain is, it can be misled and sometimes it reacts too much. That's what happened to Dr. Selye's animals and to those of Dr. Weiss and Dr. Seligman. The animals' bodies switched on the defensive process, but gradually lost the knack of turning it off again promptly enough.

If those effects in laboratory animals also apply to humans, they are enlightening and important, but do they really apply? A huge gulf of evolution separates *Homo sapiens* from the rodent species even though we too are mammals. In addition, laboratory animals typically are inbred creatures contrived by selective breeding over many generations to be uniform, predictable, and as nearly identical to each other in any one strain as possible. They are biology's interchangeable machine parts. In contrast, humans are a wild species. Except for the special case of identical twins, each one of us is substantially different from all others. Humans are anything but uniform and seldom totally predictable either by politicians or scientists. Given the differences in biology and life experience, it would be nice to have the concepts generated in artificial experiments with laboratory rats confirmed in natural populations living in the natural world.

Enter Dr. Robert Sapolsky of Stanford University. For many years he has studied groups of wild baboons and vervet monkeys in Africa. One of the objectives was precisely that of answering some of the nagging questions about how much reliance should be placed on ideas generated from the chemistry and behavior of laboratory rats. In the course of his yearly studies in Kenya, an accident of monkey overpopulation gave Dr. Sapolsky an unusual chance to see the emotional and physical effects of stress, and what stress can

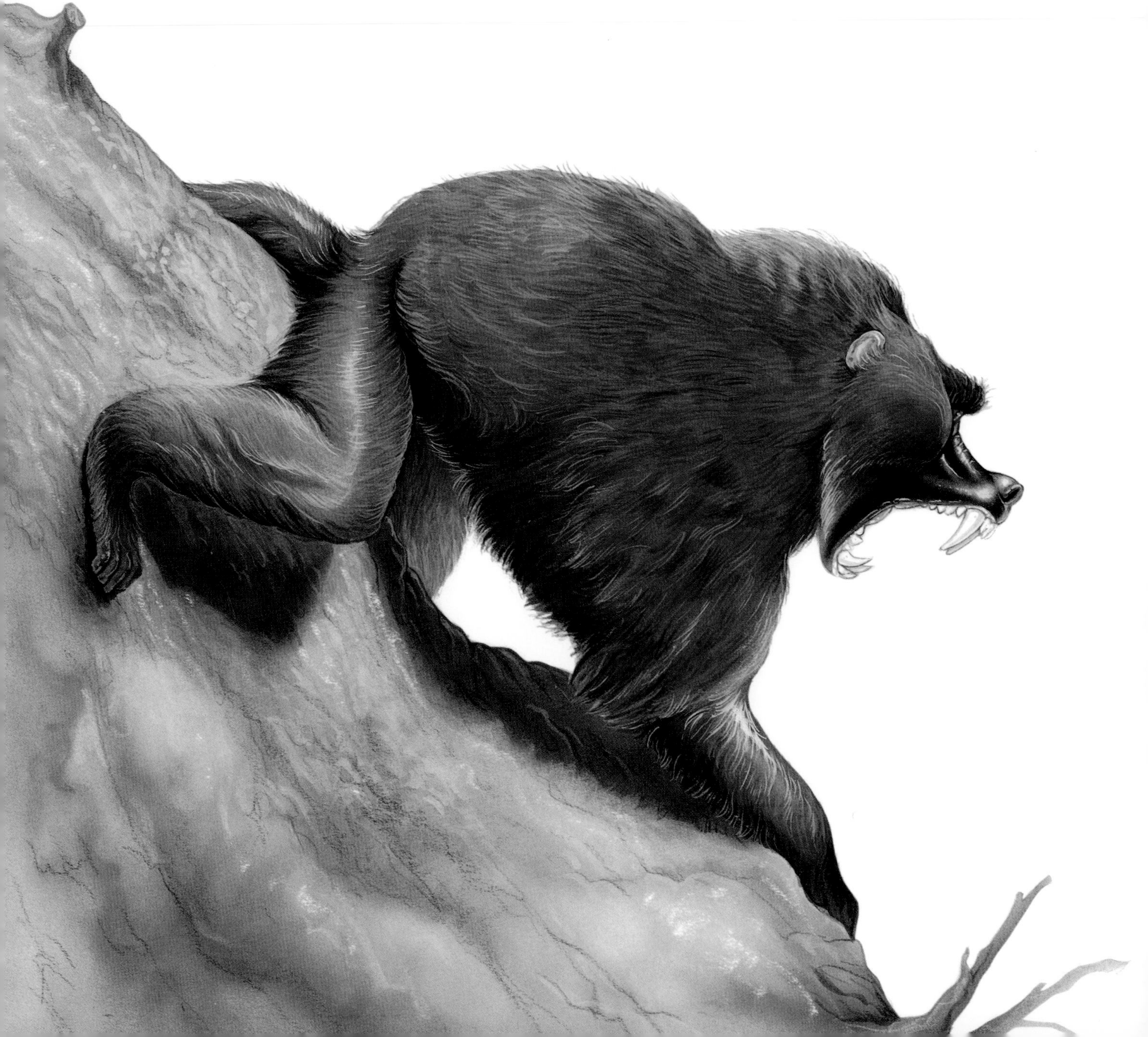

do to the adult brain. Because hordes of monkeys were destroying crops, local residents captured many of them. The animals were too valuable to be killed, so they were caged and sent to a primate center in Nairobi. But while the monkeys were living close together in captivity, some of them died. The deaths were unexpected because the animals had been in good health when they were captured. The puzzle of the deaths gave Dr. Sapolsky the opening for a particularly illuminating phase of his studies. At first it wasn't at all clear what could have killed the monkeys but he puzzled out the story from the bodies of the dead animals and the health problems of some that survived. Sherlock Holmes would have appreciated the feat.

First of all, people who study them in the wild know that baboons and monkeys tend to live in groups that have strict, unequal social structures. It is not the natural paradise imagined by the eighteenth century French philosopher, Jean Jacques Rousseau. Some of the animals dominate the others. The dominant monkeys enforce the rules of social living on their subordinates. There is no Bill of Rights. The concepts of fairness and compassion—inventions of the human brain—don't appear. When one dominant male loses a fight it is likely to go pick a fight with a less bellicose subordinate male and take out its frustrations on this victim. When the subordinate animal loses its fight it has no way to vent its anger. It is easy to imagine the ultimate roots of any kind of human despotism in these inhabitants of the natural world. In the wild, subordinate males usually stay out of the way of the dominant males, giving up the most desirable food and the most tempting females when the dominant animal appears on the scene. The arrangement works reasonably well where there is plenty of room. In a cage in captivity, however, it is not possible to keep very far out of the way. Study of the dead animals showed that they all had numerous scars from bites and the puncture wounds of other monkeys' canine teeth. From this evidence, they must have lost most of their fights. They were subordinate animals. They didn't die of the bites because most of the wounds were healed. Dr. Sapolsky concluded that they died of severe and sustained social stress. Evidently they had been caged with particularly aggressive dominant animals and had no place to run, no place to hide from the oppressor.

The dead animals all had gastric ulcers, adrenal glands that were overgrown from too much activity, colitis, and signs that their immune defenses were depressed and not functioning with normal vigor. These are all typical effects of stress in which the brain's inability to cope with the social situation creates physical problems for the rest of the body. Indeed, Dr. Sapolsky noted that a study by another scientist found that same spectrum of health disorders

Animals in the wild react to stress by changing the secretion of hormones. Dominant male baboons have a different physiological response compared with subordinate males to the same stressful event. Under stress dominant males show increased testosterone levels and subordinate males show decreased testosterone levels. They also show decreased testosterone levels in relation to being dominated and abused by the dominant male.

Based on photograph from Dr. Robert Sapolsky, Stanford University.

in monkeys known from direct observation to be subordinate animals. So it appeared quite clear that the unfortunate monkeys in the Nairobi primate center were subordinate animals who died of severe social stress. The deaths confirmed starkly the common epitaph of the overworked and underappreciated businessman: "The job killed him." The fate of the monkeys in Kenya was strong evidence that it really can happen. The monkeys' fatal constellation of health problems: ulcers, high blood pressure, kidney problems, and the rest, mimicked the whole panoply of complaints of the unhappy human who sees work and the world crowding him unmercifully. Only lacking were the peculiarly human burdens of eating too much, exercising too little, and chain-smoking cigarettes. Monkeys and baboons are not humans and their social lives bear little resemblance to ours. Nevertheless, we are far closer to them both biologically and socially than we are to laboratory rats and Dr. Sapolsky's studies deserve attention. But, in an important sense, the diagnosis of death from severe social stress only begs the question. Psychological stress is a phenomenon of the mind. It is a uniquely personal judgment about signals from the outside world. There may be obvious danger, life-threatening and immediate. There may be subtle danger, lingering, indirect but real, or sometimes only imagined. Shouts of rage from someone nearby may be stressful or totally insignificant. It all depends on the circumstances and a complicated mix of personal traits, social status, prior experience, and expectations. The person who feels too much stress may react in a host of different ways: anger and violence, fear, depression, overeating, drinking, smoking, indigestion, or harmful rises in blood pressure and heart rate. Stress can damage and kill. It is a blatant case of the brain becoming hostage to its own imaginings.

What actually happens to the brain that makes thoughts call forth this fatal damage to the rest of the body?

The monkeys who died of social stress gave some important clues here too because a dozen of their brains were saved for study. They could be compared with the brains of other monkeys that had been killed in the course of other research. The comparative brain studies gave some chilling results: severe psychological stress can damage the adult brain. To students of stress and the brain the nature of the damage was significant too. Dr. Sapolsky and his colleague, Dr. Hideo Uno, found that damage was quite selective in the brains of animals that had died of social stress. The notable damage in those animals was severe degeneration of the hippocampus. In this small area of the brain, a quarter of the animals showed degenerative changes in four-fifths of their neurons. Three-quarters of them had this kind of degeneration in one-fifth of their neurons. No comparable damage could be found in the monkeys that

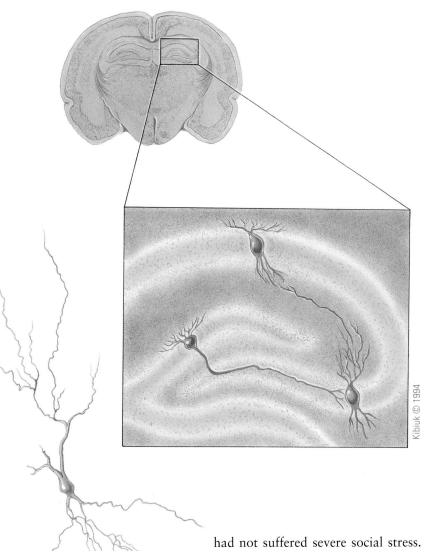

Kibiuk © 1994

The hippocampus is folded into the interior of the cerebral cortex, and it consists of two major parts, the Ammons horn and the dentate gyrus. Neurons of the hippocampus undergo shrinkage as a result of persistent stress and elevated levels of cortisol. This atrophy impairs the ability of the hippocampus to perform its normal function. If the stress or cortisol levels remain high for long periods, then permanent damage may occur and neurons are lost in the hippocampus that cannot be replaced.

had not suffered severe social stress. Dr. Sapolsky said a similar pattern of brain destruction had been seen in another species related to the monkeys and other primates, the tree shrew. Subordinate tree shrews also died of severe social stress. In these small and highly active animals it takes as little as two weeks for damage to the hippocampus to develop from severe social problems.

The hippocampus, a small formation deep in the brain, is only about two inches long. It is a part of what students of brain evolution call the "old" brain. It is known to be crucial to the processes of emotion and memory. As such it is a particularly important part of the brain in humans and other primates, although it existed long before these Johnny-come-lately species first gleamed in the everchanging rainbow of life on Earth. As part of what is called the limbic system, the hippocampus is intricately connected with everything else in the brain. Its role in the emotions makes it an obvious target for damage from excessive stress. The hippocampus monitors the brain's perceptions of the world, continually matching expectation with reality. So long as the brain registers the external realities as what it expected, the hippocampus stays quiet. The sudden impact of the unexpected jolts it into action. Stressful experiences often do that: an electric shock where the rat usually found a food pellet; a sudden attack that a monkey couldn't flee; an emotional betrayal where a man or woman thought there was love. Experiences such as those can overwork the hippocampus.

The importance of the hippocampus in the stress studies derives also from something else. It is thought to be a safety brake that holds the stress response within useful bounds. The normal sequence of events is that the brain senses a stressful situation—the attacking tiger or motorist out of control—and mobilizes blood flow, supplies of sugar, and the defense hormones for quick action. The hypothalamus, also a part of the old brain, uses its special hormones to signal the crisis to the pituitary gland. The hypothalamic hormones are called releasing hormones because they tell the pituitary to release its own hormones. Triggered by these releasing factors, the pituitary sends out its hormones as a trumpet call to action for the adrenal glands and everything else that acts in defense. It is the adrenals that produce such powerful stress hormones as adrenalin and noradrenalin, now known as epinephrine and norepinephrine. But, altogether, many hormones are involved in the process of responding to stress.

It is a cascade of events that runs a predictable course, including the automatic feedback mechanism to bring things back to normal. That is where the hippocampus is thought to play a crucial role. Soon after a sudden stress brings the emergency response into play, the hippocampus begins to rein in the exuberance of the hormones. Things have to be brought back to normal. Neither the body nor the brain is designed to withstand heavy doses of those powerful hormones on a continual basis. The feedback loop of hypothalamus, pituitary to adrenals to hippocampus, quickly restores normal balance with the help of additional chemicals that have a calming effect. That is how the system works normally and, particularly, in young animals. There has been a lot of research in rats, however, that suggests a dark side of the picture. Sometimes the emergency goes on and on, or at least the brain sees it that way. This state of persistent arousal prolongs the bath of emergency hormones. When that happens, the system apparently loses its resilience. The talent for fine-tuning the response is blunted. The emergency hormones are not turned off either sufficiently or promptly enough. The brief spurts that can be lifesaving become persistent and potentially damaging. This concept is at the heart of what brain scientists call the glucocorticoid cascade. Glucocorticoids are steroid hormones such as the familiar hydrocortisone, also known as cortisol. According to the cascade hypothesis, the feedback loop becomes distorted in an individual gripped by chronic stress. In some animals this seems to happen simply as a consequence of growing old. The safety brake stops functioning properly and abnormally high levels of cortisol continue to flood the circulation and presumably cause damage that further impairs the safety brake. A vicious circle.

The evidence from Dr. Sapolsky's monkeys seemed to fit solidly with this concept, but part of the overall idea was theory embroidering the results of brain studies in the animals. Was it really the cortisol damaging the hippocampus in these animals that was producing the bad results? The obvious way to find out was to give monkeys high doses of cortisol in amounts to be expected from extreme stress and continue these treatments for years. But this egregiously long experiment would also produce many other health effects on the monkeys, including digestive problems and, probably, severe depression as well. In describing the stress studies in monkeys in his book published in 1992, *Stress, The Aging Brain and the Mechanisms of Neuron Death*, Dr. Sapolsky said he considered it an unacceptable experiment. Instead he chose a compromise. In a few monkeys, he implanted pellets that would secrete cortisol directly into the hippocampus. He then studied the brains a year later to see whether or not there was damage to the neurons. The scientist noted several limitations on the significance of such a study. It would be hard to judge whether the doses delivered in the brain were really appropriate. They could be far too high to mimic the effects of stress or they might be too low. The study might be too brief. One year in a monkey is only the equivalent of about a month in a rat, the species in which most of the previous information had been collected. Similar treatment of rats for a month had been found too short to produce clear damage to the hippocampus.

Nevertheless, the scientist found that the brains of the monkeys in the study really were damaged. Dr. Sapolsky's conclusions were somber.

"Collectively," he said of the whole research effort, "these rather grim studies show that sustained and severe stress can damage the primate hippocampus. Moreover, glucocorticoids alone can damage both the fetal and adult hippocampus."

Homo sapiens is a primate species. Humans need to take seriously effects that occur in other primates.

It would be foolish to underestimate the differences between monkeys and humans, but if a reasonable share of what is true in them is also true of us, the implications of these studies are serious. The word Dr. Sapolsky used was "frightening."

Millions of men and women suffer prolonged and serious stress. The animal studies hint that stress of this magnitude and duration may be exacting an even higher price than anyone has yet realized. Perhaps the brain itself may be damaged by the excessive exposure to the hormones that chronic stress calls forth. Studies of concentration camp survivors and torture victims may have provided clues to understanding of the damage stress can do. Cases of severe depression, problems of thought and memory years afterward have been documented. The evidence from animals hints that the severe stress could have contributed to these long-delayed effects. Whether these victims of cruel stress also have diminished life spans as a result is harder to sort out, considering

Stress frequently activates the secretion of cortisol from the adrenal cortex that is triggered by ACTH from the pituitary. Cortisol secretion is normally "contained" by mechanisms within the brain, but under severe and persistent stress, cortisol secretion can rise above normal and this may cause a variety of damaging effects on the body.

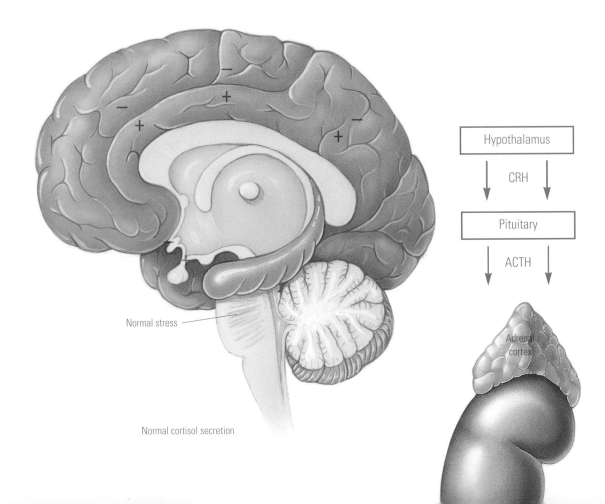

Normal stress

Normal cortisol secretion

Hypothalamus

CRH

Pituitary

ACTH

Adrenal cortex

that their ordeals involved severe physical damage and, usually, malnutrition as well as stress. In any case, the crimes of the perpetrators may be even worse than we had imagined, permanently destroying brains and personalities as well as crippling bodies.

These are plausible speculations, but they are still speculations. The evidence from animal studies shows that massive doses of stress hormones can damage the brain, but many other factors are likely to be involved in stress.

And Dr. Sapolsky said it is still not clear whether physiologically high doses, the maximum amounts the body itself can generate, are high enough in prolonged stress to damage the brain. Studies need to be done to answer that question. Meanwhile, there is another equally worrisome issue that the animal studies bring into sharp focus for the first time. Whether or not naturally produced high doses of the hormones can produce damage to the brain, it seems a good guess that steroid hormones, taken in massive doses as drugs, are capable of doing so. Millions of Americans receive substantial doses of such hormones in medical treatments for a variety of diseases. While most of

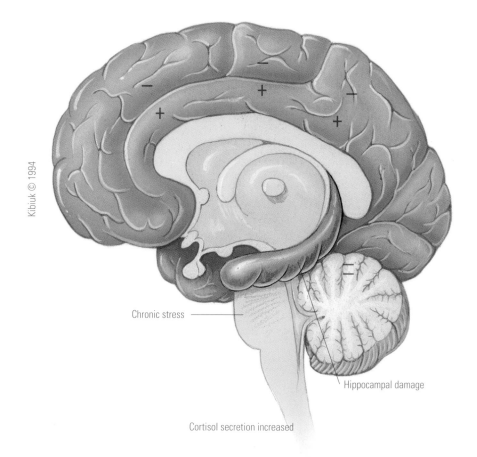

Kibiuk © 1994

Chronic stress

Hippocampal damage

Cortisol secretion increased

91

these treatments are relatively brief and carefully circumscribed there is another population of people who take various steroids in heavy doses over prolonged periods for bodybuilding. Are these bodies being built at the risk of damaging the brains that decided on that course of action? Might the price of compulsive bodybuilding in youth be an acceleration of the rate of growing old? These speculations cannot be dismissed as total fantasy. The evidence in animals appears to be beyond dispute. Seriously excessive exposure to corticoid hormones can damage the hippocampus. There is no humane way to prove that this danger does really exist for human users of hormones. The evidence that does exist in humans is still ambiguous, but frightening. Added to the many reports of personality problems in streroid abusers, there is the new animal evidence suggesting physical damage to the brain and that the damage can be permanent. It may be that the full answer won't be known until it is too late for many people who thought they were too tough or too lucky to be harmed. This is a situation in which the everchanging brain may not have a second chance to survive its own fad-generated actions.

All of the studies of the beneficial handling of young animals, stress in the laboratory, stress in wild animals, and the anecdotal evidence concerning severe stress in humans demonstrates beyond doubt that experience can change the brain at any time from fetal life through adulthood. Not surprisingly, the brain seems to be more resilient in the young than in the old. After all, the rest of the body is at its most resilient in youth too.

Furthermore, while experience changes the brain, it is clear that the brain changes everything else. One of the great sources of wonder to anyone who considers the brain is the immense power this three-pound package of tissue exerts on everything else in the body and, for that matter, on everything else in the world at large. The brain functions through chemistry and electricity, through the complex interplay of enzymes, hormones, and the balance of some of the simplest chemical compounds such as salt and water. In some particular small parts of the process, the chemistry itself has been worked out in remarkable detail. The studies of stress are an important case in point. But the most awe-inspiring part of the story comes from just what is meant by psychological stress. It is not physical. It is a matter of thought and emotion. The rats studied by Drs. Seligman and Weiss thirty years ago were not harmed by the electric shocks or any of the other physical experiences administered to them. They were harmed physically by the emotion of fear and the sense of helplessness. Dr. Sapolsky's monkeys were not killed by wounds. They died from extremes of social stress. The human brain's most powerful weapon against the world and its most serious danger to itself lie within itself. The brain can become hostage to something totally intangible: its own thoughts. They can unleash internal forces that make the final difference between health and illness, life and death.

Every person experiences something of this, but nowhere is it more stark or cataclysmic than in armed combat. In terms of war's sheer destruction of humans and things, the twentieth century has been the bloodiest hundred years in all of humanity's time on earth. In these ordeals too, the human brain has been its own strongest bulwark and its worst enemy. Many seem to have come through the stress of combat intact in both mind and body. Many have had torn bodies. In many others, the wounds have been almost entirely in the mind. But they are indisputably real wounds. Why do they occur demonstrably only in some and how can these walking wounded be helped? As a puzzle, it is probably as old as combat, but today, the doctors who treat these wounds have some new ideas that are giving the wounded new understanding and some new hope.

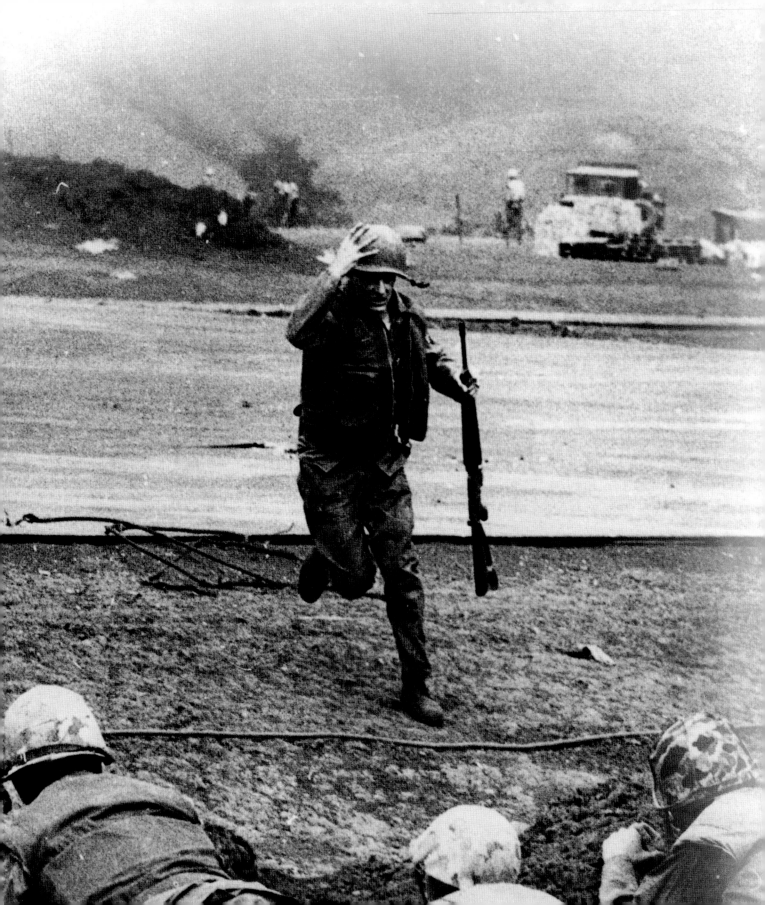

ETERNAL VIGILANCE IS THE PRICE 6

One of the bloodiest battles of the war in Vietnam was the fight for Hué City during the Tet offensive of 1968. The Vietcong had overrun the city. American troops fought house to house and street by street to drive them out. For the men who fought there, the memories are seared indelibly like scars on the mind. Explosions and the shriek of shells rocked the city and there seemed to be snipers in every building. Each house was a mortal threat; every closed door a life and death gamble. Push it open: Would the whole room explode? Would it erupt in gunfire? Or would you risk the horror of firing into a huddle of terrified women and children? One American who lived through it remembers men beside him being shot by snipers. At least one buddy died in his arms with most of his face blown away. It was terrifying. It was absolutely exhausting and it seemed to go on forever. This was stress more fierce and agonizing than most people can even imagine.

"He saw a lot of combat even apart from that," said one doctor describing a veteran of the fighting in Hué, "but that sequence of experiences was clearly the absolute worst."

This soldier came home months after Tet and thought it was all over, but it wasn't. He seldom found work and couldn't hold those jobs he did find. He drank a lot. He had nightmares. His whole life drifted downhill. Today he is receiving treatment and counseling at a Veterans Affairs center.

A U.S. Marine is rushing to cover at the end of the airstrip in Khe Sanh.
Archive Photo/Archive France

"He wakes up at night with a lot of anxiety. He has nightmares; he'll wake up sweating. He'll think he is about to bust in a door and be greeted by a hail of fire," said Dr. Terence M. Keane, a clinical psychologist at the Boston Veterans Affairs Medical Center. "He'll wake up thinking he is about to die. And he's been having these symptoms pretty much since he returned from the war."

That return was twenty-five years ago and the man's problems still persist. He suffers from what specialists now call PTSD. The letters stand for post-traumatic stress disorder. It is the same mental wound that doctors in the First World War called "shell shock" and their counterparts in World War II named "combat fatigue." The name seems to add more syllables with each new war. The changes show professionals' growing appetite for wordiness, but there is somewhat more to it than that. The first two names were labels. The third is at least an attempt to define the condition. Furthermore, the early labels referred specifically to the stress of combat. The new name is more global. It recognizes devastating life experiences that hit civilians was well as the military.

Experts say that people exposed to widely different psychological traumas—civil disasters, rape and other sexual abuse, torture, abuse in childhood, as well as heavy combat—have strikingly similar symptoms. Many also have coexisting problems such as anxiety disorders, major depression, and drug or alcohol abuse.

An Argentine writer who was tortured during the worst years of the military dictatorship said he still reacts with an unreasonable shock of terror when he sees black shoes. That was what he first saw every time his torturers entered his cell.

Nurses who care for many soldiers mangled in combat can also suffer from PTSD. Until recently they have been among the least recognized victims of the horrors of war.

Specialists who study it say PTSD can be found in civilian occupations as well as military. It is sometimes diagnosed in police and fire fighters and in the men and women who go to the rescue after airliner crashes. The troops and civilian men and women who went to Somalia to protect and feed the starving in 1992 and 1993 faced nightmare horrors too. Specialists in PTSD say it wouldn't be surprising if some of these people develop the disorder. Indeed, symptoms of PTSD have already appeared in some American veterans of Operation Desert Storm in the Middle East. From the United States' point of view, that war against Iraq's dictator was won with casualties so few as to seem miraculous. But it was a real war nevertheless and it had all of war's inevitable horrors. A National Guard medical unit saw one of their doctors and a nurse killed when the unit came under fire. The nurse was dismembered by an explosion and bled to death before she could be evacuated. Later, the same unit moved farther into Iraq where its members saw many burned, charred, and flattened human bodies and where another explosion left some members of the unit seriously wounded.

This medical group was one of two National Guard contingents studied, after they returned home, by the National Center for Post-Traumatic Stress Disorder at the West Haven VA Medical Center and Yale University in Connecticut. The team's preliminary report found full-scale PTSD uncommon. But many of the returning veterans had some symptoms from their traumatic experiences. In some of them, the symptoms persisted.

PTSD could also be a normal risk of life in some American cities. Neighborhoods in south central Los Angeles and parts of New York have been described as real combat zones where gunfire causes more deaths than auto accidents.

Civilian or military, any sensible person will be frightened in the face of sudden death, particularly if the threat is real and continues for a long time. Sometimes fear can be disabling, either then or later.

Dr. Keane said PTSD is distinct from the overwhelming and disabling fear that hits some men in the midst of heavy combat. Psychologists today call those cases combat stress reaction or CSR. They believe it is best treated as soon as possible as close to the fighting zone as possible with a quick return of the soldier to his unit. It is the same rationale as the age-old advice to anybody who has been thrown from a horse: Get up and get back on the animal as soon as you can. It is better for the mount and the rider.

But PTSD is different. By definition, it is a somewhat delayed effect that comes to the surface a month, or several months, after the events that caused it. There is a common set of symptoms: acute anxieties, nightmares, a tendency to keep recalling the experience in one's thoughts and to have flashbacks in which the victim is suddenly reliving the past horrors as though they were happening again right now. Any reminder of the experience can bring it all back in an instant: a movie scene, perhaps an aroma of Chinese food being cooked, a truck backfiring, an approaching helicopter. With these symptoms go severe difficulties in sleeping and bouts of chronic anxiety or severe depression.

For many of its victims, another hallmark of PTSD is what mental health workers call hypervigilance or hyperarousal. The person cannot relax. The effect is both mental and physical as the brain keeps the body perpetually aroused to face imagined danger. The ordinary person goes blithely through most of life assuming that nothing bad lurks beyond the next door or around the corner; in short, that nothing serious is likely to go wrong just now. The world is different for the PTSD patient. Each closed door hides a threat. There really is danger around every corner. The whole environment must be searched continually for signs. Relaxation is a skill that has to be relearned.

A serious and unusual disorder of sleep is also a hallmark of PTSD. Most people who have insomnia fall into one of two main categories: those who find it difficult to fall asleep at night and those who wake too early in the morning and can't doze off again. Dr. Keane says his PTSD patients often have problems at both ends of the night. They can't fall asleep for a long time when they go to bed. Once asleep, they wake up too early and their sleep is only fitful in between.

"It's a very unusual thing," he says. "My sense is that it is a function of the nightmares; the fear of having nightmares and the unwillingness to let one's guard down."

Another key feature of PTSD is what mental health workers call emotional numbing. The person is largely dead to joy, love, and humor. He or she feels no emotional attachment to others, or admits to none. The patient may feel anger and fear, but seldom any happy thoughts.

Can wounds this dire ever be healed? Is it possible to cure PTSD and what does the assault on the mind do to the brain itself?

Specialists say "cure" is not a meaningful word in these cases. The awful memories at the core of the problem can't be erased. But there is much that can be done to help the patient cope with the mental scars and return to relatively normal life. Religion, family support, as well as counseling and therapy by mental health professionals all help some of the patients.

Dr. Keane said relaxation training is often helpful as well as instruction in such tactics as thought-stopping—teaching the patient to turn off a painful reverie of the combat experience when it first starts to engulf him. The patient learns to remind himself that things are better now, that he really is safe, and then to shift his mind deliberately to something else.

In fact, almost every kind of behavioral, psychotherapeutic, and drug treatment thought to be useful in other mental and emotional disorders has been tried against PTSD. Some treatments seem to help, but there have been few studies of the kind needed to prove which are best.

One common finding has been that people in the long-term grip of PTSD seldom get much help from placebos, the inactive substitute pills often used in studies of a new drug's effectiveness. In such drug studies, the patients don't know at the time whether they are receiving the placebo or the real drug. Doctors have observed that many patients with anxiety disorders unrelated to PTSD, and even some with physical disorders such as high blood pressure, will get temporary relief from placebos simply because they expect the pills to help. One proof of any drug's real worth is that it produces better and more lasting therapeutic effects than the placebo. The fact that PTSD patients are not fooled by these inactive substitutes suggests that there are biological as well as psychological factors in their condition.

But why does PTSD occur in the first place? Or, to put the same question in another way, why doesn't it happen to all combat veterans? One of the prime puzzles of the condition is why some people fall victim while others seem to be spared even though they had devastating experiences too. One clue may be in the person's early life experience. Physical abuse in childhood or some other horrible experience or deprivation seems to heighten the risk. How does that work? To take a noncombat example: a woman who has been raped as a teenager may seem to recover from that trauma and yet break down years later on being mugged at knife point. The mugging brought her to the crisis point, but the rape was probably the underlying cause. In short, some set of priming experiences seems to foretell PTSD. Devastating childhood experiences, an unstable family environment, an underlying anxiety disorder or severe depression, history of drug or alcohol abuse. These are all items that pop out of the statistics.

But there is a more subtle side to the puzzle of why some people suffer from PTSD while others do not. Maybe the others haven't escaped entirely either. Dr. Keane, among others, suspects that scars are really there.

"There are a lot of people who function, objectively, just fine after these events," he said, "In other words, they can make a lot of money, become professionals, become terrific lawyers, effective businessmen, but they'll tell you that they are having a lot of symptoms. They may have nightmares. Their marriages may fall apart. They may have trouble relating to their children. They may have drinking problems."

And why are some driven to violence, drugs, and drink, while some others are driven just as hard to highly active, socially constructive lives? Anybody can think of hypotheses. Nobody knows the total answer.

Some psychiatrists still question that PTSD really exists as a totally separate entity of mental ill-health. PTSD patients are often depressed and they often suffer from terrible anxieties. Maybe those underlying problems are the central reality beneath the diagnosis. That issue can become a circular chicken-vs-egg argument. Nevertheless, many doctors who treat PTSD say there

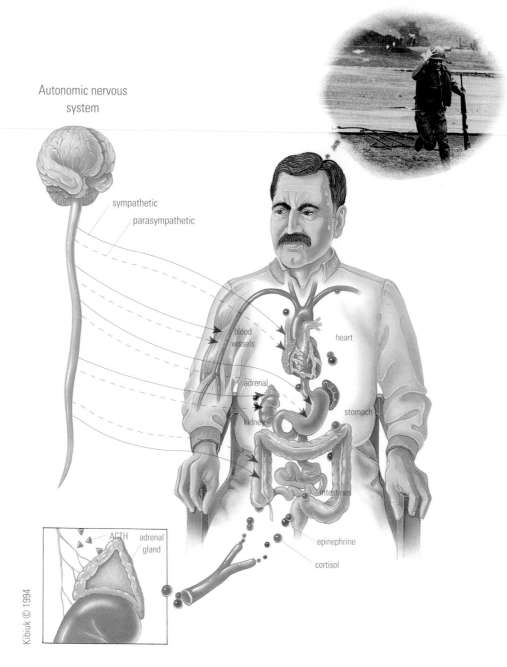

Autonomic nervous system

sympathetic
parasympathetic

blood vessels

heart

adrenal

stomach

kidney

intestines

epinephrine

cortisol

ACTH   adrenal gland

Kibiuk © 1994

A threatening event activates the "flight or fight" response. Voluntary muscles are prepared for action (1) and the sympathetic nervous system (2) dilates blood vessels and pupils of the eyes as well as increasing heart rate, in anticipation of action. Epinephrine released by the adrenal gland mobilizes immediate sources of energy (3). ACTH is released from the pituitary gland and causes a delayed reaction from the adrenal - namely, the secretion of cortisol. Cortisol acts via the receptors depicted in Fig. 4.5 to "contain" or limit the response to stress and maintain normal body function, even in the face of continuation of the stressful situation.

In states of "vigilance" that are part of PTSD, memories of threatening events can trigger the same physiological responses as real events. Moreover, the nervous system is sensitized to overreact to noises such as a car backfiring and to produce an exaggerated "startle" response as well as heightened activity of the sympathetic nervous system.
Archive Photos/Archive France

are important differences between that condition and cases of pure depression or general anxiety serious enough to require medical care.

In any case, the symptoms of PTSD are certainly real and they develop as the aftermath of terrible stress. The effects have been seen, not just for decades, but for millennia. In the bloody, violent twentieth century, it is a temptation to think our own era is the seat of all the really desperate problems. In fact, literature as far back as Homer hints at the same symptoms that today are called PTSD. Why did Achilles sulk in his tent? What was it really that prevented Odysseus from coming home to Ithaca for so many years? Some of Shakespeare's characters show scars that bring PTSD to mind and much of the poetry and fiction after the First World War could serve as a compendium of combat's late effects. *The Road Back*, Erich Maria Remarque's sequel to *All Quiet on the Western Front*, treats the matter in depth. Many of Hemingway's characters reveal that he well knew the effects. Perhaps the classic case of the man who emerged intact, but with hidden scars, was Conway, the antiheroic hero of James Hilton's novel *Lost Horizon*.

Although the concept may be ancient, the acceptance of PTSD as a psychiatric diagnosis is recent. Only in 1980 was it incorporated in the DSM III, the great current catalogue of mental disorders. (The full name of the catalogue is Diagnostic and Statistical Manual of Mental Disorders, Third Edition). Many features of PTSD are still debated. Some psychiatrists only accept grudgingly the condition's status as a definable separate entity. In a review a few years ago, Drs. Naomi Breslau and Glenn C. Davis, of the department of psychiatry at Case Western Reserve University, said the concept is based primarily on what they called "face validity." They described this as "the clinical, but untested impressions of clinicians, specifically the impression that a characteristic configuration of symptoms can be traced to an extraordinarily traumatic event."

The two scientists said there is little solid evidence to support the concept of a totally separate entity in medicine. They don't deny that many veterans of the war in Vietnam have had postwar problems. The question is whether or not combat experiences, as well as the shocks of natural disasters—extreme stressors, the doctors call them—cause effects that warrant putting them in a category totally separate from more ordinary stressors that people encounter in life in general. They said the scientific literature on disasters, civilian and wartime, doesn't support the distinction.

"Personal characteristics and the nature of the social environment modify the likelihood and form of the response of individuals to all types of stressors," they said. If PTSD is separate, it must mean that the devastating impact of the stress overwhelms all such personal differences.

"Despite its plausibility, this assumption has little empirical support," the doctors wrote.

"Thus," they said at the end of their review, "although a high proportion of Vietnam combat veterans have exhibited marital conflict, alcoholism, drug addiction or other psychiatric disorders, many veterans have demonstrated significant achievements in the occupational and political spheres." The authors conclude simply that exposure to extraordinarily stressful events, like more ordinary stresses, has "complex differential impact upon individuals."

That the effects differ incredibly from one person to another has been noticed by everyone who has studied the impact of appalling stress on the human mind. Dr. Keane of the Veterans Center in Boston estimates that a small number of people, perhaps somewhere between 10 and 20%, "take from such life experiences some very positive, growth oriented, developmental reactions; who say 'I really learned a lot from undergoing that. I learned a lot about myself and what I was capable of and what I was not capable of.' "

"You do see it," Dr. Keane added, a tinge of admiration creeping into his voice, "but, boy is it tough!"

The vagaries of the late twentieth century bring two particular concerns to the forefront of PTSD study today: the legal connotations and the scientific question of what is actually going on in the brain of the man or woman scarred by past horrors. For years, lawyers and medical specialists braced themselves figuratively for an epidemic of insanity defenses based on PTSD after Vietnam. Evidently it hasn't happened. A large-scale nationwide survey of more than eight thousand defendants who pleaded not guilty by reason of insanity during the years from 1980 through 1986 found that only twenty-eight of them had a diagnosis of PTSD. At times, the condition can certainly produce irrational violence in some patients if they believe they are suddenly under threat. For that matter, war itself can have that effect on the combatants without ever invoking the diagnosis of PTSD. Hair-trigger reflexes can be the difference between survival and death. In a time and place where mortal threats glower on all sides, it is easy to see them where they don't quite exist. Despite the pious moral certitudes of antiwar activists of the 1960s, it is a reasonable guess that some American soldiers accused of atrocities were simply ordinary people fighting a deadly but ambiguous war who were forced to perform too long too near their breaking points.

But PTSD is not an umbrella term to cover everyone who has emotional scars from the experience of combat. If that were the definition almost everyone who has ever fought in a war would be included. Instead, the diagnosis is reserved for those who are so affected that their ability to function in the post-war world is severely compromised. The same is true, of course, of those civilians who develop the condition after their own emotionally devastating experiences. In addition to treating these casualties of war and catastrophe, mental health workers and brain scientists are trying to find out just what has really happened to the victims biologically, and why.

PTSD is a diagnosis based on behavior, but behavior is governed by the brain and today's research teams search for correlates between experience and behavior on one side of the equation and neurochemistry and even the anatomy of the brain on the other side. Some of the findings have been surprising. At least one has been so surprising that many professionals simply don't believe it; or at least, not yet.

In contrast, some other surprising items of evidence do seem to help explain not only the nature of PTSD, but perhaps offer some important clues to why it afflicts some people, but seems to spare others.

One of the prime targets for study is that typographers' nightmare known to brain scientists as the hypothalamic-pituitary-adrenal (HPA) axis. In ordinary English, this HPA axis is the complex skein of chemical interactions between the hypothalamus in the brain, the pituitary gland close to the base of the brain, and the adrenal glands which function from a geographically distant perch on top of the kidneys. The HPA axis is one of the main hormonal systems the brain calls into action in responding to stress. Since PTSD is stress in capital letters, some research workers consider it worthwhile to search this axis for changes linked to PTSD that are distinct from the changes seen in other conditions. For example, abnormalities in the HPA system are a classic feature of severe depression and depression is one of the common features of PTSD. Do depression and PTSD have similar effects on the HPA system?

Study of the brain-pituitary-adrenal axis in PTSD patients should be illuminating on such questions. That was the strategy adopted by one multicenter research group. They published their conclusions not long ago in a review article in the journal *Biological Psychiatry*. There wasn't much cause for surprise when several studies they reviewed showed abnormalities in the chemistry of the HPA axis in patients who suffered from PTSD. The surprise was in the nature of those abnormalities.

Whenever the brain sounds "General Quarters!" to cope with stress, the prime function of the HPA axis is to release the stress hormone ACTH from the pituitary and glucocorticoids such as cortisol from the adrenals. The cortisol is a key feature of the feedback loop that normally keeps the response to stress from running wild. The hormone has a quieting effect on the system. In severe depression and acute, overpowering stress there is an excess of cortisol either produced or allowed to circulate. But, in contrast, several studies of PTSD patients show less cortisol action than would be expected. They seem to be in a situation in which the brain has set a new norm of heightened readiness to confront danger. That would fit the hypervigilance characteristic of PTSD.

Not all studies have shown this shift in activity of the system that releases cortisol. In most studies, the question of whether the level is up or down in PTSD patients is based on comparison with normal "controls"; that is, with people who are essentially like the PTSD patients but do not have any psychiatric problems. That raises the question of what population group could possibly be comparable to the PTSD patients in all respects save the diagnosis. College undergraduates are among the people often tapped for service as normal controls, but how could most of today's college students really be comparable to men who have seen months of heavy combat? They come from drastically different worlds. One research group decided the logical controls would be men actually serving in combat. When men in this category were compared with PTSD patients, their cortisol levels, as shown by excretion of the hormone in urine, were lower than those of the PTSD patients.

These findings seemed to show that the sufferers from PTSD had higher than normal levels of cortisol. But normal in this case meant men in fighting units. Presumably, their cortisol levels reflected the stress of combat. A separate study of a combat battalion in Vietnam in the late 1960s showed that those men had lower cortisol excretion than would be expected of other normal humans, not afflicted with mental illness and not subject to unusual stress. To understand PTSD better, the authors of the recent review said a study should be done comparing directly the HPA activity in three groups; PTSD patients, normal healthy adults whose lives were not exceptionally stressful, and soldiers in combat. The authors of the review cited several specific ways in which the so-called HPA axis performed differently in PTSD patients and in patients suffering from major depressive illness.

Regardless of differences of opinion on the nature of PTSD and its status as a distinct psychiatric entity, there is no question that the patients have real problems and need real treatment. Many things have been tried, including antipsychotic drugs, several varieties of psychotherapy and behavioral therapy, and even hypnotism.

A survey by a team from the National Institute of Mental Health found that two drug studies each lasting eight weeks showed "modest but clinically meaningful effect on PTSD" when used in combination with psychotherapy.

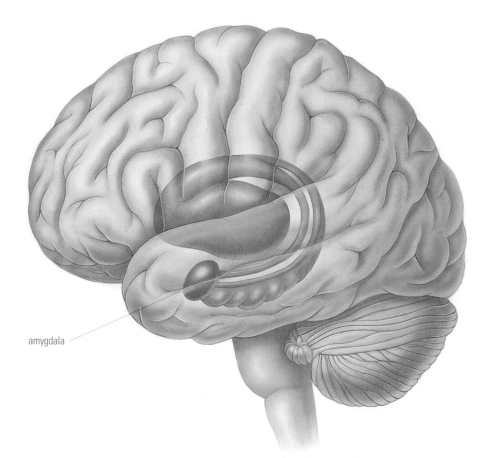

amygdala

The drugs used were phenylzine, imipramine, and amitriptyline. The survey team noted, however, that phenylzine should not be used with patients who can't maintain a prudent diet and won't abstain from substance abuse. These limitations rule out many PTSD patients.

In addition to a broad range of drugs, virtually every known form of psychotherapy has been tried on one or another group of PTSD patients. The studies analyzed in the survey showed that several types of treatment produced effects that were at least modestly beneficial. The strongest evidence favored treatments that are called behavioral. These include relaxation training and various strategies to desensitize reminders of the war experience so that patients are no longer devastated by them. From all the studies, however, the survey team came to one clear conclusion: "What these studies have demonstrated most clearly is how very much we still need to learn about the effective treatment of PTSD."

While the main focus was on the effects of combat, the survey report also offered some cogent thoughts on other causes of PTSD.

"Several kinds of traumatized populations have never been subject of a single controlled clinical trial," the researchers said. They cited particularly children who are victims of sexual and physical abuse: "Studies of children are particularly to be encouraged, since intervention at an early age holds the promise of breaking the cycle of abuse wherein child victims grow up to be themselves perpetrators of violence."

Searching the scientific literature since 1967, the survey team found 255 reports in English on treatment of PTSD. Most of the patients were combat veterans. Many of the reports were only accounts of a treatment given to a few patients without comparisons to other kinds of therapy. Such reports give some useful anecdotal evidence and hints that a given treatment might, or might not, be good. They don't provide data to estimate the comparative value of different treatments or even to compare their effects with simply doing nothing. Only a relatively few studies compared more than one type of treatment in a fashion that allowed rigorous assessment. In its final analysis, the survey by the NIMH team covered eleven studies that did meet their exacting standards. In addition to giving some useful clues as to what specific treatments are likely to be helpful for the patients, the survey offered at least indirect evidence that biology, as well as psychology, is a real factor in PTSD. Other studies have found some direct clues to these elusive biological factors.

Doctors at Mount Sinai School of Medicine in New York and Yale University and the West Haven Veterans Administration Medical Center in Connecticut found unusually high levels of the stimulant hormone adrenaline, now more commonly called epinephrine, and its companion chemical norepinephrine in the urine of PTSD patients. The same patients tended to be low in the hormone cortisol. The two hormone systems generally react together in acute stress. The research team considered the dissociation between them unusual. Indeed, this hormone picture set PTSD sufferers apart from several other kinds of psychiatric patients, including those suffering primarily from severe depression. Furthermore the PTSD patients' norepinephrine stayed high while the cortisol level stayed low throughout the patients' entire stay in the hospital and treatment with antidepressant drugs did not change the picture.

In the past, other scientists have linked high norepinephrine levels to behavior that mental health workers call "directing anger outwardly." Reaching out and hitting someone might put it in more common English. As one related example, combative prison inmates have been found to have high sustained levels of norepinephrine. In addition, high levels have also been found in normal people performing tasks that required acute states of attention and vigilance over long periods of time. These circumstances, and others, all hint at a chemical profile that fits the behavioral pattern of the PTSD patient. The brains of these men and women still seem to be paying the price of unrelieved vigilance for their overwhelming past experiences.

Studies have also shown abnormalities in the ebb and flow of important signaling chemicals in the brain. In particular, the brain circuits that depend on the neurotransmitter serotonin seem to be affected. Experts are still speculating on what the precise defect may be. In 1993, some knowledgeable physicians were turning to the use of drugs that act as serotonin inhibitors: antipsychotic chemicals such as Prozac that block uptake of the neurotransmitter in those circuits that use serotonin. Drug treatment of this kind seems to have helped at least some PTSD patients.

While many scientists have been studying the chemistry of PTSD and other severe effects of fear and anxiety, others have been looking at the geography of fear itself. The research has brought them to a small almond-shaped cluster of brain cells called the amygdala, or the amygdaloid complex. The amygdala is part of the limbic system, in evolutionary terms the most ancient and primitive region of the human brain. It is considered a heritage of evolution from the age of the reptiles. In keeping with its ancient origins, the limbic system is important in some of the body's largely automatic functions such as heart rate and breathing. It is also the main arbiter of the sense of smell, a sense that was vital to survival in our earliest mammalian ancestors. The limbic system and the amygdala are particularly important in shaping and expressing emotions and some kinds of memories. Dr. Paul D. MacLean, an authority on brain evolution, at the National Institute of Mental Health, has described the limbic system as the "feeling brain" as contrasted with the cerebral cortex, which he calls the brain of "knowing."

But recent studies have added a new dimension to this picture of the amygdala as part of the "brain of feeling." It is also the prime generator of fear. Rats in which the amygdala has been taken out of the circuit walk up to sleeping cats and nibble their ears. Birds similarly treated seem to lose their fear of humans.

In describing new research in this field, Dr. Michael Davis, of the Department of Psychiatry, Yale University School of Medicine, described the amygdala and its many projections to other brain regions as "a central fear system." He said it is involved in both the expression and acquisition of conditioned fear. This is exactly the kind of fear and anxiety that erupts in the PTSD patient who hears the deep bass chatter of a helicopter flying low and suddenly imagines himself back in Vietnam fighting for his life. He knows the

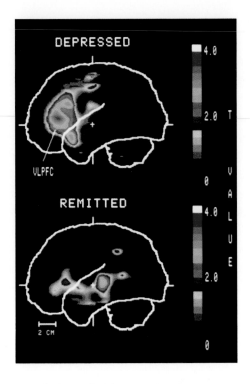

DEPRESSED

VLPFC

REMITTED

2 CM

VALUE

helicopter no longer signifies any danger. It is probably carrying passengers from the airport to downtown, but the combat veteran's brain circuits are almost permanently conditioned to respond drastically to that sound.

Hints of the amygdala's role in hair-raising emotions were seen more than a decade ago in studies of epilepsy patients. Feelings of fear, dread, and foreboding often preceded epileptic seizures when those seizures were marked by abnormal electrical activity in the amygdala. It is also well known that the amygdala has copious nerve connections to other areas of the brain, such as the brain stem, the hypothalamus, and the cerebral cortex. In short, the amygdala is connected to key regions of the brain that can produce thoughts of fear and anxiety, as well as many of the important outward signs of those emotions: rapid heart beat and breathing, rise in blood pressure, dilation of pupils, changes in hormone flow, and what specialists call "an increased startle response" to sudden sounds. It is the kind of response a layman might describe by saying "he nearly jumped out of his skin."

In animals, electrical stimulation of the amygdala produces effects that are typical outward signs of fear, such as the racing heart and rapid breathing. Humans who had direct electrical stimulation of the amygdala reported immediate feelings of fear and anxiety.

"The highly correlated set of behaviors seen during fear may result from activation of a single area of the brain (the amygdala, especially its central nucleus), which then projects to a variety of target areas, each of which is critical for specific symptoms of fear and the perception of anxiety," said Dr. Davis.

Fear, at the right time, is vital to survival. In neither humans nor laboratory animals does it take any previous fear conditioning to achieve these quick effects. Evolution must have already hard wired the fear circuits into the brain. What does have to be conditioned, however, is the kind of response that turns something neutral like the helicopter sound into an immediate signal for panic. The evidence suggests that, in PTSD patients, the fear circuits somehow become frozen in the "on" state. It may be akin to the hypervigilance that is also a feature of the condition.

Something similar was discovered by Wayne C. Drevets and Marcus E. Raichle, of Washington University of Medicine, St. Louis, in a different illness —one form of serious depression. Doing PET scan studies of patients, the medical scientists found increased blood flow—meaning increased brain activity—in the left prefrontal cortex, the amygdala, and the medial thalamus. These are all connected areas likely to be involved in emotional states. Even more interesting, their data led Drs. Drevets and Raichle to suspect that key brain circuits may be kept active in depressed patients by abnormal reverberations that maintain the thought processes and emotions of severe depression.

The wide-ranging studies of the amygdala's role in fear may also be producing useful dividends for treatment of patients suffering from PTSD. The central nucleus of the amygdala has a high density of opiate receptors and also many receptors for drugs of the benzodiazepine class. In fact, laboratory animals can be saved from developing symptoms of conditioned fear by infusions of opiates or benzodiazepines. The evidence may prove useful in the development of new drugs and new treatments for human patients. In any case, study of the amygdala is continuing to reveal new features of the brain's ancient, but still operative, circuits for producing fear.

One of the most tantalizing findings linked to PTSD in the early 1990s had to do with a closely related part of the limbic system—the hippocampus— in the brains of sufferers from PTSD. This tiny, cornucopia-shaped structure deep in the brain is intimately involved with memory and emotion. One study found the hippocampus formations in a sample of PTSD patients to be unusually small. The finding was startling, but festooned with question marks. It was not a controlled study; that is, it did not directly compare the brains of patients with otherwise comparable normal people. In addition, the number of patients was small, the data came from one part of a single study by one laboratory, and the finding would hardly fit into the mainstream of expert thinking on PTSD. Nevertheless, it might prove true. As of 1993, many specialists in PTSD were waiting to see if another study would confirm the finding. This was no aspersion on the scientists who made the original finding. It is simply the way science works. Any discovery has to be confirmed by someone else before it is accepted. Many a tempting hypothesis has fallen because no second study could confirm the original study results.

"There are a lot of people who are seriously questioning whether that is a real finding," said Dr. Keane of Boston. "If it is true that PTSD causes a reduction in hippocampus, it is going to be huge news, I mean just huge news. There is another possibility with that same research study. That is: people who have smaller hippocampuses wind up getting PTSD, but in either case this would be huge news and we would have to rethink a lot of how the brain functions as a result of it."

He said he was curious about the finding, but was not prepared to believe it quite yet.

In the final analysis, PTSD arises from the brain's sense of the dangers that lurk everywhere in the universe beyond the body's nerve endings. Whether the dangers are real or imagined, the brain changes and reacts powerfully to its own perceptions. The brain is master of its own thoughts, but hostage to them too. Its chemistry can shield the body from harm. The brain can also kill the body. Nowhere is that truth more perplexing than in PTSD. Research in animals shows that too much stress and too much vigilance can damage the heart and other vital organs. It would be no surprise if this happened in humans too, but the issue is hard to resolve. Many PTSD patients, because of their mental condition, eat too much of the wrong foods, drink too much, and exercise too little. Who can say whether a patient's high cholesterol level results from chronic hypervigilance or self-destructive life style? Perhaps it doesn't matter. In either case, it is the all-too-human brain that calls the tune.

Everything that has gone before and lies ahead in these chapters shows that the genetic system, the language of DNA and RNA, is at the heart of life. But within the constraints of that great, pliant system are others of incredible complexity. Most important is the central nervous system consisting of the brain and its galaxy of related cells and circuits. The brain changes continually and changes everything else too. That is one of the main themes of the entire story. Nowhere is this more apparent than in stress, a tale the brain contrives to bring the outside world into focus for self defense.

One of the clearest lessons of stress research is the multiple effects it can have on other systems—on the rhapsody of hormones, as we have already seen, and on the immune defenses. Immunity protects the body against disease, distinguishes native tissues from everything foreign. It sends messages from cell to cell and tissue to tissue. The immune system affects the brain and the brain can hamper immunity. The many infections to which PTSD patients are prone may reflect this. Study of the brain can never be complete without study of immunity and the effects the two systems have on each other. The basics of immunity may seem free from the brain's incessant meddling, but some case histories turn that notion magically on its head.

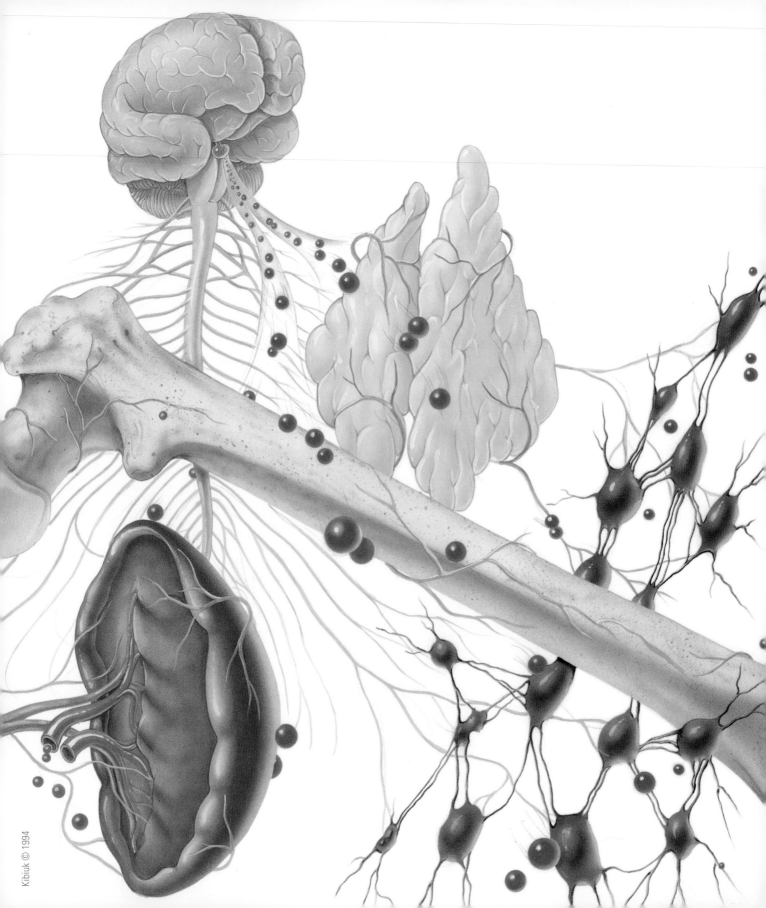

THE OTHER GREAT LANGUAGE——IMMUNOLOGY

A twenty-eight-year old Filipino woman was feeling weak and ill. She had an idea what the trouble was and it was serious. At the time, she was living in the state of Washington where medical care has a reputation for excellence and high sophistication. The young woman went to a doctor.

The physician found multiple symptoms beyond her feeling of weakness. Among other things, her liver and some of her lymph nodes were enlarged, a strong hint of inflammation. The doctor agreed that it might be serious and referred her to specialists. They added to the list of symptoms and, after thorough testing, diagnosed her illness as systemic lupus erythematosus, a serious disorder of the immune system. It strikes women predominantly, can erupt suddenly, but sometimes develops only slowly. No one knows exactly what causes it and the outcome of any case is hard to predict. Commonly, systemic lupus becomes chronic and is subject to relapses after long periods of symptom-free life. In a few rare cases it kills within weeks.

The doctors prescribed several drugs, including prednisone, a corticosteroid hormone. Before long the young woman felt well again, but that didn't last. In fact, the situation got worse. She developed kidney problems—the doctors said it was lupus nephritis. She also showed signs of fluid accumulation (edema). Her thyroid function was disturbingly low (a condition called myxedema) as contrasted with

The thymus, bone marrow, spleen, and lymph nodes are the major organs of the immune system. Each of them receives a supply of nerves and is sensitive to a variety of circulating hormones. Thus the immune system is influenced by the brain through both direct nervous system activity as well as by way of circulating hormones.

normal thyroid function which doctors call euthyroidism. In addition, the woman began to have episodes of irrationality, a problem that sometimes arises when thyroid function is poor. The doctors did more tests and reaffirmed the diagnosis of systemic lupus erythematosus. They tried other drugs and prepared to do a set of more radical treatments that are used in the most serious cases.

But at that point, the young woman packed up and went home to the Philippines, returning to the village where she had been born. Nobody in the States, particularly her doctors, expected to see her alive again.

They were all amazed three weeks later when she returned, happy and apparently healthy. And she stayed that way. She explained that the American diagnosis had been wrong. The real problem was that a rejected suitor had put a curse on her. The witch doctor in her native village understood this and removed the curse. She was cured. Two years later, she gave birth to a normal, healthy daughter. After that, she vanished from the medical annals, apparently still healthy five years after she first went to the doctor.

And where was this strange case reported; in a supermarket tabloid, or some far-out antiestablishment healer's propaganda? Guess again. It was a case report in the *Journal of the American Medical Association*. The author cited the case as powerful, if mysterious, testimony to the influence of the human mind over the human immune defense system. The doctor said he was aware of evidence that witch doctors can cause death if the victim believes in the witch's power. But this seemed even more strange and difficult to explain.

"... by what mechanism," the American physician asked, "did the machinations of an Asian medicine man cure active lupus nephritis, change myxedema into euthyroidism, and allow precipitous withdrawal from corticosteroid treatment without symptoms of adrenal insufficiency?" He had no answers.

Most stories of seemingly miraculous cures are suspect because the details are fuzzy and probably colored by wishful thinking. There is seldom much evidence to prove what illness the patient really had, if any, before the "miracle." This case was different. There were copious records, some of them made just before the woman left for the Philippines. The woman did have lupus and she did come back healthy.

Cases of this sort are rare, a tantalizing trickle in a torrent of dubious claims. In most cases, the cures are all too evanescent and the original disease, whatever it was, reappears after all the congratulations and hoopla have abated. But this is not always the case. Sometimes there are lasting effects that even go beyond the fortunate individual patient.

Dr. Steven Rosenberg, chief surgeon of the National Cancer Institute, recalled one such occurrence that had a powerful influence on his own career. It began before he became a doctor: a man with stomach cancer was being treated at Harvard's Peter Bent Brigham Hospital in Boston. The treatment wasn't halting the cancer. In fact the malignancy spread to his liver, a grave turn for the worse that is almost always fatal. The man didn't want to die in the hospital, so he went home with, at best, a few months to live. End of case.

Years later, when Dr. Rosenberg was a young resident physician at the same hospital, a patient turned up in need of treatment for a noncancerous problem with his spleen. A check of the records astounded the doctors. It was the same man who had gone home to die of stomach cancer years before. The cancer had totally disappeared. For reasons that are still a mystery, the man's own immune defenses apparently counterattacked the cancer and destroyed it. Like the case on the West Coast, this incredible story was no rumor. The doctors had before-and-after evidence and the amazingly living man to prove it. The experience planted a permanent seed in Dr. Rosenberg's mind. He has gone on to make important advances in treating human cancer by manipulating the patients' immune systems. Indeed he is the prime originator of an entire new field in that kind of experimental medicine.

Unlike the case on the West Coast, there was nothing in the stomach cancer episode to link the cure to any direct effects by the thinking brain, but there is a lot of anecdotal evidence showing that the brain can influence immunity and that this can influence the course of disease. It is no great surprise that group therapy can help cancer patients adjust psychologically to their illness. That adjustment, after all, is the province of the mind. But cancer survival is something else entirely. Or should one say almost entirely?

A research team from Stanford University and University of California, Berkeley, raised that question in studying the effects of supportive group therapy on the well-being of cancer patients. The primary aim was to see how useful the group sessions would be in improving the patients' quality of life. To explore this, eighty-six women with breast cancer were recruited after their tumors had metastasized. By the time cancer has spread in that way to distant parts of the body the future is usually grim. One of the motives for doing the study was to throw the cold light of a scientific study on a subject that has been too often pockmarked by extravagant claims: the notion that the right mental attitude will help cancer patients conquer their disease.

"We expected to improve the quality of life without affecting its quantity," the research team reported.

In the first year after their cancer spread was discovered, the patients who agreed to take part in the project were divided at random into two groups. All of the women received good medical care and anticancer treatment. Fifty of them also embarked on a year-long course of supportive group therapy and instruction in self-hypnosis to make their pain more bearable. The women were not offered any prescriptions for fighting cancer with mental attitude nor were they led to expect any improvements of that kind. The intent was to follow all surviving patients for ten years to see what effects the group therapy had on their lives.

For the women, the emphasis was put on "living as fully as possible, improving communication with family members and doctors, facing and mastering fears about death and dying, and controlling pain and other symptoms."

The once-a-week group sessions were held during the study's first year. The number of survivors in the entire panel dropped steadily from the start and, not surprisingly, all but three of the eighty-six women died during the ten years of follow-up study.

The research did produce one big surprise: a marked difference in survival between those who took part in group therapy and those who did not. This trend didn't become apparent until almost a year after the group sessions ended. Thereafter, the difference became more and more striking as the years went by. Altogether, those in the group support program lived twice as long on the average as the others. By the end of the study's first three years, all of the women who had not taken the group therapy sessions were dead. When the entire ten-year period of follow-up was over, three women were still alive. All of them had participated in the group sessions.

How did the group therapy sessions help? The question is certainly important, but answers are mostly speculation. The authors of the study said social support is important in helping people cope with stress. They suggested that involvement in the group may have helped the women mobilize their resources, perhaps helped them comply best with their medical treatment programs, and may even have improved their appetite and diet by reducing depression and helping control pain.

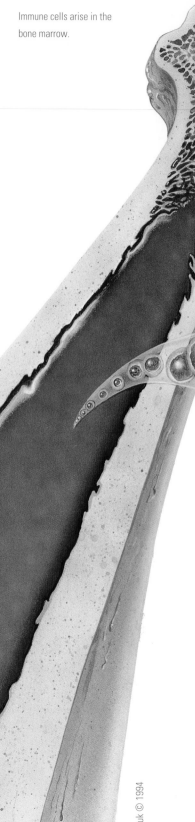

Immune cells arise in the bone marrow.

bone marrow

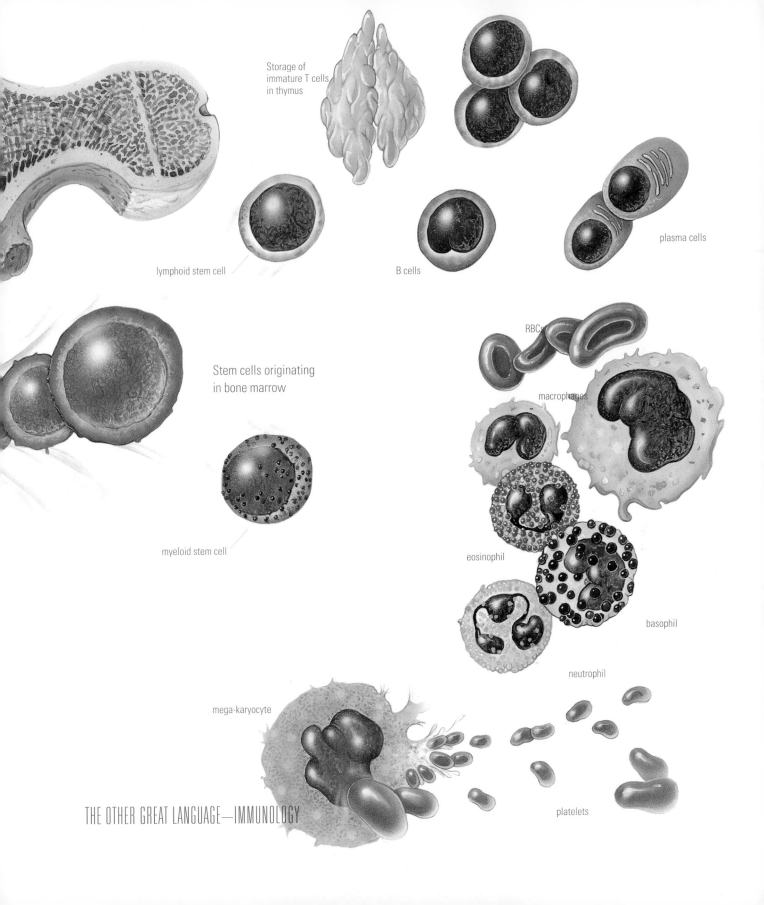

Storage of
immature T cells
in thymus

plasma cells

lymphoid stem cell

B cells

RBCs

Stem cells originating
in bone marrow

macrophages

myeloid stem cell

eosinophil

basophil

neutrophil

mega-karyocyte

THE OTHER GREAT LANGUAGE—IMMUNOLOGY

platelets

The authors cited other studies showing that married cancer patients survive longer than singles, even though this did not seem to be true of their own project. They suggested that the group sessions gave the patients a place to belong and to express their feelings. The research team also said the neuroendocrine and immune systems "may be a major link" between emotional processes and the course of cancer.

There is no doubt that the brain and mind can be taken hostage in many strange ways by disease. It is tempting to think that the support of family and friends can sometimes help the brain achieve a rescue.

The immune system is the body's main chemical bulwark against an aggressive and everchanging outside world. If the genetic system is the great language of life, the immune system could be called the great communicator of self-defense. Neither the genetic nor the immune system employs a language at all like the brain's, but both systems involve highly sophisticated communications—the continual passage of messages to and from a multitude of cells and tissues.

In a broad fashion, the nervous and immune systems complement each other in manifold ways. The genetic system's imperative role, from primordial time to the present, is to get its own genes reproduced and perpetuated. The brain arose as the master strategist of that task. The immune system provides defense to keep the body alive and intact until that transfer of genes to a new generation is accomplished. After that, its essential work is done. That, perhaps, is why autoimmune diseases and other failures of the immune system occur more frequently in the later years of life. These mistakes don't matter, except to the individual. As the body becomes old, the immune system gradually loses its potency. Inflammatory diseases occur and there is less capacity to defend quickly and strongly against infections. Immune defense against cancer is less vigilant.

The brain too is concerned with passing forward the genes, but it has also acquired another agenda as defender and promoter of the individual as well as the species.

Like everything else in the human body, the immune system is controlled ultimately by the brain, but immunity seems to have so much autonomy and to be so powerful in its own independent mechanisms that brain-immunity links are often overlooked. The illusion of total independence has been strengthened by the fact that many immune reactions will take place in the test tube with the brain totally out of the circuit. But these laboratory experiments do not reflect the whole integrated system. In that, the brain has the final word.

118

In fact, nerve fibers of the autonomic nervous system are braided through all of the organs of immunity. There is strong evidence that this semi-independent branch of the nervous system is deeply involved in governance of immunity. The autonomic nervous system regulates most of the involuntary functions of the body including heart beat, breathing, digestion, constriction and dilation of blood vessels, and the function of glands.

A few cells that will give rise to the immune system first appear in the human embryo about nine weeks after conception. By the time the baby is born, the immune system has settled its headquarters on a few organs, notably the bone marrow and the thymus gland. At the heart of the immune defenses are two broad classes of white blood cells, also called lymphocytes, that circulate in the blood and the lymphatic system. The two classes are called T cells and B cells. They work together in a multitude of ways. They are exquisitely primed to distinguish "self" from "nonself" in every cell and tissue and to mobilize a variety of attacks against everything foreign; everything nonself.

All of these cells arise from what are called stem cells in the bone marrow and in the fetal liver and spleen. Those cells that will become various kinds of T cells pass first through the thymus gland where they are processed and educated for their specialized life work.

Immunologists sometimes pay little attention to the brain's role in these functions, but anatomy alone suggests it is crucial. Regions of the thymus gland are richly endowed with nerve fibers of the autonomic system. The thymus also produces hormones that affect nerve functions and also affect the functions of the hypothalamus of the brain. Some of the brain's nerve signal substances, the neurotransmitters, can apparently affect lymphocytes and their production directly.

Karen Bulloch of University of California, San Diego, notes that several types of nerve terminals and receptor complexes have been found in the thymus. Their structure suggests that they have functions in governing the secretion of products and in the regulation of blood vessel constriction and relaxation among other things. Nerve fibers to the bone marrow, studied in animals, suggest a role for the nervous system in production of the stem cells on which the entire immune system depends.

The white blood cells called B cells, which have far different functions from those of T cells, do not pass through the thymus gland. B cells give rise to antibodies, the multitude of defensive proteins that might be viewed as the infantry of the immune defense system. They are educated for their roles elsewhere, but it is not entirely certain just where and how. In fact, the name B cell is something of an embarrassment to immunologists. The equivalent of B

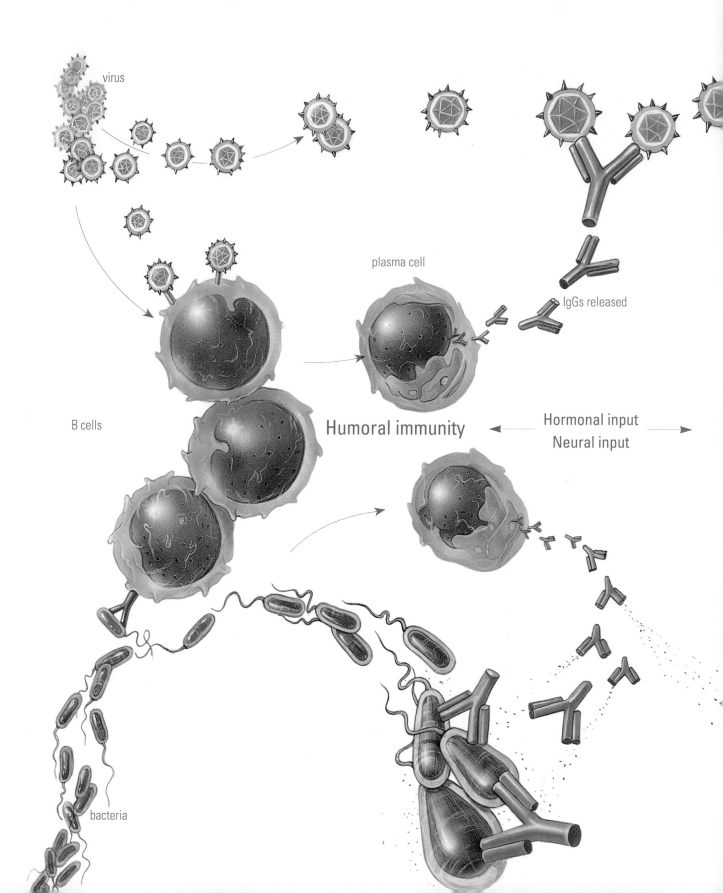

virus

plasma cell

IgGs released

B cells

Humoral immunity

Hormonal input

Neural input

bacteria

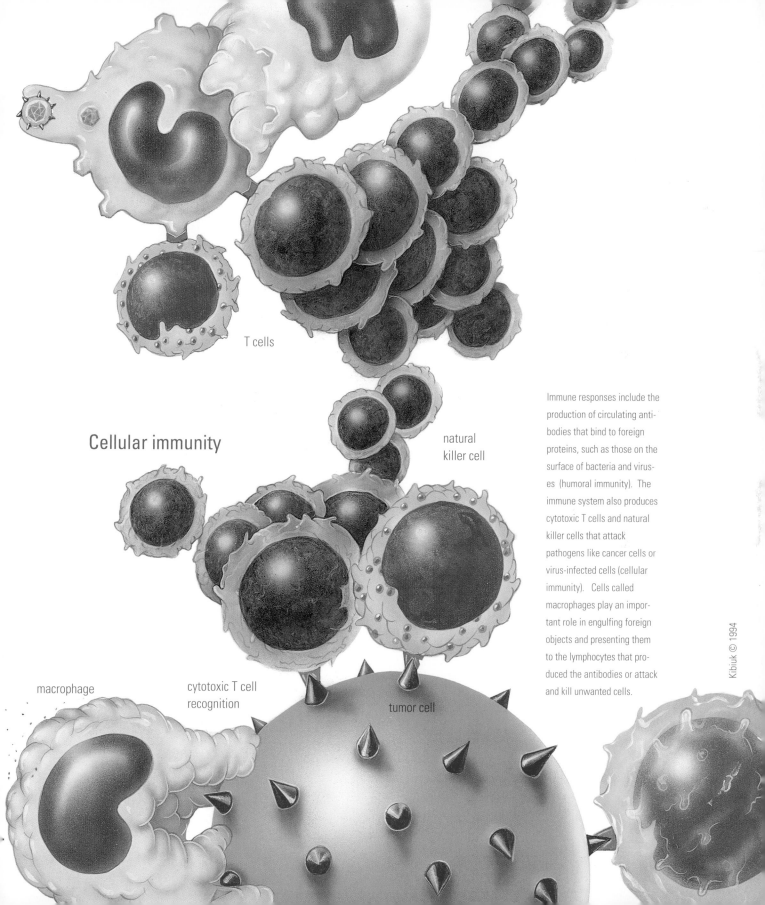

Cellular immunity

T cells

natural
killer cell

macrophage

cytotoxic T cell
recognition

tumor cell

Immune responses include the
production of circulating antibodies that bind to foreign
proteins, such as those on the
surface of bacteria and viruses (humoral immunity). The
immune system also produces
cytotoxic T cells and natural
killer cells that attack
pathogens like cancer cells or
virus-infected cells (cellular
immunity).   Cells called
macrophages play an important role in engulfing foreign
objects and presenting them
to the lymphocytes that produced the antibodies or attack
and kill unwanted cells.

Kibiuk © 1994

cells in chickens are processed in an organ called the bursa of Fabricius, and were named B, for the bursa, many years ago. It was assumed that the bursa equivalent in humans would be discovered in short order, but it still hasn't been found.

In contrast to the brain and the genetic system, which influence every aspect of human life, the immune defenses are remarkably single-minded. Immunity's whole function is to protect the body, including the brain, from invasion from the outside and treachery from within. To put it in more biological terms, immunity protects against infections of almost countless kinds, including bacteria, viruses, and parasites, and such accidents as stepping on a dirty nail or getting a transfusion with the wrong type of blood. The treacheries are of a more subtle kind. The worst of them is cancer. T cells are believed to patrol every tissue of the body continually to find and destroy parasites and any native cells that have escaped their normal restraints and have begun to grow dangerously without discipline. Given time, these rogue cells would become cancers. Most of the time in most individuals, the immune system prevents that.

Unfortunately, cancer cells do not flaunt any obvious universal tag to alert either the patient's body or the physician. But there are subtle differences from the normal and the immune surveillance system is thought to find and destroy those abnormal cells that are so marked. At least, that is what it does most of the time. This is one of the jobs of what is called cellular immunity, the province of T cells acting in concert with B cells, with the scavenger cells called macrophages and all the powerful substances those cells produce to destroy all manner of enemies. But these defenses are not foolproof; otherwise, cancers would never arise. Furthermore, the defense can be too aggressive as well as too weak. Sometimes immunity declares war on the body's own tissues in an aberration called autoimmunity. There are many diseases known to do their damage through autoimmune processes and still others are under suspicion. Even some disorders of human behavior may be linked to autoimmune processes.

Like the brain, the immune system is sensitive to the world it encounters. During pregnancy it changes to protect both the mother and the "foreign" individual in the uterus. It changes in the face of stress and it differs in some respects between males and females. Like the brain, the immune system functions through communication. Its language cannot match the incredible flights of fancy of the brain's, and its mechanisms are far different, but it does have its own internal language, neverthe-

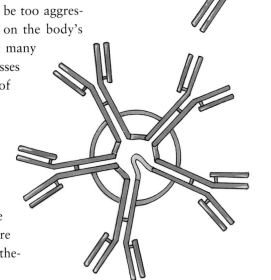

The immune system produces many types of antibody molecules, each of which serves a specific function.

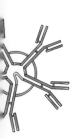

less. It is a sophisticated message system in which cells signal to one another continually in a conversation that spells the difference between health and illness, life and death. Also like the brain, the immune system is remarkable for the tenacity of its memory. Immune memory is far different from the brain's memory both in function and biological method. Nevertheless some of the crucial functions of the immune system are best described as a kind of memory.

Immune memory plays a crucial role in keeping most of us healthy most of the time. Once exposed to a dangerous invader, the system can sound the alarm to bring prompt defeat to that same enemy many years later. One of the most familiar examples is the measles virus. One exposure to the virus usually gives lifelong immunity. That is why measles vaccine works so well. The vaccine is a concoction of carefully rebuilt measles viruses that are harmless to the person, but unmistakably recognizable as measles virus to the immune system. Decades after first exposure to the virus, the normal immune defenses can still call up from its deep memory the idea of the measles virus and quickly blow the whistle on any attempted new invasion by that enemy.

Antibodies are crucial to the counterattack against disease-causing viruses, bacteria, and other microbes. One of the amazing things about antibodies is what scientists call their specificity. One antibody recognizes only one target and ignores virtually everything else. This too is familiar from the experience of vaccines. Measles vaccine protects against measles, but not any of the multitude of other viruses. There are three main types of poliovirus and each of the three has to be incorporated in polio vaccine because vaccine against one type is useless against the other two even though all three viruses are closely similar to each other. Vaccine against influenza is changed every year because the viruses that cause that widespread disease are so changeable. They often mutate enough to fool the vaccine of the previous year.

The hallmarks of the immune system are diversity and precision. In both of these elements, the talents of the immune system seem downright incredible. The system does its defense work by generating diversity on a scale so vast that the idea was once dismissed as impossible. The diversity is most notable in the swarm of defensive antibodies. They are called into action quickly and under a wide variety of conditions. An antibody chooses its target by matching a shape on the enemy corresponding to a shape on the antibody. Once it attaches to an enemy, it calls forth a variety of defensive actions by other components of immunity. Antibodies are so various that one or another of them will fit a matching shape on any invading germ even if the body has never encountered that germ before. The analogy of locks and keys is often used to describe this matching of shapes, but that hardly does justice to the system. It is not so much like being given the key to the city, but being endowed with every key that ever has, or ever will be, used to fit any lock in that city. But the antibodies are not the system, just one class of important products of that system. The overall system is intricate. Its control by the brain is complicated too, and far from being totally understood today.

Difficult as it is to sort out the specific ways in which the brain exercises control over the immune defense system, there has been a wealth of evidence that it actually does so. The anecdote of the woman on the West Coast diagnosed as having lupus is an example. The stomach cancer patient in Boston is another.

Unfortunately, some of the most consistent evidence linking brain and immunity shows the brain dampening the immune defenses, not adding to their strength. The effects of stress are the most obvious example. Indeed, studies have shown that animals put under severe and continued stress have lowered resistance to experimentally produced cancers. There is a logic to the stress examples that show the immune system being weakened by the brain's influence. It can be seen in Dr. Robert M. Sapolsky's concept of stress being a force that defers until a later, safer time, the "optimistic" long-term functions of the living system. Immunity is one of those expensive functions that is worth the effort only if there really is a future. It is a defense the body often puts on the back burner at times of crisis. But the body can't survive this strategy if cancer is part of the problem. Cancer is a long-term crisis. That is among the reasons why studies of cancer immunity and studies of the brain are mutually reinforcing. They have crucial elements in common.

Appreciating the links between those two great systems, brain and immunity, is not exactly a unique triumph of modern science. The Greek physician Galen observed two thousand years ago that "melancholic" women were more prone than "sanguine" women to develop cancer. Galen had never heard of immunology, T cells, or B cells, but he could interpret what he saw.

Modern science goes far beyond even the most shrewd observations of the ancients. On chemical evidence, some scientists have argued that the internally produced opiates, the body's natural painkillers that the brain evokes during stress, may have effects in suppressing the immune defense system. Not only some of the natural painkillers, usually called endogenous opioids, but also morphine itself, a plant substance derived from the opium poppy, seems to suppress immunity. Morphine even seems to help cancers, according to some studies in animals, an unsettling piece of evidence considering how many patients in the late stages of cancer are given morphine to deaden their pain.

But the evidence is not all on one side. Some of the body's natural painkillers may bolster immunity while others depress it.

Some years ago, Dr. John Liebeskind, of the University of California, Los Angeles, even found a difference between avoidable and unavoidable shock in the effects they had on animals' immune defenses. The inescapable form of stress—the worst kind—did suppress a key element of immunity, the activity of the defense cells called natural killer cells, while shocks from which the animal could escape did not suppress immunity at all.

Given that cancer is a growth process aided by failures in immunity, studies of malignancy offer some tantalizing hints to the links between the brain and the immune system. For example, some studies have shown that people who are depressed have a somewhat heightened risk of cancer. That is just what Galen thought, but the case is not closed. Some other modern studies have found no such link between depression and cancer. Still others have found that a positive, even combative mental attitude toward the illness can have good biological effects.

A new study that started out far afield from any thoughts of the brain's influence on disease has added another suggestive question mark to the forest of perplexities. Scientists in Canada, pursuing an intracellular receptor called the antiestrogen binding site, followed a research trail that led to surprising evidence in an entirely different field. They found that some of the antidepressant drugs widely used by humans have cancer-promoting effects in mice and rats. Understandably, cancer is likely to cause depression and patients use drugs to cope with the grim knowledge of their disease. Could effects of the drugs on cancer growth put an unexpected spin on the results of studies that explore links between cancer and mental state?

Clearly, the influence of the brain on immunity is not a one-way street. Along with the evidence that the brain affects immunity, there is also evidence that the immune system can have effects on the brain.

In recent years a whole realm of science has developed to explore the links among three of the most intimately connected and powerful working systems of the human body: the brain, the endocrine system, and immunity. The brain is very much involved in the flow of hormones and hormonelike substances that are crucial to the immune defense system. The central nervous system has direct and multiple connections to the major organs of immunity such as the bone marrow and the thymus.

Research teams today are making a big effort to understand the natural defenses of immunity better and to find new ways to enhance their natural powers against cancer or reduce their excesses in cases of autoimmune disease.

Not surprisingly, the multiple ingredients of immunity are intimately connected with the brain. Some of the links between the two systems are direct nerve fiber connections between the nervous system and the organs of immunity such as thymus and bone marrow. Sometimes the messages are passed by circulating substances that are like hormones but, at the same time, like neurotransmitters, the signaling substances of the brain and central nervous system.

Given all of those connecting links, it should be possible, at least in principle, to use the brain to bolster the immune system if anyone can figure out how to do it. There are tantalizing hints that this sometimes happens. The rare spontaneous remissions of cancer may be examples. Additional hints are the occasional studies that seem to show that a belligerent and unquenchably hopeful attitude helps some cancer patients fight longer against their cancers. Other studies, as we have seen, suggest that members of mutual support groups among cancer patients do better in the long run than patients who have no such bolstering of the mental defenses against disaster.

But "tantalizing" and "hints" are the operative words here. The self-help and mutual reinforcement strategies are no guarantee of better outcome. Some people are helped, sometimes. That seems indisputable. But the statistics of cancer are also indisputable and these statistics make it painfully clear that the power of any kind of positive thinking hardly makes a blip on the overall mortality charts. For almost all cancer patients, the best hope lies in the growing roster of anticancer drugs, including those new ones that act through immunology, and on the older traditional weapons, surgery and radiation. The cases in which thinking really does turn the tide are all too rare. Yet there ought to be hope of doing better because links between immunity and the brain are indisputable and the details of how this interconnection works are being discovered in ever-increasing detail. Many scientists are approaching the problem from the side of immunity, while others focus on the brain's side of the equation.

The influence extends both ways. The brain receives signals from the immune system. Hormones of the thymus gland affect the pituitary. Some of the immune system's own signaling substances, the interleukins, help bring sleep as well as fever in fighting illness. The higher temperature helps kill the invader, while sleep helps the body restore its strength. The immune system makes some hormones, such as ACTH, and some other hormones present in the brain can also be found in the thymus. The brain, endocrine and immune systems all work together.

The nervous system, the endocrine system and the immune system, all communicate with each other by way of chemical messengers, including hormones, neurotransmitters, and the cytokines or immune cell growth factors. (1) Hormones from the pituitary gland stimulate secretion of hormones from endocrine glands like the thyroid, gonads, and adrenals. (2) Activity of neurons regulate hormone secretion as well as affecting directly the immune system. (3) Hormones from the thyroid, gonads, and adrenals affect the brain in various ways. (4) Hormones also affect immune system cells. (5) Chemical messengers from the immune system, such as cytokines and hormones produced by the thymus gland, regulate production of certain hormones. (6) Chemical messengers from the immune system, such as cytokines, have direct and indirect influences on the brain. (7) Immune cells migrate through the circulation and lymphatic ducts and performance surveillance to detect, intercept, and destroy tumor cells and pathogens such as bacteria and viruses. (8) Injury, inflammations, and toxins from infection stimulate immunity as well as cytokine production. (9) Injury, inflammations, and toxins also signal the brain and pituitary gland, often acting through the production of cytokines, as in 6.

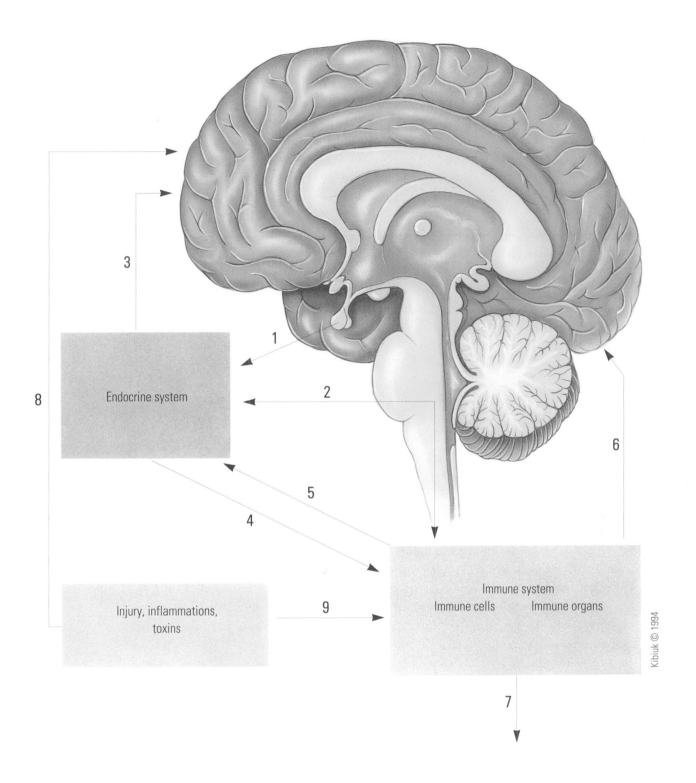

Endocrine system

Immune system
Immune cells   Immune organs

Injury, inflammations,
toxins

1
2
3
4
5
6
7
8
9

Kibiuk © 1994

Today, biologists are beginning to appreciate that even the subjective circumstance of feeling sick is not just the body's reflection of harm caused by an infection. Instead, the symptoms are a real feature of the body's fight to heal itself. This is a process in which brain and immune defenses work together in subtle but remarkable ways. Explorers of this defense process see "sickness behavior" as a set of symptoms that includes loss of appetite, diminished mental and physical activity, a tendency to sleep a lot, a general feeling of listlessness and lack of interest in other people and outside events, even failure to perform rudimentary self-care. In the conventional view, most of this is simply the cumulative effect of being debilitated by illness.

The new view is that the behavior is an energy-saving feature of the counterattack by body and brain against infection. Prime agents of the counterattack are some of the substances called cytokines that cells produce to influence themselves and their neighbors. The immune system uses these signal substances, such as the interleukins 1 and 6, tumor necrosis factor alpha, and interferon alpha to push the defensive fight. Part of that process is to tell the brain to hold off on some of the energy-expensive actions it controls and to maximize useful effects, such as high temperature, that make things difficult for infectious microbes. One research team said fever and sickness behavior are as useful in fighting infection as arousal and fear are in mobilizing the body against sudden physical threat. Similarly, of course, the reactions can get out of hand. But the whole process bespeaks the brain's close interaction with the immune defenses.

A vital player in that brain-immunity alliance is the hypothalamus, a deceptively small region of the brain that plays many crucial roles. It is central to the links that empower the nervous system to work closely with the immune system and with the endocrine system. It is a key to memory and emotion. It has close and pervasive links to the cerebral cortex, the main organ of the thinking brain. Appreciating those multiple links makes it easier to understand how the immune defenses and the ebb and flow of hormones can impinge so much on thoughts and emotions. Similarly, the links make plausible the powerful effects the thinking and "feeling" brain can have on the chemical worlds of immunity and endocrinology.

A site of primary communications between the nervous system and the immune system is the thymus, which is a master gland of the immune system, just as the pituitary is the master gland of the endocrine system and the brain is the master organ that governs those two and everything else. More than a decade ago, scientists discovered that the thymus gland produces a hormone. It was given the name thymosin. Today, students of immunity know that thymosin is not a single entity but a large family of substances that have a variety of overlapping functions. They are peptides, which means that each substance consists of a relatively short chain of amino acids. Peptide hormones are a diverse and widespread class. Research continues to reveal new functions of such hormones produced by a variety of the body's tissues and organs. So it is with the thymosins.

For example, the report of a conference several years ago on links between immunity, nervous system, and the endocrine system, noted that thymosins act on T cells of the immune system in ways that stimulate the production of yet another family of hormonelike peptides called lymphokines. Many of the lymphokines have effects on both the immune and nervous systems. A report of the conference was published as a book under the title *The Neuro-Immune-Endocrine Connection*. Many of the thymosins act in the development and maturation of T cells. But some of the thymosins have also been found in the brain, specifically in those tissues of the hypothalamus that are thought to be important in regulating the pituitary–adrenal axis; that is, the hormonal system that uses and regulates the flow of hormones from both the pituitary gland and the adrenal glands. These links, via the thymus, between the immune system and the brain are by no means the whole story. Even macrophages, the immune system's powerfully defensive scavenger cells, are involved. Macrophages produce substances of their own that seem to influence both glial cells, the brain's "housekeeping" cells, and neurons, the brain cells that do the fundamental work of signaling, creating memories, and all the other higher functions of the brain.

Many lines of research support the idea that the nervous system and the immune defense system communicate with each other closely and that each influences the other. There is little doubt that the two key systems coordinate the body's defense against infections and attacks by parasites and cancers. Studies by many research teams have also made it clear that the brain's response to crisis can harm the immune system's power to defend.

But what of the other side of that equation: can problems of the immune system exact a price from the brain? In one respect, it has been clear for many years that this can happen. Infectious diseases such as meningitis and encephalitis, arising from many different causes, can damage the brain, sometimes fatally. These disasters occur when an invading virus or bacterium evades the vigilance of the immune system and the blood-brain barrier to attack the brain. The disease AIDS is one of the most tragic of contemporary examples. The full name of AIDS, after all, is acquired immunodeficiency syndrome. It is a disorder of immunity, caused by the virus named HIV (human immunodeficiency virus). It often damages the nervous system. Many victims of AIDS suffer from memory loss, confusion, and dementia before the end. In addition, scientists of San Francisco General Hospital found that AIDS patients who suffered from depression in the early stage of the disease lost ground faster than other AIDS patients and tended to die sooner. The doctors collected data on more than 300 men in the San Francisco Men's Health Study from 1985 to 1991 and compared those AIDS patients who suffered from serious depression with those who did not. A particular kind of T cell, called the CD-4 cell, that is the particular target of the AIDS virus declined more each year among the depressed patients than among the others. It is impossible to say how much of the effect on patient survival was related to depression's effects on immunity, but the possibility comes quickly to mind.

There are also more subtle, yet devastating problems of the brain and mind that seem to have their roots in derangements of the immune defense system. In some of these disorders, problems of memory, perception, judgment, and the whole gamut of things called behavior are believed to stem from abnormal traffic between the brain and the immune defenses. Sometimes the problem is linked to disorders of early development. Sometimes it is acquired in childhood or adult life.

As a matter of history, Albert M. Galaburda, of Harvard Medical School, traces one such condition back to an outbreak of polio in 1934 in Los Angeles. Doctors there became aware of a bizarre illness that was much like polio in some respects, but far different in others. Several research teams have documented more recent outbreaks in later decades. Most of the patients had previous virus infections often with flulike symptoms. In other cases, specific viruses were implicated, including rubella, coxsackie virus, which used to be confused with poliovirus although the symptoms it produced were milder; and varicella zoster, viruses most widely known as the cause of chickenpox and shingles.

The symptoms that made this strange illness notable, however, were far different from any of those of the familiar virus infections. The condition is now called postviral fatigue syndrome. But fatigue was only a minor part of the problem. Patients complained of hypersensitivity to light and noise, frightening hallucinations that occurred when the person was sleepy, difficulty with memory of recent events, depression, hair-trigger emotions, and a tendency to become hysterical. Some patients even became paranoid.

Given those symptoms, many of the victims of this strange disorder went to psychiatrists and the links to virus infection were overlooked.

Dr. Peter Behan's research team at Institute of Neurological Sciences, University of Glasgow, Scotland, has studied the most patients and has provided the most detailed picture of this illness. Among them, Dr. Behan found a common occurrence of chemical abnormalities in muscles and evidence that pointed clearly to abnormalities in the immune system. Circulating white blood cells were deficient in their production of proteins in a standard test and the patients generally had noticeable amounts of antibodies circulating in their blood that were targeted against their own tissues—autoantibodies. This is usually an important clue that something has gone awry in the immune defense system. Furthermore, more than half of the patients showed evidence that they were suffering from chronic virus infections.

Dr. Carl Cotman, of the University of California, Irvine, sees an important concept emerging from the research. That is the possibility that a hitherto unrecognized group of diseases exists in which serious neurological and behavioral symptoms—the hallucinations, hysteria, and worse—appeared in patients who also had immune disturbances and persistent virus infections too subtle to be picked up in routine testing. Experienced research workers know better than to assume that just because two conditions occur in the same patient that one causes the other. But they also know better than to discount that possibility altogether. The evidence, dating back all the way to the middle 1930s, is interesting specifically because it hints that the disturbances of immunity may be factors in the serious mental aberrations.

Meanwhile, the modern evidence on disorders of immunity makes a compelling case for the notion that immunity and the endocrine system affect the brain in ways that are important, sometimes crippling, but today only dimly understood. One of the clearest lessons that emerges at every point in the story is the brain's marvelous complexity. This is made even more a source of wonder by understanding that the brain, the immune system, and the endocrine system all influence one another while they are all being influenced by the multitude of effects that come from the outside world. There are many ways in which the brain can be taken hostage. Everything that affects the body impinges on the brain: the cold and heat, floods and droughts, food and famine, viruses, bacteria, parasites, and everything the brain defines as joy or sadness, tranquility or stress.

But woven into this tapestry of life, there is a whole separate category of influences that also have profound effects; an influence that animals don't ignore and humans ignore only at their peril. These factors, quite simply, are the time of day, the day of the month, and the season of the year. Those too can be shaping forces in health and illness and the smooth or tortured functioning of the mind. They are ancient rhythms of life that make another new and important chapter in the story of the hostage brain.

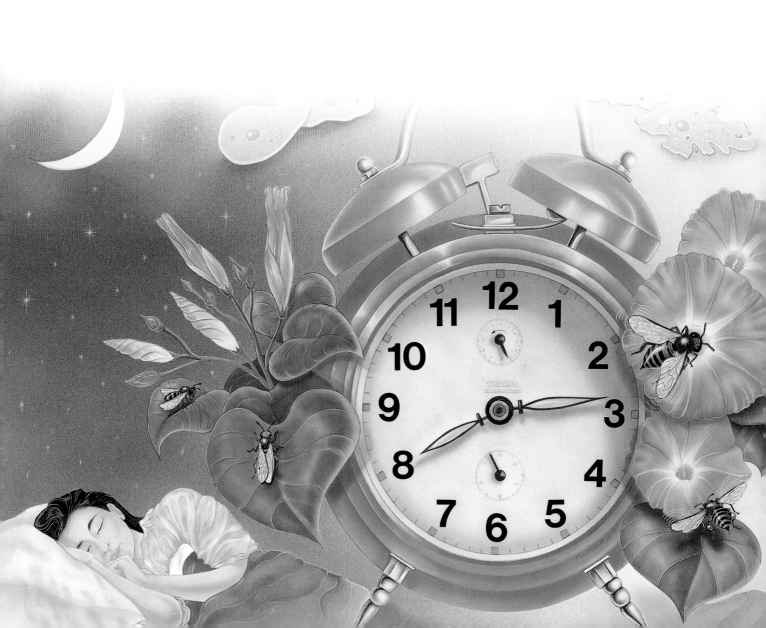

TO EVERY THING THERE IS A SEASON   8

Sunrise and sunset have always shaped our lives. We tend to forget this in the electric glare of the late twentieth century. But the modern era, driven by clocks and man-made timetables, is just an eye-flick of time; an afterthought following the millions of years in which the sun, the moon, and the seasons were almost the only timekeepers. The word "almost" is important here because all of us have internal clocks of our own. The first of these biological clocks began ticking in the early days of life on earth and still keeps living creatures in tune with the world and the heavens.

Today a new appreciation of these internal clocks is dawning. Great strides are being made in understanding how the brain keeps time, where the internal clocks are actually located, and how timekeeping affects brain function, health, and well-being. Scientists and physicians are becoming more conscious of the internal clocks that measure roughly the space of a day as well as the clocks of other cycles of life; some measured in seconds, some in months, others in seasons. These clocks all make a difference in how we feel, how we perform, who we are, and how long we live.

Maybe it is just a matter of relearning ancient truths, but it is no longer considered foolish to ask what time of day one should take a pill or schedule an operation or what time of year to take an exam. Scientists are beginning to understand why a lift of the spirits comes from switching on extra lights during the dark days of winter. They are more appreciative of the primeval rhythms of life that still influence every living thing.

Most creatures have their own biological clocks that enable them to adapt to cycles of night and day.

133

Biological clocks are more than simple responses to the cycle of light and dark, but the idea that they do have a measure of autonomy was long derided. It flew in the face of logic and daily observation. For countless millennia humans have realized that all manner of living things respond to light and darkness, heat and cold. Plants lift their leaves to the sun and close their petals when the light fades. Since the retreat of the last great Ice Age, humans have seen birds flock and go south as winter approaches and come back unerringly next spring. Animals grow new coats of fur for the winter and shed them when the seasons change. Many civilizations have worshipped the sun as a god. It isn't surprising that humans, animals, and plants pay homage to that flaming source of all light and life. But it doesn't take a clock to feel the cold bite of an October morning or see the early flood of light in June. So why should there be biological clocks? It is simpler to imagine that all living creatures just follow the sun.

It could be as simple as that, but it isn't. There is more to the rhythms of life than sun worship. As early as 1729, a French astronomer, Jean Jacques d'Ortous de Mairan, took a step toward proving this, but hardly anyone believed him. He wondered what would happen to a plant that opened and shut its leaves and petals in response to the sun if there was no sunlight. Putting his plants in a dark room he found that they opened and closed on a roughly twenty-four-hour schedule anyway. They must have an internal sense of time. His fellow scientists scoffed. How could something as simple as a plant tell time? Obviously, light was leaking into the room somehow. The plants were still responding to the sun. Mairan suggested that others try experiments to settle the issue, but most ignored him. The all-pervading influence of the sun was sufficient and all too obvious.

But was it? The question surfaced again two centuries later because a Swiss physician, August Forel, was annoyed by bees at breakfast. In a book, *The Clocks that Time Us*, recent historians of the subject described that scene:

"When he and his family were taking breakfast one morning on the terrace of his summer home in the Swiss Alps, Forel noticed a few worker bees from a hive located about 125 meters from the house arrived to sample some marmalade on the table. After a few days, he found that the bees often appeared on the terrace just before breakfast was served, as if they knew it was time for the food to arrive. Finally, finding it impossible to eat outside, the family moved inside, only to notice that for several days, the bees continued to arrive outside exactly at breakfast time and walk around the terrace table as though they expected to find food."

The bees didn't waste any other time of day looking for food on that particular table. The observant doctor concluded that the bees must have some kind of memory for time. That was in 1910. Later studies showed that within certain limits bees can tell time with rather sharp precision. Why that talent should have evolved in bees is the important question. They can't have marshaled the forces of evolution to profit from a human breakfast menu.

A large part of the answer was already available from another source, the great eighteenth century Swedish botanist, Carolus Linnaeus. He had noticed that various flowering plants opened their petals at different specific times of day from dawn to nightfall. The timing was so predictable that Linneaus even thought of making a garden clock in which the hours could actually be told by the performances of a dozen or so different flowers.

Bees knew about the flowers' schedules long before Linnaeus discovered them and the bees' innate sense of timing goes a long way toward explaining the value of internal clocks. Timekeeping saves energy and that can make the difference between survival and death. Being able to tell time, bees avoid the dangerous waste of their strength that would come from flying to distant flowers that weren't in a receptive posture when they arrived. The bees' clocks allow them to reach flowers just at the time the petals open. Modern studies have shown that timekeeping is an art shared by an incredible range of living things. Algae do it. So do mollusks. Even bread mold seems to have its own daily rhythm. The proverbial early bird uses its internal clocks to get its worm. Internal clocks give birds a wake up call just before the cues of light and rising temperature appear with the dawn. As any farmer knows, cocks start crowing while the dawn is still faint. But what do all these facts about molds and clams and flowers and the birds and the bees have to do with the human brain? A lot.

Ancient peoples who worshiped the sun saw that a plant, lifting its leaves to the light, was self-evidently paying homage to the same god. Ancient Greek myth explained the rise and fall of the leaves of the heliotrope in just that way. The plant was the reincarnation of a Babylonian princess who had loved the sun god Helios.

Casting aside these "primitive" ideas, we have lost a measure of respect for time. Modern humans have the illusion that we are its masters just because we have learned how to count it. But some features of modern life have begun to correct this arrogance. Not only do internal clocks influence the best time of day to take medicine; they impinge on all manner of subtle things including the effects of stress, the best time of year to take examinations, and the perils of being too avid a member of the jet set. In all of these, the role of the everchanging brain is only now coming powerfully to light.

Biological clocks developed, presumably, because we live on a rotating planet that circles the sun, our ultimate source of life. There is a powerful advantage in keeping tuned to the cycles of day and night, the months and the seasons. But, as the bees demonstrate, there is also profit in keeping your own time. Our internal clocks are reset punctually by the sun, the seasons, and other cues, but they are not simple reflections of the solar cycles. They have a surprising measure of independence from those timesetting cues. Only in recent years have the details of that independence come to light along with appreciation of the vital importance of biological clocks to human health and performance. Within roughly the past decade, malfunctions of the circadian timing system have become the focus of an important medical discipline. Scientists are learning what happens when biological clocks are disturbed. They see the benefits of being more respectful of the rhythms of life, particularly those called circadian because their cycles are approximately twenty-four hours long. The word comes from "circa" meaning "about" and "dies" for a day. Circadian rhythms are such a pervasive factor in human biology that they have required a rethinking of much diagnosis and treatment.

One deceptively simple exercise in statistics a few years ago put the issue sharply. Scientists at Harvard Medical School showed that there is a particular span of hours of the day when people are most likely to have heart attacks: 6:00 a.m. to noon. The discovery was more than just a matter of curiosity. It suggested a mechanism and a potentially valuable course of action. Heart attacks (myocardial infarctions) occur when one or more of the heart's coronary arteries become blocked, thus starving part of the heart muscle of the oxygen-rich blood it must have. The blockage is called thrombosis. The medical team at Harvard, reporting in the *New England Journal of Medicine*, said their findings suggest the tendency to thrombosis may vary in a circadian rhythm and that this knowledge might prove lifesaving: "If the rhythmic processes which drive the circadian rhythm of myocardial infarction onset can be identified, their modification might delay, or prevent, the occurrence of infarction."

The influence of circadian rhythms on the timing of heart attacks is only one feature of the links between internal clocks and health. Many years ago other medical scientists noticed daily rhythms in the occurrence of deaths in both surgical and nonsurgical patients. In animal experiments, chemicals that are deadly at one time of day are only moderately toxic when an animal's internal clocks are in a different phase. Studies in several fields have bolstered the argument that biological clocks are as important to modern humans as they are to the much-celebrated swallows that come back to Capistrano.

There has been a major effort, and considerable progress, in finding the actual clocks within the human brain as well as the chemistry that makes the clocks tick and keeps their figurative hands moving.

The fact that the clocks exist is no longer in dispute, nor is there any doubt that problems with timekeeping can have serious consequences. An important aspect of the new medical discipline focused on clocks and time keeping has to do with diagnosis. For example, Addison's disease and Cushing's disease are two important disorders of hormone balance. Their diagnosis depends in part on the levels of cortisol in the patient's blood. Yet studies have shown there is a large normal variation depending on time of day. Diagnosticians now know they must take this into account in interpreting a patient's blood cortisol.

Another variation, seemingly bizarre, but potentially important to specialists, has to do with asthma. The patient's frightening attacks of breathlessness arise in large part from constriction of the bronchial airways. In asthmatics, unlike nonsufferers, there is often a greatly exaggerated circadian rhythm in the tendency of the airways to constrict. In one study, patients' maximal constriction was found to come around 6:00 a.m. In those patients the crisis of respiratory arrest was also most likely to come early in the morning. Discussing this finding, one team of specialists said it was not clear whether the dangerous rhythm caused the disease or arose from it, but they saw an important lesson in the evidence: "In either case," they said, "the relation suggests the advisability of concentrating therapy and observation at the predictable times of increased risk."

Studies in several animal species have shown that both the curative and killing effects of powerful drugs vary according to time of day. This has suggested that anticancer treatment might profit from this circadian rhythmicity. If the tumor tissue obeys a somewhat different rhythm than the normal body, or could be pushed into a different phase, the effectiveness of anticancer drugs might be maximized. Doses could be timed to kill the cancer yet spare normal tissue.

Today cancer specialists are embroiled in debate on another issue: is there a best time of month to operate on a woman for breast cancer? New studies at Memorial Sloan-Kettering Cancer Center in New York have found that premenopausal women survive significantly longer when their surgery for breast cancer is performed during the second half of the monthly cycle. The doctors involved in the study think there is a biochemical mechanism at work, perhaps helping to kill cancer cells distant from the main tumor. Some other doctors think it is all superstition. It may take years to settle this issue, but women have long been unhappy with male doctors who almost automatically dismiss connections between the menstrual cycle and anything else as "all in the mind."

While new attention is being placed on ways in which biological time-keeping can contribute to disease or its treatment, there are also many circumstances in which disturbances in the rhythm itself are the problem. One of the most obvious examples is jet lag.

Everyone who has flown from continent to continent or even from coast to coast, knows the feeling; the sense of having been up all night while the world around you is just hitting its morning stride. But there is more to it than that. Jet lag does violence to human circadian timekeeping. It has potential risks including temporary amnesia, bouts of severe depression in those who are susceptible, and even a somewhat elevated risk of heart attack because the experience of jet lag tends to raise blood pressure and the blood's cargo of fats (blood lipids).

Jet lag didn't exist when speed was gauged by how fast a horse could gallop or a ship could sail. No one traveled fast enough to upset a biological clock. The development of jet aircraft changed our relationships to time. Even today only astronauts in orbit can circle the earth more rapidly than the earth rotates, but jet aircraft fly at a substantial fraction of the rotational speed and humans often arrive on a new continent in the morning when their clocks tell them it is bedtime. Many thousands of travelers have experienced jet lag. Often the effects are trivial; a passing discomfort and mental sluggishness. But sometimes the effects are serious.

A whole pharmacopoeia of nostrums and remedies has been promoted to cure jet lag. Predictably, some of the remedies produce problems of their own. One obvious idea is to use a sleeping pill and maybe a little alcohol to help relax. Most people don't bother to analyze the results, but a few years ago three neurologists tried that strategy on themselves. They weren't looking for scientific data, but neurologists are trained to note specifics and to think about consequences. The results of the efforts to head off jet lag were so surprising that they surfaced in a report to the *Journal of the American Medical Association.*

The first of these self-medicating jet laggards was a healthy forty-three-year-old doctor who flew from New York to Stockholm with his wife, who was also a neurologist. He had three glasses of champagne and a small glass of port wine during the flight and also took a modest half-milligram dose of triazolam, a benzodiazapine drug that had been rumored useful in minimizing jet lag. Its commercial name is Halcion. The couple arrived in Stockholm in the morning, local time, but 2:30 a.m. New York time, and had a busy, evi-

When we move rapidly from New York to Paris by jet airplane, our biological rhythms stay behind and take a number of days to catch up. For example, the early morning elevation of cortisol reaches its peak on the first day after travel at the same time as in New York, which happens to be midmorning in Paris. This delay contributes to feelings of confusion, delayed hunger, and dysphoria. In contrast to cortisol, melatonin secretion is almost immediately inhibited by early daylight in Paris, and this begins to signal a gradual resetting of the biological clock.

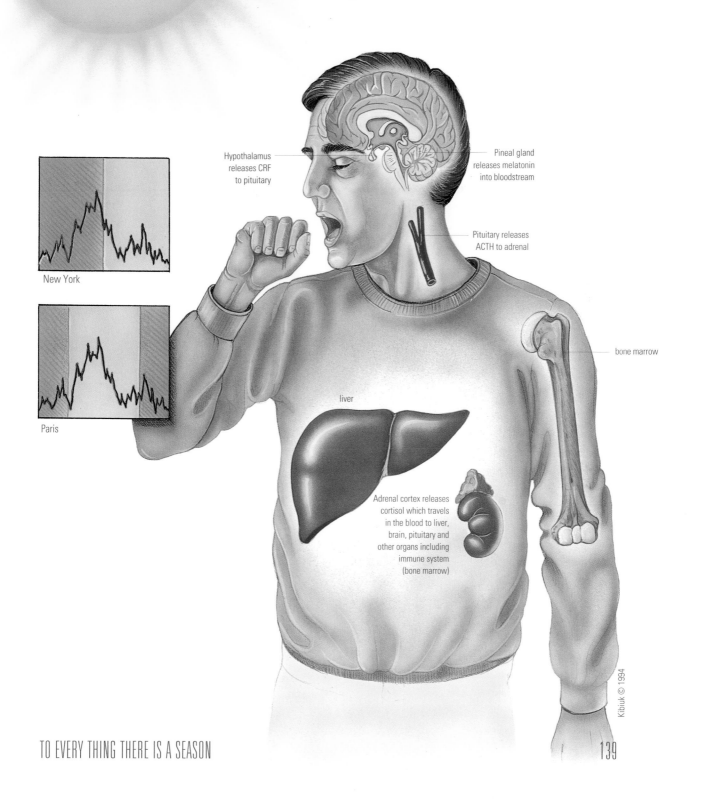

Hypothalamus
releases CRF
to pituitary

Pineal gland
releases melatonin
into bloodstream

Pituitary releases
ACTH to adrenal

bone marrow

New York

Paris

liver

Adrenal cortex releases
cortisol which travels
in the blood to liver,
brain, pituitary and
other organs including
immune system
(bone marrow)

Kibiuk © 1994

TO EVERY THING THERE IS A SEASON

139

dently pleasant, social day. The surprise came later.

"On the next day," the report said, "his wife asked a couple of questions about the previous morning, which he did not remember. She astutely quizzed him more closely and found he did not remember landing in Stockholm, going through the airport, reaching downtown, checking into the hotel, taking pictures or having coffee."

A period of several hours had gone blank in his memory.

The second neurologist, also a man of early middle age, had one glass of wine and also the half-milligram dose of triazolam during a flight to Germany. His memory lapse included going through customs in Frankfurt, changing planes for a flight to Munich, meeting a German neurologist friend in that city and having lunch.

The third neurologist, a woman in her thirties, drank one beer with dinner during a flight from New York to Frankfurt and took the same modest dose of the sedative as the other two. There was a baggage mix-up in Frankfurt. She waited more than an hour for the next plane in hopes that her bags might be on it. Then she went to the airline office for help. To her great surprise, the clerk already knew her name, address, telephone number, and destination. She had totally forgotten her first visit to the same office earlier that morning.

In a later issue of the same medical journal other doctors reported similar cases some of which involved mental confusion as well as transient loss of memory.

The original article said the practical lessons are clear: "Travelers (and others) should be cautious about taking triazolam (and presumably other benzodiazapines) to prevent jet lag. They should probably be especially cautious if any amount of ethyl alcohol will be consumed."

Other studies of the same drug showed similar ill-effects on the brain's ability to store memories. The problems included confusion, hallucinations, and even delirium, some linked to jet lag, others not. In some people, triazolam can be a danger to short-term memory by itself. In fact, the drug has become a subject of considerable controversy because of its reported effects on human behavior. In 1992 a court in Texas awarded a family substantial damages in a suit against the maker of Halcion because of a murder allegedly committed under the influence of the drug.

Nonetheless, jet lag can have memory-erasing effects without any drugs and memory loss is only one of the effects. An example of the most serious ill-effects of jet lag came to light more than a decade ago when a young resident physician returned to his hospital in the U.S. after a two-week vacation in Japan. He was scheduled to work alternating days and nights and one

140

exhausting thirty-six-hour shift in the hospital's intensive care unit. He went into a serious state of depression. He had suffered previous bouts of depression and review of his case showed that all of them followed long distance travel that traversed many time zones. They all appeared to be instances of what doctors call endogenous depression meaning that there seemed to be no personal tragedy or social loss at the root of the episode. Said the doctor who reported the case in the *American Journal of Psychiatry*:

"We should pay more attention to the influence of jet lag on endogenous depression, especially when individuals return from a trip and their circadian rhythm is further disturbed by an irregular schedule of day and night work." So, the larger lesson is also clear: be respectful of all the drugs you take, but never disregard the needs of your circadian clocks.

Many cases of severe depression do arise after tragic personal losses, but disruptions of biological clocks often contribute to the problem. A few years ago, Drs. Cindy L. Ehlers, Ellen Frank and David J. Kupfer, suggested a hypothesis using the evidence concerning the brain's biological clocks as a way of bridging the gap between theories of depression as a biological problem and as a response to personal tragedies of various kinds.

They suggested that serious personal losses could upset the individual's biological timekeeping and thus, through emotional and psychological distress, could trigger instability of biological rhythms. The end result would be the biological and chemical effects of clock disruption that generate serious depression.

While jet lag is a relatively new and trendy means of upsetting biological time keeping, there is a more common cause of disruption that afflicts people who never take to the air. Potentially, it is even more harmful to brain and body than jet lag. This is the increasing use of shift work. It is a much older problem than jet lag, but it too has increased in recent years because of the imperatives of industrial production and the increasingly around-the-clock nature of travel, entertainment, and services of many kinds. A Federal study more than a decade ago estimated that over a quarter of male workers and 16 percent of female workers had jobs in which they had to rotate between day and night shifts.

The human circadian clock does not keep time precisely according to earth's rotation. If left on its own without time cues, it settles into a rhythm of a little more than twenty-four hours, or sometimes a little less. But sunrise and sunset in addition to many social cues keep it tied neatly to the world's twenty-four-hour timetable. Specialists would say it is entrained by these ever-present time cues. The clock is somewhat flexible and does adjust to conditions, but there are limits to this and much of shift work goes beyond the limits. By one estimate over 80% of shift workers suffer from insomnia at home and sleepiness at work because of this. There is also evidence that increased risks of heart disease and gastrointestinal disorders are frequent in such workers. Studies of the effects of sailors' watch schedules on nuclear submarines add emotional disturbances and impaired physical coordination to the hazards.

The naval watch schedule, six hours on duty and twelve hours off, is too much for the circadian clock to take in its normal stride. The same is true of the common industrial shift arrangement of one week on night shift, one week on evenings, and one on days. Drs. Martin C. Moore-Ede and Charles A. Czeisler of Harvard, internationally known experts on biological time-keeping, estimate that, at best, the human circadian clock can reset itself by only one or two hours a day. That means the facts of shift work and watchkeeping force the individual to spend all week catching up with time and then have to start all over again in the next week when the rules are changed again.

Not surprisingly, upsets in biological timekeeping also disturb the normal daily pattern of temperature rise and fall and the rhythm of hormone production by the adrenals and other glands. These are ultimately controlled by the brain and the brain is intimately concerned with time. Jet travel and shift work are known to have bad effects on mental performance including vigilance, discrimination, learning, and memory during those periods when the rhythms of temperature and hormone production are desynchronized. Some aspects of adreno-cortical hormone rhythm become readjusted within a few days after a quick trip across five or six time zones while others take weeks to adapt fully. Of course, there are ups and downs of performance even when the daily rhythms are well coordinated.

To give one thoroughly documented item: the period of greatest mental alertness begins shortly after the body reaches its peak in secretion of the glucocorticoid hormones and this depends on the person's internal clocks. Some of the hormone effects are remarkably specific: administration of synthetic adrenal hormones in one study produced increased errors of commission in a verbal memory task, but did not increase errors of omission. Stress and the hormones it calls into play can impair learning and memory. With items of evidence such as these, scientists believe it is important to dissect thoroughly the role of intrinsic biological rhythms and cycles of hormone signaling within the body and the changes in mental function that follow them.

The armed services have become aware of these factors of stress, hormone flow, and cyclical rhythms in general and have solicited research proposals

A tiny group of nerve cells in the hypothalamus called the suprachiasmatic nucleus contains a biological clock that provides the hamster with a basic rhythm of body functions, including locomotor activity. If this nucleus is destroyed, and the suprachiasmatic nucleus of another hamster with a different rhythm (e. g. 22 h rather than 24 h) is transplanted into the brain, then the recipient animal shows the rhythm conferred by the donor's tissue.

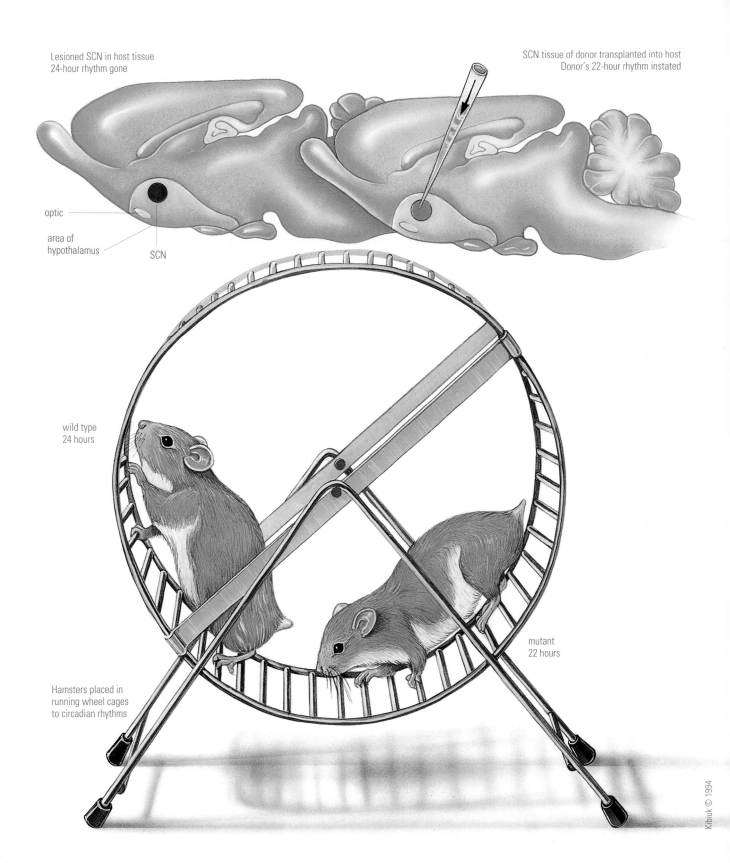

Lesioned SCN in host tissue
24-hour rhythm gone

SCN tissue of donor transplanted into host
Donor's 22-hour rhythm instated

optic

area of
hypothalamus

SCN

wild type
24 hours

mutant
22 hours

Hamsters placed in
running wheel cages
to circadian rhythms

Kibiuk © 1994

designed to clarify the problems. They are also much interested in the possibilities of raising human performance to the maximum when this is most needed. The recent experiences of war in the Persian Gulf and the troop deployment to Somalia underscore these needs powerfully, because troops and military technicians had to perform at peak levels under severe stress after abrupt travel from Western Hemisphere time zones to those of the distant Middle East.

The problems of industrial shift work are minor compared with those of the military who may have to face armed combat after flying a third of the way around the world. But that fact is no excuse for ignoring the problems of shift work. Indeed, demonstration projects designed to adjust shift work to fit the limits of the workers ability to reset their clocks have resulted in better worker health, marked increase in productivity, and reduced worker turnover.

The pineal gland lies deep within the brain and yet is responsive to light reaching it through the eyes and also directly through the skull. Light regulates formation of the pineal hormone, melatonin, which has a number of effects in the brain, pituitary gland, and organs of the body.

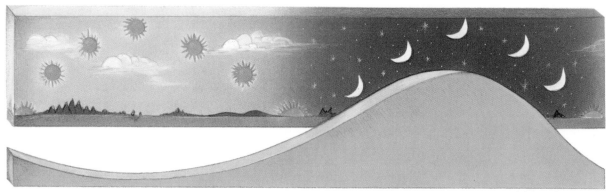

Melatonin secretion

Biological clocks in the everchanging brain are not to be ignored. Even the process of growing old has consequences. Some studies have shown that most older adults are "morning people," who function better before the afternoon hours, while most young adults are either "night people" or neutral in that respect.

In mammals, including humans, the physical elements of the main circadian clock appear to be housed in a small region on each side of the brain, the suprachiasmatic nuclei of the hypothalamus. Animal experiments in which these cell clusters were actually transplanted from one animal to another showed this clearly. When the cells were transplanted into animals that were out of rhythm because their own clusters had been destroyed, they quickly picked up the biological rhythms of the transplanted tissues. In certain birds such as sparrows and some other vertebrate species, the pineal gland functions as the clock that governs daily rhythms. It is the "circadian pacemaker." The

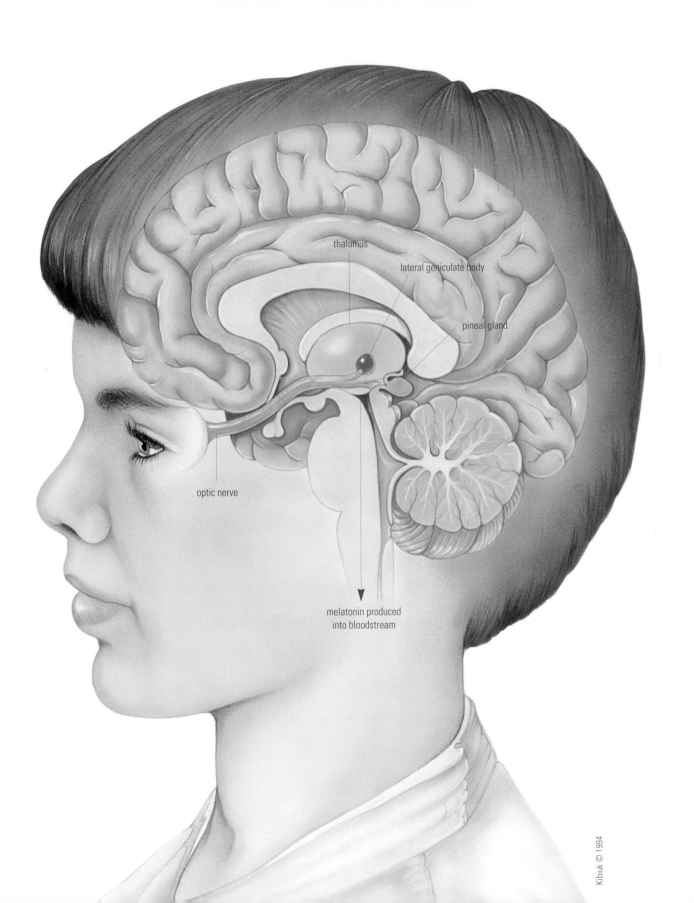

thalamus

lateral geniculate body

pineal gland

optic nerve

melatonin produced
into bloodstream

Kibiuk © 1994

pineal gland is housed on the top of the brain, gets most of its signals from the outside world via the eyes, and has a copious supply of blood vessels to send its hormones to other parts of the brain. This hormone flow is important to the time sense of mammals including humans.

Many studies have shown that a major element of the chemistry of internal time keeping is the hormone melatonin, a product of the pineal gland. But there are other factors too and the search for complete understanding has not been easy. The frustration sometimes shows through even in the circumspect language of a scientific report. Here is what two research workers of Brandeis University had to say on that issue:

"Sometimes it seems that for every experiment in one organism that implicates a certain process or molecule in clock function there is, in another system, a result tending to eliminate the same process or molecule from consideration."

This isn't surprising. Biology is complex and brains are usually the most complex feature. That is certainly true of the human brain. The internal circadian clock has to reset itself regularly with the outside world, yet be somewhat independent of that world and all its manifold influences on brain and body. In any case, the frustrations in the search for the clock itself are related to efforts to pin down the actual working parts of the clocks. There is no doubt that clocks exist or that they are important.

Melatonin, a hormone produced by the pineal gland primarily at night, seems to be crucially important. Some scientists think it may act as a synchronizer that brings several different body rhythms into harmony. If that is true, shouldn't it follow that melatonin might help alleviate the symptoms of jet lag? Medical scientists in New Zealand set out to test that idea with the help of eight women and twelve men who were experienced transcontinental travelers. The test was a round trip by air from Auckland to London and back. Half of the volunteers took doses of melatonin in gelatin capsules before the long journey, during their outbound flights, and for several days after arrival in London. The others took inactive gelatin capsules on the same schedule. None of them knew which they received, but the doses were reversed on the return journey. When the research team sorted out the effects and the travelers' accounts, they found a sharp disparity. The men and women who took melatonin had less feelings of jet lag, took fewer days than the others to reestablish normal sleep patterns, and recuperated sooner from feelings of daytime tiredness. The researchers concluded that melatonin can indeed alleviate jet lag and the feelings of fatigue that follow long-haul flights.

Other scientists have found that exposure to bright light can speed up the recovery from crossing many time zones in a short period and there is much evidence that extra bright illumination in home and office can help some people avoid feelings of severe depression during the winter months. Light is known to be one of the prime cues that help reset internal clocks to keep them synchronized with sun time. As to melatonin, some health food stores in the U. S. have begun to sell products described as containing it or likely to bolster its action. As of mid-1994, however, the Food and Drug Administration has not approved any melatonin preparation for use against jet lag.

Much has been debated concerning variations in female performance and behavior that match the stages of the menstrual cycle. Such variations have been explored in medical and psychological studies and have been contested in more than a few court cases. But possible effects on males have had much less scrutiny. Men do not have the obvious monthly cycle that women undergo, but there are other cycles.

Research by scientists in Canada shows that certain mental talents in males tend to be seasonal; more acute in the spring than in the fall. It is clearly a biological rhythm and, not surprisingly, the controlling element appears to be hormones. One element of mental performance in which males seem to do better than females, on the average, is in spatial concepts, tasks in solid geometry for example. This proficiency appears to be linked to male sex hormones. Just why the hormones should have this particularly subtle effect on brain function is not clear, but there appears to be an optimum level of testosterone for this kind of mental agility. The optimum is somewhat above the average found normally in females and somewhat below the average for males. In adults, the hormone levels appear to be quite stable, but there is a normal variation through the seasons. It seemed reasonable to Dr. Doreen Kimura of University of Western Ontario, that some of this variation would be reflected in performance on mental tasks. She and her colleagues tested young men and young women on a variety of mental tasks in spring and fall. None of the comparisons showed any seasonal differences in skills except one: the males were better in spatial tasks in the spring than in the fall. Significantly, the levels of testosterone measured in the males' saliva were also closest to the optimum during the spring.

Dr. Kimura has contributed much to the understanding of hormone effects on the brain and on the differences in development, function, and anatomy of the brains of men and women. It is largely through these studies that she has also helped advance scientists' knowledge of the rhythms, circadian, seasonal, and others that shape many of the brain's responses to the outside world.

This multiplicity of causes, effects, and relationships is one of the essential themes required for understanding the dynamic human brain. The intertwined ingredients include genetics, chemistry, environment, experience, and, finally, anatomy. Tissues transplanted between animals can change the clock rhythms of the brain. Brain tissue transplanted between humans can have powerful effects on brain chemistry and behavior, as Chapter 11 will show.

Human biological clocks are a matter of chemistry, but also clearly a matter of anatomy. In the modern era of molecular biology, one sometimes forgets how important anatomy is to function. Yet accidents that cause physical injuries to the brain can also cause profound changes. From some of these accidents that distort small details of anatomy, scientists have gleaned some of their most important insights. That is where the story leads us next: to the strange memory lapses of a man whose brain was damaged when he almost died of heart disease.

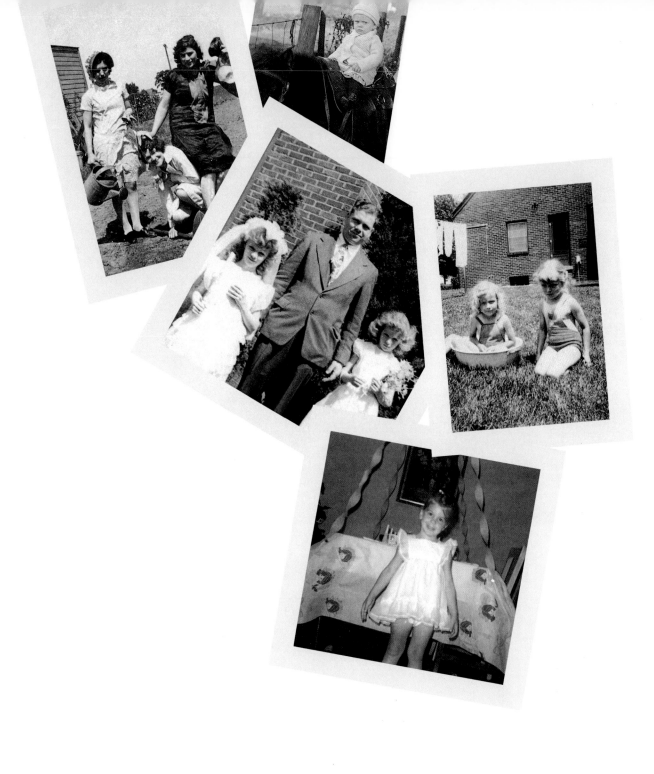

ANATOMY OF THE MIND   9

The fifty-two-year-old postal worker, known today as "R.B.", was in the hospital for open heart surgery. During the night after his operation, he suffered one of those mishaps that are the nightmare of doctors and patients everywhere. His newly repaired heart muscle ripped and began to bleed; a sudden catastrophe. An alert medical staff saved his life. It took massive transfusions and days of harried, anxious work to bring him back safely to the world of the living. At the time, everybody was thankful that he lived. Nobody expected him to become famous. But, when he finally awoke after the ordeal, his world had been changed. Human understanding of the brain changed too.

"He was resuscitated and stabilized over a period of several days," said Dr. Larry R. Squire, a brain scientist who studied R. B. after the surgery, "but as he stabilized, it became clear that he had some kind of memory problem."

Loss of blood is damaging to almost any part of the human body, but for the brain it is disaster. The time limit varies with individual circumstances, but, generally, the adult human brain can only survive about ten minutes without circulating blood to bring oxygen to its cells. R. B.'s emergency did not deprive his whole brain for even that brief time, but part was starved and damaged.

R. B. was treated at the Veterans Affairs Medical Center in San Diego, California, an institution where study of the brain is a specialty. Dr. Squire, a scientist at the VA and a professor at the nearby University of California

School of Medicine, San Diego, soon became involved in R. B.'s case. During the weeks and months that followed the heart operation, it became clear that the patient's memory problem was scientifically intriguing. R. B. had no detectable loss of intellect and he remembered his past life with no difficulty at all. But in the world of the present, he suffered from a profound forgetfulness. He could hold a new telephone number in his mind as long as he kept his attention on it, but if he was distracted even briefly, the number was gone and he couldn't get it back. The memory was lost forever in the shadows of the past. Somehow, his ability to convert immediate thoughts into durable memory was ruined. It wasn't, like some of the other famous cases, a situation in which memories flashed away second by second, slipping from the mind as fast as the experiences occurred. It seemed that R. B. had an impairment that was not quite so drastic, but did leave his memories without any permanent trace. Most everything disappeared from hour to hour and day to day. Twenty minutes after reading a passage of prose it was gone from his memory. If he talked with his children on the telephone he forgot, a day later, that he had done so. The memory loss intruded seriously on R. B.'s life. His problem was also interesting to scientists because it was so sharply defined. R. B. had lost only the ability to form new durable memories.

Nothing else. It was as though a circuit had been broken so that the experiences of the moment could not lay down any permanent record. He lived for five more years and then, in 1983, died of heart disease. The family knew how devastating the memory problem had been to him and hoped his brain might help scientists cope better with other patients' problems in the future. They allowed doctors at the hospital to take R.B's brain.

Dr. Squire's group had studied the man during his last years of life and the brain offered a rare opportunity to match a particular memory defect to a flaw in anatomy, if they could find that flaw. The team studied the brain intensively, examining its every region in a search for changes from the nor-

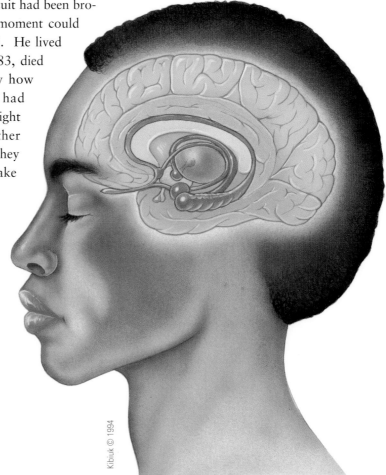

View into the human brain showing the location of the temporal lobe and the amygdala and hippocampus. Inset shows that damage to the brain of R. B. (see text) was localized to the hippocampus. In this diagram, the lesion is represented as a dashed line in the area called CA1 (4), which is part of a circuit that begins at (1) and connects via (2) to (3) and then to (4). The disruption of (4) prevents any information from traveling to (5). *Inset of R. B. hippocampus courtesy of Dr. Stuart Zola-Morgan, University of California, San Diego.*

Kibiuk © 1994

mal that might offer clues.

"What is interesting in retrospect is that we didn't have a theory to guide our examination," Dr. Squire recalls. They had "candidate brain areas" certainly, but no prime target in the search.

It took two years to document and prove conclusively the injury's location. After they did find what they were seeking, it seemed downright obvious. The damage was in that deep-seated part of the "old" brain called the hippocampus. It is a tube-shaped structure a little less than two inches long. It extends through the central region of the brain and scientists have long believed that it has functions in emotion, stress, and memory. But the brain is intricately interconnected. Nerve fibers from one part of the organ fan out to link other distant parts. It was far from obvious before they found it where the damage lurked that rendered R. B. incapable of forming new memories. Once the scientists knew where to look, the damage was there beyond question.

"You could actually see the pathology with the naked eye," Dr. Squire said. "You see the gray matter of the cortex coming around into the medial part of the brain and as you fold into the hippocampus area, suddenly this cell

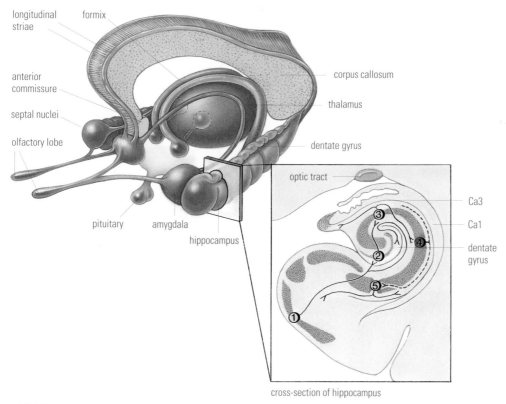

cross-section of hippocampus

field just collapses into nothing. It goes like that for a few millimeters and then it appears again."

The gap was a place where nerve cells had died. The damage was found throughout the hippocampus in a particular region called the CA-1 field. All the nerve cells in that field appeared to be lost. Because of what they already knew of the anatomy of the hippocampus, it was obvious at once that a loss like that would break a circuit of nerve signals that normally flowed through that small part of the brain. R. B.'s loss of one cluster of cells interrupted an important chain that the brain used to process incoming information.

"R. B. was really the case that established that the hippocampus itself is the critical component of the system," Dr. Squire said. It had been suspected for years, but never so clearly proved. R. B.'s tragedy opened an important new window for the understanding of the brain.

It is through accidents more or less like R. B.'s catastrophic bleeding episode that much of the information has been gathered concerning the functions of important parts of the human brain. A great deal has also been learned from animal research.

Considering all the natural difficulties of studying the brain, it is remarkable how long ago some of the basic facts were known. The Greek physician, Hippocrates, often called the "Father of Medicine," evidently appreciated the brain nearly 400 years before the birth of Christ. Dr. Wilder Penfield, one of the twentieth century's most famous neurosurgeons, said that only one Hippocratic statement on the brain has survived, but that "his discussion constitutes the finest treatise on the brain and the mind that was to appear in medical literature until well after the discovery of electricity." In short, it was unmatched for two thousand years.

In his last book, published in 1975, Dr. Penfield quoted from that lecture by the Greek physician of the third century B.C. as it has come down to us in translation:

"Some people say that the heart is the organ with which we think and that it feels pain and anxiety. But it is not so. Men ought to know that from the brain and from the brain only arise our pleasures, joys, laughter, and tears. Through it, in particular, we think, see, hear, and distinguish the ugly from the beautiful, the bad from the good, the pleasant from the unpleasant ... To consciousness the brain is messenger."

Dr. Penfield, a pioneer in the study and treatment of epilepsy, was also impressed by Hippocrates' simple and accurate remark on that serious disease; that it comes from the brain "when it is not normal."

In the Hellenistic era, a century or so after Hippocrates, the physician-anatomist Herophilus of Chalcedon founded a medical school in Alexandria. He too is known to have judged correctly that the brain, not the heart, was the center of the nervous system. Herophilus was one of the first physicians to learn from autopsies of the human body. A particular feature of the dura mater, the tough membrane covering the human brain, is still called torcular Herophili in his honor.

These items don't signify, by any means, that the true functions of the brain have been accepted without question since antiquity. Aristotle, although he made immense contributions to logic, astronomy, mathematics, and the development of observational science itself, was in grievous error on many points of biology. One of his major errors had to do with the brain. He imagined that its prime function was to cool the blood and that the heart was the seat of consciousness and the soul. His teachings became revered as dogma in the Middle Ages and some of his errors took many centuries to correct.

The misconception concerning the heart was certainly not Aristotle's alone. The error has a durable logic that persists in our thoughts and speech today. After all, the heart does beat faster in the throes of hate, fear, and love. Unconsciousness and death come almost instantly when the heart stops beating. It takes experiment, not any feat of pure logic, to prove that the heart is just following the brain's instructions and that the heart's only role in the mind is to serve as the pump that keeps the brain alive. Only in recent decades has death been defined in terms of the brain rather than the beating heart. We still celebrate love and St. Valentine's day with symbols of the heart, not the brain, and use such expressions as "heartsick" and "heartfelt" to describe other emotions that arise in the brain. Shakespeare played it both ways, invoking "the brain which some suppose the soul's frail dwelling house" and yet having Othello, in his rage, growl "My heart is turn'd to stone."

The shrewd insights of Hippocrates and others among the ancient Greeks seem even more remarkable when one considers that the brain is not easy to study even with all the tools of modern science. The brain has no internal skeleton to keep its parts in order, nor even muscles, tendons, or ligaments. It is a heavy mass of tissue with sizeable cavities (the ventricles) and a bewildering outer surface that seems like a mountain range of folds, fissures, and convolutions. Its functions depend on an incredible maze of interconnected networks. There are an estimated 100 billion individual nerve cells (neurons) although no one has ever counted them. The cell bodies of the neurons are clustered together in clumps and thick sheets called "gray matter." Each neuron has a hundred to a thousand or more dendrites that make an all-but-unimaginable profusion of connections among the nerve cells. The vast skein of nerve fibers are the "white matter." The legendary Gordian knot that Alexander severed was a simple cat's cradle compared with the human brain.

Nevertheless, scientists have made much progress in sorting out most of the anatomy, the electrical signaling, some of the chemistry, and even some of the highest functions of this sentient marvel that has evolved during hundreds of millions of years.

General improvements in medical care over the past few centuries have contributed to better understanding of the brain because people whose brains were damaged by injury or wounds of war were more likely to survive, enabling doctors to observe the effects their different injuries had on behavior, thought processes, and memory. In recent years, the unfolding knowledge has been accelerated by brain surgery designed, sometimes neither wisely nor responsibly, to cope with grave cases of epilepsy and even intractable behavioral problems. Some of the operations cut off large portions of the brain from the rest. The operations did change behavior, but not always in the way intended and sometimes with serious damage to the processes of memory, the ability to learn, and to the person's total personality.

As a product of evolution, the human brain still contains, and depends on, structures and networks that probably arose in the age of the dinosaurs if not earlier. Dr. Paul D. MacLean, of the National Institute of Mental Health, used the term triune brain to define this ancient legacy that we carry around inside our skulls. Today some neuroanatomists think his imagery of the brain old-fashioned, but it still offers a useful reminder of our ancient heritage and our links to many species both ancient and contemporary.

In Dr. MacLean's view, the oldest portion of the brain, which he called the proto-reptilian brain, consists of the basic structure of the brainstem and spinal cord by which the brain controls such life-sustaining basics as blood pressure, muscular reflexes, the compulsion to drink water, and the body's reaction to temperature changes.

Next in order in Dr. MacLean's three-part package is the old cortex, which surrounds the brain stem and seems to have been added to it during the evolution of mammals. He called elements of this old mammalian brain the paleomammalian forebrain and the limbic system. He saw this portion of the brain as important to emotional feeling and expressive states vital to self preservation—the search for food, feeding, fighting, and self protection. This ancient invention of mammals, the old cortex, contributed such things as maternal nursing behavior and the deeply ingrained instinct in females to care for the young. It is possible to imagine the roots of human behavior in many of these elements. Vocal communication and urgent response to those sounds helped mother and infant avoid dangerous separations. Emotional distress on separation is helpful in keeping the brood safely together. Play behavior in the young may promote harmony in the nest and perhaps contribute to a lifetime of community actions.

The final, largest, and most indisputably human, part of the brain is the new cortex or neocortex, which Dr. MacLean described succinctly as "the brain of reading, writing, and arithmetic." He might have added: music, compassion, and awe at the wonders of the universe and of the brain itself. The neocortex, the most human part of the human brain, has important functions in controlling all the voluntary muscles that allow us to run, swim, and dance. Above all it is the integrative master control of the brain that allows the whole to function as a single governing organ for the whole body. A portion of the neocortex—the forward part, called the prefrontal cortex—is known today as an important site of some of the most human of brain processes. These include insight, mental abstractions, self-awareness, and also the particularly human kinds of memory.

Anatomically, the neocortex is the feature that sets the human brain apart from all other brains. In most species the cerebral cortex is a modest structure dwarfed by other features such as those that govern the ability to control muscles or to translate the senses of vision or smell. In humans, the cerebral cortex has grown to be 80% of the whole brain and neither consciousness nor memory would exist without its huge network of interrelated cells.

While it is convenient to discuss these three components of the triune brain as separate, they actually function in close and continual concert in the normal human. And all of the three parts have evolved to become the new whole. In humans, the "thinking" brain orchestrates everything, but sometimes seems to be in less than complete control. Emotions arise to a large extent in the old cortex. Although their origins may be ancient, it is hard to deny that emotions often rule. Another ancient part of the human cortex that can easily be observed at work today is the olfactory cortex, concerned with sense of smell. It is a legacy from the early evolution of mammals when the small, furtive progenitors of mastodons, whales, and humans depended for survival on a highly refined sense of smell. Rats and mice still retain that sophistication in reading the world from its odors. Even human infants learn early to identify important odors, such as their mothers'. Some aspects of factual learning in humans seems to be analogous to olfactory learning in rodents.

Drs. Gary S. Lynch and Carl W. Cotman of University of California, Irvine, have found that one of the earliest signs of Alzheimer's disease is impairment in the sense of smell. They are hopeful that this discovery can be turned into a useful clinical test.

To add to the complications of brain study, the organ violates the rules of structural symmetry that seem so pervasive in most of nature. There are two sides to the brain—the right and left hemispheres—and their functions are anything but symmetrical. It was once thought that they did match, but it is now known that the two hemispheres have their own specializations and that the two are far from being mirror images of each other. They differ not only in function, but in structure. The specializations are important. Some students of evolution believe the differences contributed to the emergence of the uniquely human brain.

In most humans, including right-handed people who make up about 90% of the population, the left hemisphere is a major processor of information in phonetics, sequential analysis of information, and similar analytical thinking. Because language is based so greatly on these analytical elements, it too is a predominantly left hemisphere function. The right hemisphere is thought to be the place where such innate talents as perception of form, spatial relationships, and some important aspects of music reside. Because of its special functions, the right hemisphere has entered the popular imagination in oversimplified terms as the hemisphere of artistic creativity. But, of course, in the normal human brain the two hemispheres work closely together to create the personality.

Nevertheless, the hemispheres are capable of functioning with a large degree of autonomy. The two are connected by the thick cable of nerve fibers called the corpus callosum. After operations for severe epilepsy or injuries in which this great nerve cable is completely cut, the two sides of the thinking brain can each continue to operate in total ignorance of what the other is up to.

Human skills in learning and memory offer some of the most dramatic insights to the brain's everchanging nature and its mysteries. It is a common experience among us to glance at an old group photograph and pick out one half-obscured face and recall instantly the person's name, identity, habits of speech, and taste in music after a lapse of decades. Although computers can calculate with dizzying speed, no machine today can match these marvels that the brain achieves with such apparent ease. Our amazing feats of memory are also proof that, somewhere in the brain, some kind of trace has been laid down that can be called up many years later. The sheer magnitude of the task is all but beyond imagining. A psychologist tested college students on their ability to recognize particular photographs among many thousands after a one day lapse and found that they performed incredibly well. Another scientist, calculating how many "bits" of information would have to be marked and stored to accomplish what the students did, came up with the figure of approximately 10 to the eleventh power; that is, 10 followed by eleven zeros. Few computers can surpass that with the "real time" agility of the human brain.

The human mind is the human personality and most people think of both as immutable. For centuries, philosophers and scientists have debated whether the mind is somehow separate and distinct from the brain, but no one has found anything else in the body that could be the seat of the mind. In Hippocrates' words "... from the brain only arise our pleasures, joys, laughter, and tears."

Although humans like to think of their personalities and minds as permanent, the brain's function and structure do change. The brain uses clues from the environment continually to better the chances of survival. The brain can also be held hostage by influences from the outside world.

"It is now clear that the environment and even learning of skills impacts on brain structure throughout life, and particularly during development," said Drs. Cotman and Lynch in a presentation to a conference at the National Institutes of Health.

Even today, the mechanisms of human memory are still full of mystery. It is certain, however, that learning and memory depend intimately on each other and that memories are effects of the outside world on the brain. The mental impacts of the outside world do cause physical changes in the brain. Dendrites, the connecting threads that grow from neurons, and the synapses, the actual nerve connections that join cells into complex networks, change with experience. Animals raised in "enriched" environments, where there is plenty of stimulation for the brain, showed more dendrite branching and more complex dendritic trees than animals raised in the boring conditions of the ordinary laboratory.

There is evidence that synapses may be lost and replaced and that their numbers and quality may be subject to continual turnover, not only during embryonic development, but throughout life. Day by day we are always learning, and day by day the brain changes as it learns.

Of course, not all of the changes are for the good. Cases such as that of R. B. show that the ability to create memories can be destroyed by damage to remarkably small portions of the brain, notably the hippocampus. Yet that vital part of the brain is not the long-sought storehouse for memory. Damage to the hippocampus leaves existing remote memories intact. The search for the anatomy of the mind is not that easy. It would be a mistake to infer too much from any shopping list of parts of the brain that are seen to be involved in remembering. Memory cannot be attributed to any single part of the brain alone. While the hippocampus in the "old brain" may be vital to some aspects of memory formation, the complexities of human memories and our incredible ability to store and recall them certainly depend on the "new" cerebral cortex and probably on other features of the brain as well.

The very concept of memory is deceptively oversimple. The word brings to mind seemingly simple feats such as recalling a date, a telephone number, or the first line of a poem. In fact, memory is probably the most complicated set of functions of the incomparably complex human brain. No other species has anything like the memory of our species. It is a large part of what makes us human. What most of us think of simply as memory is the realm many scientists call declarative memory. This is stored information about words and numbers, facts and faces, scenes, events, noises and odors. These are all items of conscious memory that can be recalled, sometimes with conscious effort, sometimes with incredible speed and sophistication. Memories may also float to the surface of the conscious mind unbidden. Two words recall a whole passage from a book; a few notes bring back a whole symphony and a whole orchestra playing it. A waft of fragrance on a chance summer breeze can suddenly fill an adult's mind with a complete scene from childhood; picking blueberries in a pine woods, playing stickball on the hot macadam of a city street or baseball on fresh cut grass.

This is all declarative memory, a vast and important mental territory. It contributes to humans' most brilliant insights and also to the commonplace operational needs of grocery shopping, carpentry, cooking, ocean fishing, and the myriad forms of office routines. To be useful, declarative memory has to function in gear with the closely related system of the "working memory" which helps in the useful storage, short-term recall, and manipulation of declarative memories.

There is another whole broad category of memory that is nonconscious and expressed only through performance. This is a matter of learned skills and habits. It is sometimes called implicit, procedural, or nondeclarative memory. A tennis serve, golf stroke, or the ability to throw a spear so well learned as to seem instinctive are examples of this kind of memory. It too is vital to the effective functioning that makes human life possible. More important, it seems to be entirely separate from declarative memory. Conscious memories can be destroyed with no damage to the unconsciously memorized skills. The conscious declarative kind of memory appears to be processed by brain systems different from the other kind and these systems are more easily disturbed than are the mechanisms of the seemingly automatic procedural kind. This may help explain why a victim of Alzheimer's disease may continue to play the piano skillfully for a time even after the disorder has gravely damaged the capacity to remember dates and people and has devoured most of the person's personality.

Amnesia is also a result of harm to the systems of declarative memory. An amnesia victim may forget who he is and where he lives, but can still play the sport he had already learned. He will have many of the old habits that defined his personality in the preamnesic past. Furthermore, amnesia that leaves a person incapable of storing factual memories need not prevent the learning of new skills. Patients have demonstrated this by learning new skills, but being unable to remember going through the training.

Can a blow to the head produce amnesia as many novels and movies would have us believe? Probably, but it is not at all clear just how this happens and it is not by any means the only road to amnesia. Dr. Squire recalls one case in which a patient came to his hospital complaining that he had completely forgotten his identity and his past after such a blow. Several days later, the man admitted he had been lying. He had faked amnesia to gain admission to the hospital. What about the blow to the head? The patient admitted that he had put that into his script because he thought it was how amnesia always began.

Because the human brain is so incomparably complex, we have always had difficulty in finding a good metaphor. In the eighteenth and nineteenth centuries, the brain was often likened to an ultrasophisticated hydraulic machine. In the early twentieth, it was an electrical device, sometimes a telephone switchboard, and now, toward the end of our century, it seems natural to describe brain function in terms of tape recorders or the latest computers or even holograms. But none of these ingenious artifacts of the human brain can do what the brain itself can do.

Today some of the newest developments in medical diagnosis are contributing marvelous detail to our understanding of the wonders and the problems of the human brain. Magnetic resonance imaging (MRI) and the widely used CAT scan technique (computed axial tomography) have added much including the observation that there are structural differences between the brains of normal people and sufferers from schizophrenia or autism, and still other differences between heterosexuals and homosexuals. Whether such differences are causes or effects of the mental conditions they accompany is still unknown.

The even newer method of visualizing the brain, called positron emission tomography (the PET scan), actually makes it possible to eavesdrop on the brain as it works and thinks. The technique reveals patterns of blood flow to different parts of the brain as the brain uses blood-borne oxygen to fuel the intellectual machinery. The flow of blood shows which portions of the brain are most active in various aspects of performance. The PET scan's color images show distinctly different parts of the brain in action even in such seemingly similar functions as hearing words, seeing words in print, repeating words aloud, and generating words.

One of the most persistent and teasing questions about the human brain has always been the nature and the geography of stored memories. The progress that is being made today has been hammered out after a profusion of unproductive clues and many hypotheses that seemed brilliant, but turned out to be wrong.

A startling experience that seemed to be related to memory occurred during a surgical exploration of the human brain by the neurosurgeon, Dr. Wilder Penfield. He was American born, but generally regarded as a Canadian scientist because much of his career was spent as director of the Montreal Neurological Institute, formed in the early 1930s by scientists at McGill

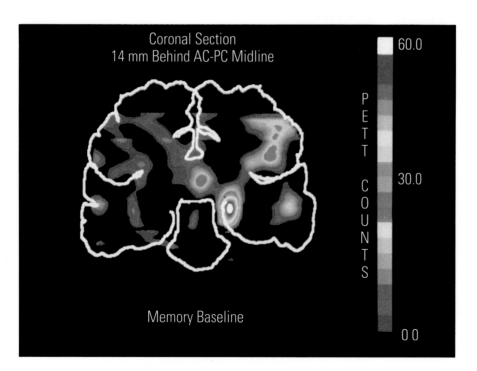

PET images showing regional blood flow activated by a memory task in the right medial temporal lobe region including the hippocampus and parahippocampal gyrus. *Courtesy of Dr. Larry Squire, University of California, San Diego, and Dr. Marcus Raichle, Washington University, St. Louis.*

University. Dr. Penfield, the institute's first director, was a pioneer in treating certain cases of epilepsy by removing small damaged portions of the brain's cerebral cortex that were the foci of epileptic seizures. The treatment was sometimes dramatically effective, but success depended on being able to find the abnormal spot of brain tissue. Epilepsy is part of the down side of the everchanging nature of the brain. Brain function can be impaired by scars in its own tissues. Epileptic seizures are caused by sudden, paroxysmal disturbances in the electrical activity of the brain. Some cases arise because of brain damage and can be treated surgically by destroying the damaged tissue when it is limited to a sufficiently small and circumscribed area. One of the early ways of finding these danger spots was to open the skull and explore the surface of the cortex with an electrical probe. The mild pulse of electricity could sometimes reveal the disordered tissue by evoking abnormal electrical activity in that part of the brain. Dr. Penfield used that technique in his early years.

One of the strange things about the infinitely mysterious master organ of the human body is that the brain itself feels no pain. Headaches may seem to be seated in the brain, but in fact, their pains comes from the nerves of the blood vessels in the head. The brain senses pain everywhere else in the body, but brain tissue itself has no pain receptors at all. This lack of pain was an important advantage to the study and treatment of epilepsy because it meant that the surgeon could open the skull under local anesthetic and explore the surface of the brain while the patient was awake and able to respond. Patients could aid in their own diagnoses by telling the surgeon their sensations when mild electrical stimulation was applied to points on the surface of the cortex. Often a patient could feel a sensation developing that was just like the customary seizures. That meant the probe had found the right place. But sometimes the surgeon got a different and startling response.

It first happened to Dr. Penfield in 1930, according to a biography by his grandson Jefferson Lewis. The neurosurgeon was exploring the brain surface of a middle-aged woman who suffered from epileptic seizures. Such attacks sometimes arise in one of the temporal lobes, located at the sides of the forward part of the brain. The limbic system and the hippocampus are deep in the central brain behind the surface of the temporal cortex of each hemisphere. Dr. Penfield was starting to explore this region of cortex in his patient. Mr. Lewis described the scene:

"When he touched the temporal lobe she suddenly spoke: 'I seem to see myself as I was when I was having my baby.' Though surprised at her reaction, Wilder simply made a note of it and continued his probing elsewhere, thinking it could have resulted from the trauma of surgery, or the drugs, or any of a number of other causes."

Being a good scientist, Dr. Penfield didn't forget the incident. The case took on greater significance when he encountered others of the same kind, always involving the temporal lobes:

A young French Canadian woman heard an orchestra playing. When the surgeon held the probe in place she could hum along with the song verse by verse. When he pulled the probe away, the song stopped.

"Not only could she hear the music," Dr. Penfield's biographer wrote, "she felt the same excitement and pleasure as when she had heard the tune played in a concert hall."

Dr. Penfield reported other cases in his own last book, *The Mystery of the Mind*. A mother told him she was suddenly in her kitchen, listening to the voice of her little boy who was playing outside in the yard.

Another patient, a young man, was transported instantly to a baseball game, years ago, where he was sitting in the stands watching a little boy crawl under the fence.

Still another man was in a concert hall listening to an orchestra and was able to hear each different instrument as it played.

"All these were unimportant events but recalled with complete detail," Dr. Penfield wrote.

It seemed that the surgeon had stumbled on the ultimate seat of memory. These mental images that his probing evoked were sharp and "real." They didn't shift wildly the way dreams do, or drift in fantasy like hallucinations. To Dr. Penfield and his colleague Herbert Jasper, they seemed like fragments of reality recorded somehow in the brain.

"When Penfield and Jasper considered their results, it appeared that the brain held an untold number of film clips, each with sound and picture, of vivid events from the patient's past. The replaying would evoke, as well, the emotions that accompanied the original experiences," Mr. Lewis wrote of his grandfather's work.

Dr. Penfield was a remarkable man, neurosurgeon, scientist, philosopher, author of many technical works and two historical novels, one on the patriarch Abraham, the other on Hippocrates. During his career as a surgeon he pursued the strange evocations of memory-like images through the 1930s and after World War II. In 1963 he published an account of all 1,132 cases in which he explored the living human brain in the course of diagnosis and treatment of epilepsy. Among the 520 that involved explorations of the temporal lobes, there were 40 in which the mild electrical stimulation evoked images and scenes evidently from memory. Dr. Penfield called these "experiential responses." He published all the details of the patients' brain conditions and their responses to stimulation, "so others might judge their meaning for themselves."

Dr. Penfield noted that he changed his mind on one important aspect of the cases.

"In 1951, I had proposed that certain parts of the temporal cortex should be called 'memory cortex,' and suggested that the neuronal record was located there in the cortex near the points at which the stimulating electrode may call forth an experiential response. This was a mistake."

He knew there were discordant facts. Sometimes patients picked up the same mental image again and again when a single point on the cortex was touched repeatedly. In other cases, different "memories" were evoked from repeated stimulations at a single site. Some of the scenes were dreamlike fantasies. While some seemed sharp enough to suggest they were records of events, others were impossibilities such as apparently hearing both sides of someone else's telephone conversation, or being confronted with robbers carrying guns even though the patient had never really had that experience.

Dr. Penfield finally concluded that the record of past events is not stored in neat packets in the temporal cortex near the places where he stimulated the surface of his patients' brains. Nor was the memory mechanism all in one place. The issues were much more complicated than he had once hoped. Today, in the light of much research since Dr. Penfield's time, it is clear that the complexities are prodigious. In commenting on the Penfield studies, Dr. Squire of University of California put it this way:

"Memory for whole events is stored widely, not in a single location; literal or biologic forgetting can occur, so that a recollection of past events is a reconstruction from fragments." He said it is nothing like a literal playback of past events.

While Dr. Penfield originally thought the "memories" he was evoking by mild electrical stimulation were coming from the tissues directly beneath the cortex, in fact, they were apparently sparked by electrical discharges from the hippocampus and another deep-seated brain structure called the amygdala. This is a small almond-shaped cluster of cells near the hippocampus deep in the brain. The amygdala is thought important in shaping emotional behavior and in creating emotional memories, such as fear of a particular dark corner where one has been mugged. It functions also in some of the seemingly automatic activities of the autonomic nervous system such as heartbeat, muscular actions of the digestive tract, and the functioning of glands. It is also believed to have a role in higher mental functions and in memory.

The sum of evidence today favors the concept that declarative memories involve multiple areas of the cortex activated through portions of the limbic system: the old brain structures, including the hippocampus and the amygdala. Furthermore, it is at least a plausible idea that different aspects of the same memory may be held in different parts of the brain and must be integrated by still other brain systems before they emerge in conscious thought. The goal of finding any place in the nervous system that is the storage place of any aspect of memory remains a formidable task. A different kind of search for the physical basis of memory broke on the scene after Dr. Penfield's work and was quite unrelated to it. This new quest was spawned in part by the greatest scientific triumph of the mid-twentieth century, the revolution in molecular biology and the chemistry of genetics—the rapidly unfolding world of genes and chromosomes and DNA.

The so-called central dogma of molecular biology holds that DNA is the ultimate archive of genetic information and that the messages of the DNA are translated into the related form of RNA and the proteins produced according to the working blueprints of RNA. The sequence of events in which all genetic information is passed forward is DNA-to-RNA-to-protein. Above all, DNA, RNA, and protein are all part of an incredibly potent information scheme. Probably the greatest single wonder of the language of genetics is its memory. It carries the records of heredity not only from cell to cell and creature to creature, but spans evolution from one species to another and may carry at least traces of its memories back to the origin of life itself. Given so powerful a system that developed once in the evolution of life, would it not be natural for the brain to store its memories in this same great language?

As soon as this concept of molecular genetics as a memory system was understood, some brain specialists wondered if it was not also a key to unlock some of the puzzles of their own research. Perhaps the brain's memory system too was stored directly in the DNA and RNA. An early explorer of this idea was Dr. Georges Ungar who tried to put it to the test of experiment. Working at Baylor in the 1960s, he startled the world by grinding up the brains of rats that had gone through a behavioral experiment, injecting some of the material into others and, lo and behold, the naive, inexperienced rats performed as though they too had received the treatment. Specifically, it was an experiment in habituation. The treated rats were subjected to the sound of gongs often enough to reduce the sound's ability to startle them. The naive rats that received brain injections seemed to have picked up that same ability to stay calm in the noise. Some experiments with simpler animals, worms and similar invertebrates, also suggested that physical transplantation of memory might be possible. But Dr. Ungar's studies carried the idea into a compelling new phase. If it could be done in mammals, the concept probably had meaning for understanding the human brain.

Rats are naturally creatures of the dark, feeling comfortable and protected away from the glow of light. Dr. Ungar trained some of them to have an unnatural aversion to the dark. It was their brains that he minced to find a protein he called scotophobin. When he injected it into other rats they too seemed to avoid the dark. This was a sensational finding. Many others tried similar experiments and many got similar results. Scotophobin was a small protein, a string of just fifteen amino acids, and yet it appeared to confer fear of the dark. At least, the experiments could be explained that way. But, from the start, there were many skeptics who doubted that interpretation. Maybe the substance was simply making the animals more active and fidgety so that they ventured forth from the dark more often than usual. There seemed to be many possible explanations that had nothing to do with direct effects on the memories, or the emotions, of the brain.

As Dr. Squire noted in his book *Memory and Brain*, there were hundreds of experiments in the 1960s devoted to attempts to show a chemical transfer of learning. A substantial number of laboratories were involved and there were many "successes." But it was never really clear that these experiments did demonstrate chemical transfer of learning. There were always other plausible explanations.

At one point early in the long controversy over this issue, a group of seven research teams took the unusual step of sending a letter to the journal *Science* saying that they had all tried to reproduce important results cited by the proponents of learning transfer and had all been unable to do so. Such a wholesale failure to confirm a research result is usually taken as damning evidence that the original work was not valid. Dr. Ungar died in 1977 with the jury still out on this issue. But the concept that memory could be transferred chemically did not survive long after his death. The idea had lost too much ground to other explanations of memory storage in the brain. If memory was actually encoded in protein or RNA, as Dr. Ungar supposed, his experiments were plausible. Today, however, it is most widely believed that memories are laid down as physical changes in the network of connections between nerve axons and dendrites. If that is true, the process of chopping up a brain would certainly destroy its memories. Most of the intriguing aura of the transfer studies has faded eventually into the never-never land of experimental results that could not be repeated and confirmed.

The transfer experiments and the interpretations of the scenes evoked by electrical stimulation of the cortex had stalled in trying to decipher the complexities of the human brain. This is neither surprising nor an indictment of the scientists who did the work. The human brain seldom announces simple answers to its own riddles. But the riddles are important and need to be solved so that we will understand better who we are and how we can best cope with the problems of life. The physics, chemistry, and anatomy of memory are crucial to this quest for understanding. A great deal of progress has been made in understanding the complexities of memory and in matching them with electrical and chemical activity in the brain.

As Drs. Cotman and Lynch noted in their report to the conference at the NIH:

"The ability to encode, catalogue, and recall a vast number of facts and experiences is one of the definitive characteristics of humans and one that distinguishes us as individuals."

Memories are a key feature of human personality and the human mind. Each person is a unique tapestry formed from the combined influences of what used to be called nature and nurture. Like most other traits, memory is a subtle combination of those two factors. Memories arise from experience and therefore must be listed in the nurture column. But the richness with which any person lays down and recalls memories is influenced by the innate gene-determined biology of the brain—nature. Like every other living thing, the human brain is an amalgam of influences both of nature and of nurture. Unfortunately for the human condition, we often seem determined to find either/or solutions to our problems. Nowhere has that been more dangerous than in the old debate over nature vs nurture. That is where the story goes next.

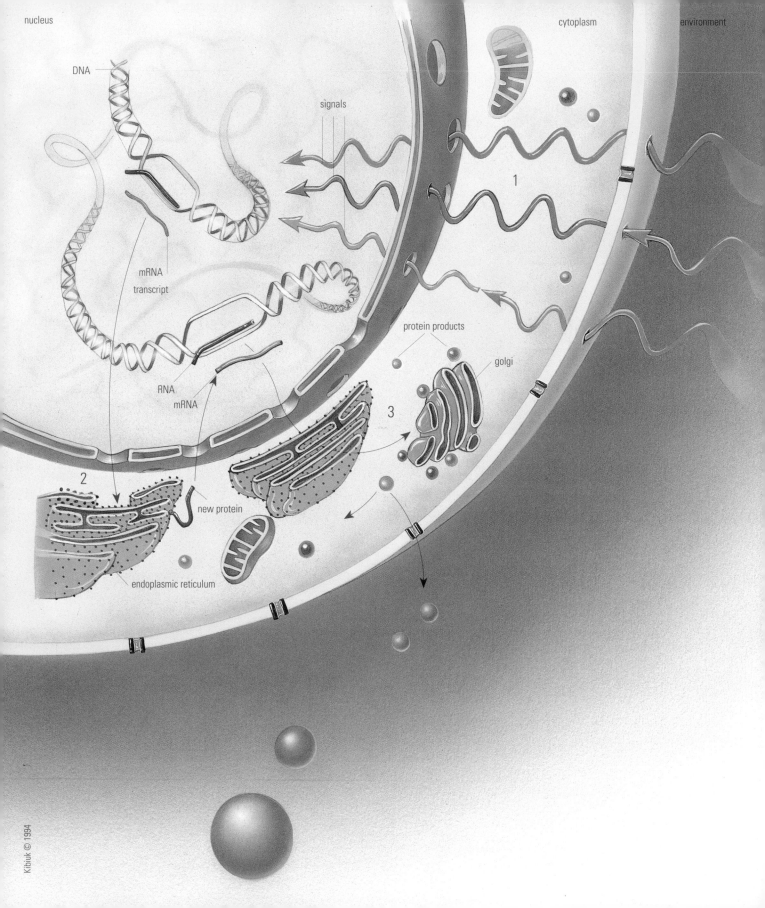

nucleus

cytoplasm

environment

DNA

signals

mRNA

RNA

mRNA

protein products

golgi

new protein

endoplasmic reticulum

1

2

3

Kibiuk © 1994

NATURE VS NURTURE VS KNOWLEDGE   10

The disorder called autism is one of the most dreadful afflictions that can assault a child and a family. The autistic child seems totally withdrawn from life; strangely indifferent to joy or love; drastically stunted in behavior.

A normal child can have dizzying swings of mood; talkative one moment, silent the next; filled with affection, laughter, tears, anger, clouds, and sunshine. The hallmark of normal childhood is irrepressible curiosity with ever-expanding horizons. In grim contrast, an autistic child may seem like a robot, or even less than that. In severe cases, the child does not speak and hardly communicates in any other detectable way. The main activities are repetitive, stereotyped movements—routines that seem to have no purpose. There is no detectable affection, scant response to affection, seemingly no personality at all.

What causes this terrible lack of normal childhood effervescence? Is it nature or nurture to use the old words, or some combination of those forces? Is something, or someone, to blame? There have been many hypotheses, but no one knows what exactly causes the condition. Some of the theories have shown the old nature-nurture debate in its most destructive form. In the classic sense nature simply meant heredity and nurture meant everything else: every aspect of personal experience, environment in its broadest sense.

Not long ago, "the experts" in the field of psychiatry and mental health placed the blame for autism squarely on the parents' behavior. It was a

The environment outside of each cell sends signals that stimulate genes inside of the cell nucleus to change their activity. (1) Signals may enter the nucleus and affect it directly, as do steroid hormones (Chapter 4); or they may stimulate a second messenger at the cell membrane or in the cytoplasm, which then sends signals to the nucleus. (2) Some genes that are activated by these external signals (called immediate early genes) produce proteins that re-enter the nucleus and activate other genes. (3) The genes that are activated by steroids, second messengers, or immediate early genes then produce products which are either secreted by the cell or perform functions within the cell.

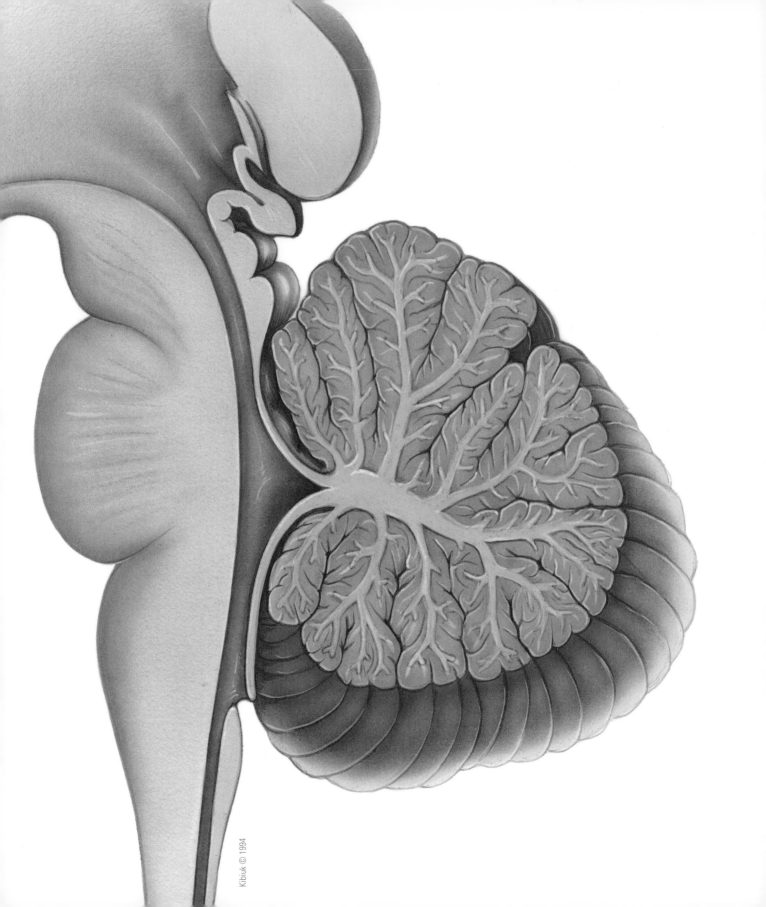

failure of Nurture with a capital N.

"In 1955, parents would likely have been told about their pathogenic role in triggering their child's disorder," said the authors of an authoritative handbook on autism and developmental disorders. "Years of personal therapy for the parents would have been suggested, and the child would have been engaged in protracted psychotherapy, generally with little specific benefit. Parents often felt, sometimes as a result of the direct suggestion of professionals, that they were responsible for their child's problems."

The results of this "professional advice" were often catastrophic. A young couple already shattered by their child's terrifying nullity were not helped by being told it was all their fault. It was particularly cruel and destructive arrogance from professionals who, to put it bluntly, didn't know what they were talking about. It was theory about psychological and emotional nurture spun from conjectures supported by altogether too little fact. Today, the idea that the parents are to blame has been discarded. The failure of that theory shows the risks of assuming there is always some behavioral cause for behavioral symptoms. The truth is more elusive. The brain is the organ of behavior. It changes continually from a wide variety of causes and behavior can change with it. A rubella infection in the pregnant woman can do her developing child as much harm as emotional neglect after that child is born.

For at least a decade, scientists have been finding evidence of some physical differences between the brains of autistic children and normal children of the same age. In particular, the autistic child's brainstem and the cerebellum, or part of it, are likely to be somewhat smaller than normal. How this could produce the complex symptoms of the disorder is still a puzzle. Regions of the brainstem control breathing, blood pressure, and similar automatic vital functions. The cerebellum is the main arbiter of muscle tone, body posture, and such skills as the coordination of hand and eye movements. All of these items seem far removed from the highest human mental capabilities. But no such list of particulars reveals the total functions of any part of the human brain. The immense powers of that organ stem from the multitude of connections among its regions and its circuits. Problems with brainstem function have long been suspected in autism. There is also recent evidence that the cerebellum has more influence than was previously suspected on the brain's talent for thinking and for communicating with others.

But these new items of physical evidence and the failure to pin the blame on upbringing don't prove that the fault in autism lies only in hereditary nature. Like many other grave problems, autism simply cannot be explained in

The cerebellum is one brain structure that may be affected in autism, but it is not clear what the nature of the damage is to this brain structure.

terms of the nature-nurture debate. There are probably multiple causes, possibly including such insults to the developing brain as a fetal virus infection or some disruption in fetal nourishment at a key time in the brain's growth. The educated guessing today is that autism is a problem in biology; some train of events gone awry in the development of the brain. Often it is difficult to match such biological causes with their sometimes subtle effects. Some autistic children are mentally retarded. Others evidently are not. Parents' response to the problem can be helpful or the reverse, but autism is not a result of "bad parenting." It has taken a long time to correct the error of placing the blame there and it might be rash, even now, to assume the correction has been universal.

These tragic cases are a valuable warning against too glib certainties and there are many other issues of mental health in which absolute alternatives of nature or nurture have been destructive. More often than not, the harm was done by too ready leaps to the conclusion that a problem was of nature acting independently from nurture. For a long time, many moralists and policy makers had a bias toward blaming heredity ("bad blood," it used to be called) for many of society's ills.

The paired terms nature and nurture can be traced at least as far back as Shakespeare, who used them in *The Tempest*. The magician Prospero made it clear that nature, was the governing influence as he denounced his treacherous servant, Caliban:

> "A devil, a born devil, on whose nature
> Nurture can never stick; on whom my pains
> Humanely taken, all, all lost, quite lost"

Centuries later, reformers spoke of "the criminal classes" as though all people who broke the law were hereditary misfits and hoodlums. The English social experiment that populated Australia began in 1787 as an effort to rid the British Isles of that same imagined criminal class by shipping as many as possible to the other end of the world. Altogether, 160,000 unfortunate men and women were transported over a span of many decades. Through their children and grandchildren, incidentally, the survivors disproved the idea that it was bad genes that led them into conflict with the law. Australian descendants of these "dregs of the criminal class" have made their country one of the shining lights of civilization and democracy of the British Commonwealth and the world. But long after that point had been thoroughly demonstrated in Australia, the eugenics movement in the United States led many states to enact compulsory sterilization laws designed to prevent "undesirables" from breeding and contaminating the gene pool. Some of the laws legalized compulsory sterilization for such assertedly "hereditary defects" as habitual criminal behavior and "moral perversion" as well as schizophrenia, feeble-mindedness, serious manic depressive illness, and epilepsy. By 1931 there were various laws of this kind in twenty-seven states. Fortunately they were seldom enforced in most states. But by 1935 when the bloom began to fade from this idea, similar laws had been passed in Denmark, Switzerland, Germany, and Sweden.

The horrors of Nazi racial policies dealt the final blow to the social acceptability of such eugenic measures. It is difficult to deny that there is any role at all for a genetic factor in some of the most antisocial human behavior. Genes, after all, are involved in almost every aspect of life. But the variations from person to person in any cluster of people are far greater than the variations from group to group. There is no rationale for social policies based on asserted group differences. There is grave danger and potential harm in assuming that such group differences exist.

Today the pendulum of opinion has swung far in the other direction. The very suggestion that there might be a genetic component in any criminal behavior is enough to spark violent denunciation. In 1992, the University of Maryland planned a conference on the broad issue of "Genetic Factors in Crime: Findings, Uses, and Implications." It was one of several planned conferences on the potential effects of the Human Genome Project, which seeks to map and identify all of the roughly 100,000 human genes. The National Institutes of Health, main sponsor of the Genome Project and originally the main sponsor of the meeting in Maryland, withdrew its support after an outcry by opponents. The protesters denounced the entire idea as racist, socially disruptive, and likely to promote "biological and psychiatric intrusions upon presumably dangerous people." In a letter to organizers of the conference, Dr. John W. Diggs, a deputy director of the NIH, wrote that the conference brochure "touts genetic research as offering the prospect of identifying individuals who may be predisposed to certain kinds of conduct." He said statements like that "inflamed public opinion." In rebuttal, David Wasserman, of the University of Maryland, declared the program to be a legitimate airing of important issues. He said the freeze on funding by the NIH was illegal and "politically motivated" and that it "has hampered our efforts to address important issues about the social impact of behavioral genetic research."

Professor Wasserman said the conference intended to address "many of the questions its opponents are now raising. Do genetic explanations of

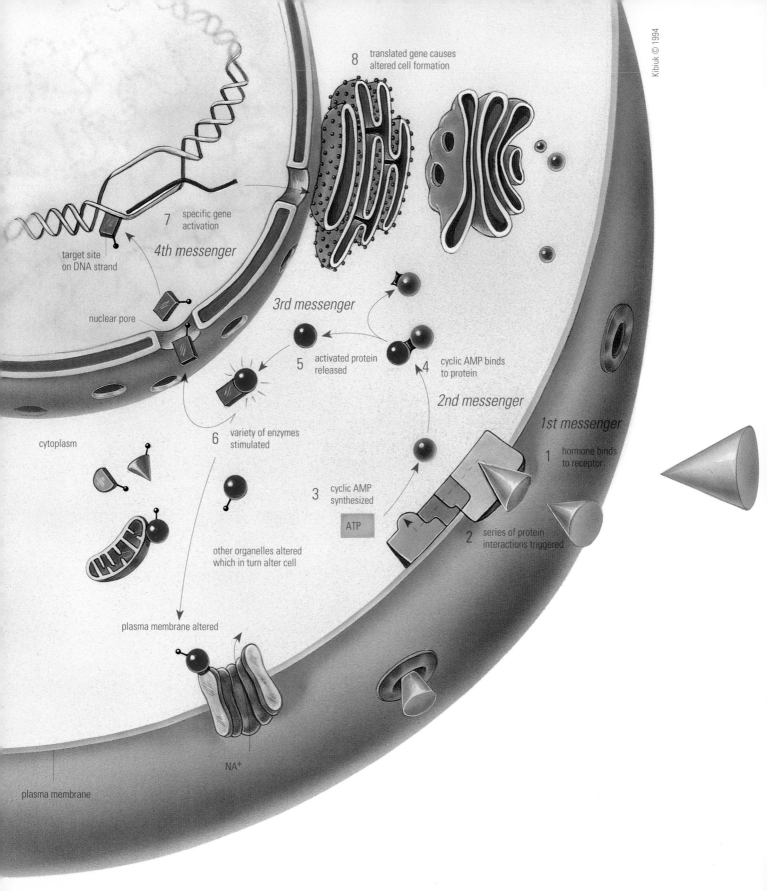

8 translated gene causes altered cell formation

7 specific gene activation

4th messenger

target site on DNA strand

nuclear pore

3rd messenger

5 activated protein released

4 cyclic AMP binds to protein

2nd messenger

1st messenger

cytoplasm

6 variety of enzymes stimulated

1 hormone binds to receptor

3 cyclic AMP synthesized

ATP

2 series of protein interactions triggered

other organelles altered which in turn alter cell

plasma membrane altered

NA+

plasma membrane

Kibiuk © 1994

behavior undermine or refine environmental explanations? Does genetic research focus on some kinds of crime to the exclusion of others? Will that research divert attention from social causes of crime? How can genetic factors explain socially defined behavior? What uses will be made by the criminal and juvenile justice systems of the claims of genetic influence and genetic predisposition likely to emerge from current research? And how will those claims affect public perceptions and broader social policy?"

Late in 1993, it appeared that the NIH withdrawal of support would probably be reversed and the conference might yet be held.

The controversy shows how charged with emotion many aspects of genetic research and the issues of heredity versus environment have become. In fact, the bulk of scientific evidence today shows nature and nurture to be biological forces that are closely intertwined from early embryonic life all the way to the final horizon of old age. Nowhere is this more apparent, or more charged with consequences, than in the brain. To think otherwise would be like trying to blame one part of an equation exclusively for everything that comes after the equals sign. Each human brain is the joint product of its genes and its behavioral responses to the world. Those two categories of cause are everywhere commingled. The truth of that proposition can even be seen in the functioning of the genes. Sometimes genes can be turned on or off in response to hormones or neurotransmitters that have, themselves, been activated by the brain. Furthermore, all genes are called into action selectively, not wholesale.

Even though each living cell in the body has the same complete set of genes, different tissues and organs vary widely in which of these tens of thousands of genes are allowed to act. In most cells only relatively few genes are ever activated. Most stay silent. Like the huge pipe organ in a cathedral, the music of life is made not by hitting all the keys and stops, but by creative playing on the possibilities. This creativity is the province of, and the essence of, the everchanging brain. The brain is continually reshaped by its own actions, even by its own thoughts and certainly by its emotions. Trying to make a rigid separation between nature and nurture in this orchestration is meaningless.

Nor is it just philosophy that labels the brain everchanging and potential hostage to its own interactions with the world. This view is the inescapable conclusion from the bulk of research. Several major themes run throughout the story of the hostage

steroid hormone released
into bloodstream

Other hormones bind to receptors on the surface of cells and activate a chain reaction. The first step is production of a second messenger, e. g., cyclic AMP. Cyclic AMP stimulates third messengers, which in turn activate fourth messengers. One type of fourth messenger is a protein that binds to DNA and activates gene expression in a manner much like the steroid hormone receptors.

177

brain. These include the complex process of development, the effects of stress and aging, and the universal influence of hormones in modulating the brain and helping protect it while sometimes making it captive to assaults from the outside world. Hormones are the messengers and the messages that evoke all manner of changes.

Important among these messengers of change are those hormones produced by the thyroid and adrenal glands and the sex hormones—the gonadal hormones of both men and women. The brain is their orchestrator because these various hormones are all secreted at the brain's orders. The endocrine glands release their hormones in response to the messages of other hormones that come from the pituitary gland. In turn, these pituitary hormones are regulated, deep inside the brain, by the hypothalamus. The causation doesn't stop there. The chemical activity of the hypothalamus is influenced by the emotions and even the rational thoughts that emanate from higher brain centers involving the cerebral cortex.

This whole brain-controlled system also reacts and changes in response to experience as the brain senses the outside world through vision, smell, taste, sound, and other physical signals that we know as heat, cold, pain, pressure, and a world of other physical impacts ranging from blasts to feather touches.

While the brain uses all of these to play its own intricate fugues and rhapsodies, the master organ also serves as a chemical thermostat to guard the whole system from blowout. Today's favored term is feedback. The hormone flow from all the endocrine glands is initiated by the brain, but it also feeds back to the brain and all the other organs where the hormones act. The continual feedback governs processes in cells that, in turn, control hormone output. Since the brain is at the center of this subtle ebb and flow, the feedback loop also influences moods and behavior: fear, anger, love, and laughter. These, in turn, have powerful effects on the hormone output that is ultimately governed by the brain.

All this means that, while the brain evokes hormones and their multitude of effects, the tide of hormones affects the brain too. The implications are profound: individual differences in experience are translated into differences in brain function, even brain structure. That is what makes the situation so complex, so difficult to resolve into such tidy simplicities as nature vs nurture. Early life experiences and the hormone exposures that are determined by the brain's reactions to those experiences provide cues that will change the way the brain responds to new experiences in the future. Heredity puts outer limits on how the brain can perform, but there is immense room for variation within those limits. Nature and nurture do not work separately and apart from each other.

Modern research in brain chemistry has supplied a surprising amount of detail to the generalities of how the good and bad nurture of the environment shapes the nature of the functioning human brain.

An important dimension was added to the story more than twenty years ago with the discovery of the receptors in the brain for all of the classes of steroid hormones, including the sex hormones and those of the adrenals and thyroid glands.

These discoveries led to understanding of a direct link between the environmental effects of hormones and the brain's control over the functioning of its own genes. Receptors are the connecting links through which hormones deliver their messages to individual cells. To put the matter more concretely: the receptors are proteins whose twists and strands and folded sheets include shapings where parts of the hormone molecule fit like a hand in its glove. Another piece of that same receptor protein is designed to fit with the detailed shape and chemistry of a particular piece of DNA. When the hormone comes to rest in its glovelike target, it causes a new twist in the DNA so that a key part of a gene is exposed in a way that makes it accessible to another part of the whole store of DNA that geneticists call the genome (the totality of the genes). Specifically, the hormone makes a particular piece of the genetic material accessible to activating pieces of DNA called enhancers. The link between the enhancer and a special part of a gene's structure completes the hormone's message. Depending on the identities of the hormone, the cell, the gene, and the enhancer, this chemical waltz of the shapes either increases or decreases the gene's opportunity to be transcribed into the form of RNA.

Only when a gene in the total archive of DNA is translated into the form of RNA can it go into action. The gene in its RNA form is the working blueprint that is shipped to the cell's manufacturing center. There, in the typical case, it directs the assembly of another protein that the cell or the body needs.

Through this neat bit of nature-coupled-to-nurture activity, the brain influences the activity of its genes and the manufacturing efforts of its billions of cells. One of the pioneers in making this point clear was Holger Hyden, who first showed that the RNA content of neurons and glial cells in the brain was modified as a result of activity and learning.

To sum up the conclusions that arise from much research: the steroid hormones of the gonads and adrenal glands are messengers sent by signals originating in the brain to coordinate and regulate events in many organs of the body, including the brain itself. And they do this by acting on the genome. This goes on throughout life in a multitude of hormone effects. But the nature of those effects changes as the brain matures and ages. During early development, the actions of hormones cause permanent changes in neuronal growth and differentiation in embryo and fetus. This is most obvious in the hormones' crucial role in sexual differentiation. Later in life, hormone actions on the mature neurons modulate gene expression, but the effects are typically reversible, not permanent.

The steroid hormones are almost universal actors in this life drama, but they aren't the only agents that affect the activity of genes in the brain. Neurotransmitters also change the activity of genes through a cascade of changes starting at the surface of the cell and triggering the formation of second and third messengers which carry the message into the cell nucleus.

All of these findings concerning hormones, neurotransmitters, and brain function have been immensely significant both to philosophy and to science. As we have seen, there are many kinds of learning. Nevertheless, in some of its forms, whether the process be in rats, chipmunks, or humans, learning is a mental function. Yet this mental activity can alter the functions of genes in the brain. By doing so, learning can alter both the chemistry and the structure of the brain while it alters that brain's outlook on life.

This concept, so alien to our earlier culture, is now well appreciated even in musical comedy. Sky Masterson, the gambler in *Guys and Dolls*, the musical based on Damon Runyon's stories, says he will leave his choice of love to "chance and chemistry."

But for scientists who try to sort out the subtle effects of chemistry on behavior, humans can be hard to study. Because of that, many of the important concepts have come to light through research with laboratory animals. Some important revelations of nature's scheme of things have also come from studies of birds, squirrels, and other wild animals. In some wild species, the hippocampus is larger in males than females, and these seem to be species in which the males have to spend more time outside in the world, worrying about their own territory and knowing its boundaries. Among other things, this puts particular emphasis on the hippocampus, one of the brain structures most important to memory. The males apparently rise to the occasion by growth of that part of the brain.

The hippocampus is also enlarged in species that store food for the winter. They have to choose storage spaces and remember their locations to prevent starvation during the cold, snow-covered winter months. The clear implication is that evolution has produced adaptations in such qualities as the strength of spatial memory to cope with some of these problems. There appear to be seasonal variations in some of this plasticity of the brain. In hibernating species of ground squirrels dendrites in part of the hippocampus will actually retract during hibernation. Evidently these threads that connect nerve cells are not much used during the long winter sleep.

But this effect can be reversed with amazing quickness. Within several hours of coming out of hibernation, those dendrites grow out again, giving the brain new scope for making neuron-to-neuron connections that are thought to be vital to new learning and new memories.

This regrowth happens within several hours after the animal has awakened from hibernation. The regeneration is so rapid that it challenges scientists' current ideas of how that kind of regrowth can occur. There is at least tentative evidence that the brains of adult animals in some species may actually produce new neurons under these circumstances and destroy neurons when the seasons change. The plasticity may go beyond forming new dendrites to forming new nerve cells as well.

Scientists at The Rockefeller University have found evidence that adrenal steroid hormones can exercise some control over both the destruction and the production of nerve cells in the brains of adult animals in some species. It is a reasonable guess, although still a tentative one, that a reason for this control is to allow the brain to produce and destroy neurons to cope with seasonal change.

Adding to the interest of the puzzle, dendrites in the hippocampal brain region in hibernating animals have been found to atrophy under the assault of repeated stress. Perhaps the stresses overwork brain circuits that have other natural functions. Thus do the concepts of nature and nurture come ever closer together through the knowledge that new research supplies.

It is worth reemphasizing that the coming together is a matter of both brain chemistry and brain anatomy. Accumulating evidence for the anatomical changes has come as a series of shocking surprises to many brain scientists. Everyone knew that some changes must occur when the brain lays down permanent memories. But beyond that, the well-established dogma had been that the brain was the immutable, unchanging black box. It had no business revising its circuitry to keep up with the times or to develop new skills. But the dogma was wrong.

One scientist who has demonstrated this with striking clarity is Dr. Michael Merzenich of University of California, San Francisco. In the 1970s he was a major contributor to studies of the human auditory system which led to important advances in hearing aids for the severely deaf. In recent years his laboratory has drawn international attention through studies that have shown dramatically how plastic and changeable the adult cerebral cortex can really

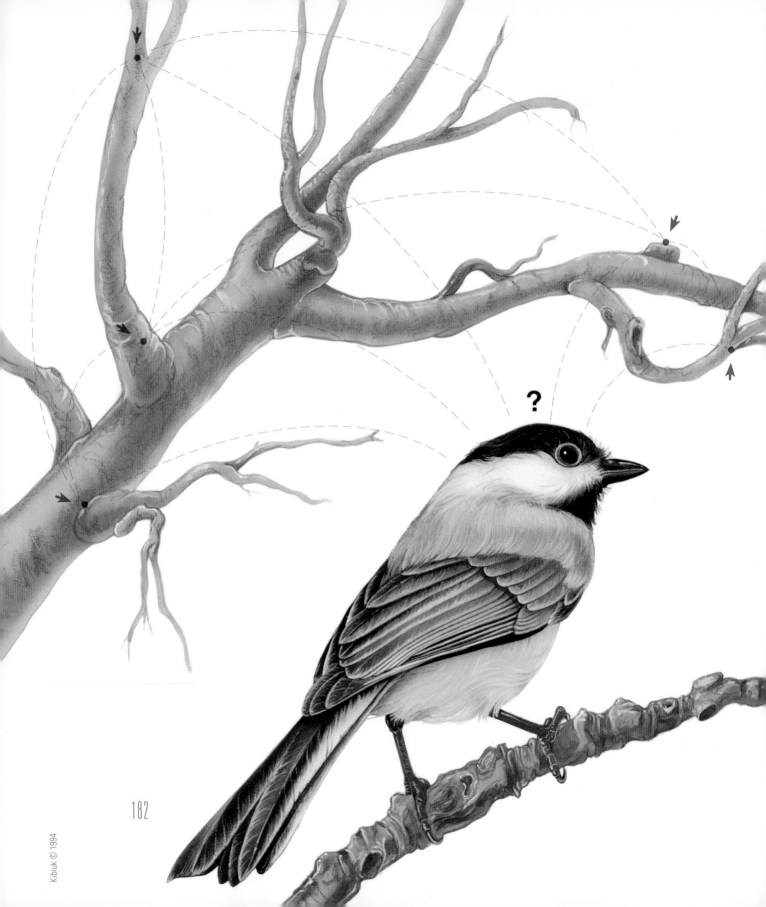

?

Kibiuk © 1994

be. The research has been mainly in adult monkeys, but there are important implications for humans who suffer nerve damage and even for understanding how it is that such subtle physical skills as violin or piano playing or expert use of a typewriter keyboard can become so finely honed as to seem instinctive.

Dr. Merzenich is a map maker, but his maps are of the cerebral cortex, the part of the brain, more than any other, that makes humans uniquely human. His research has concentrated on what is called the somatosensory area of the cortex. This is the area where the brain registers the physical sensations of touch in various parts of the skin surface. Brain scientists make highly detailed maps of this region, showing, for example, the specific part of the cortex to which the peripheral nerves send signals from the lips, each toe on each foot, and the fingers of each hand. It is done with microelectrodes that penetrate the cortex and reveal brain signals there when a specific part of the body surface is touched or otherwise stimulated.

Dr. Merzenich's maps are incredibly detailed, but it isn't just the detail that is amazing. It is how the maps mirror the animal's experiences throughout life.

The classical view of these maps was that they were established early as the nerve cells and their web of connections matured. Once established, it was thought, the circuits were stable. Dr. Merzenich has demolished that comfortable faith in the status quo. In fact, he finds that the maps are remodeled continually, mirroring the animal's interactions with the world. Even more surprising, the map region that registers sensations from a much used part of the body actually expands at the expense of less used parts. Workers in his laboratory trained a monkey to do a simple task that involved much use of one fingertip. Over a period of three months, the cortex map registering that fingertip was enlarged fivefold from its original territory.

Similarly, a person who has lost a finger or a whole limb through accident or disease, would have the cortex map of that region diminish from lack of

Food-storing birds such as the black-capped chickadee use their hippocampus to locate stored food throughout their habitat. Food-storing birds have a larger hippocampus than birds that do not store food in this manner. Damaging the hippocampus causes the birds to make mistakes in locating the places where they had stored food.

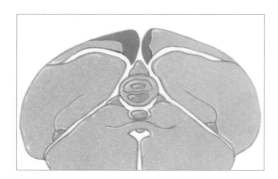

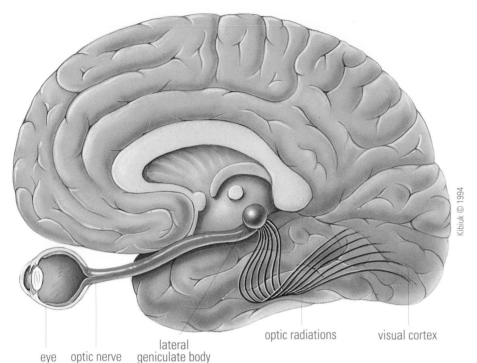

eye   optic nerve   lateral geniculate body   optic radiations   visual cortex

Kibiuk © 1994

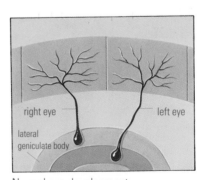

Normal eye development

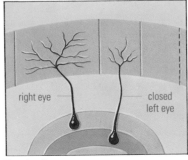

Deprivation

During a critical period of early development, there are permanent effects of monocular visual deprivation produced by covering one eye with a patch that prevents shapes and patterns, but not light itself, from reaching the retina. This prevents the normal development of the ocular dominance columns of the visual receiving area of the cerebral cortex. Normally, both eyes contribute equally, each eye to adjacent columns. In the monocular deprived condition, the normal eye columns take over more and more neurons in the visual cortex, while the covered-eye columns shrink. After this critical period of development ends, this damage is irreversible and the closed eye will never again regain normal sight.

Original art used by the Society for Neuroscience in June 1994 "Brain Briefings".

184

use while other parts of the body would encroach on that unused territory in the brain.

Dr. Merzenich believes this same kind of plasticity and remodeling of the brain accounts for at least part of the learned skills and artistries and the wealth of behavioral possibilities that are the signature of our species.

So nurture, in the sense of experience, builds usefully upon nature. Parts of the brain are remodeled in the perfection of skills. But deprivation too is an aspect of nurture and it can have tragic effects. Evidence of this began to emerge many years ago. Two scientists at Harvard University made a landmark discovery when they wondered about the sad fate of children who had congenital cataracts. Why didn't the children quickly develop full vision when their sight-clouding cataracts were removed?

Cataracts are opaque spots in the lens of the eye. Most develop in middle age or later, but sometimes they are present at birth. These are called congenital cataracts and doctors have learned that they must be removed early in infancy. When it is not done soon enough the delay can be disastrous. Vision may be seriously and permanently impaired, even though the eye and retina now functioned normally. A similar problem was discovered in animal experiments in which cats or monkeys were reared through infancy in total darkness. They suffered serious and persistent loss in vision even though there was nothing at all wrong with their eyes.

These unexpected findings addressed a crucial question that had plagued philosophers at least as far back at Rene Descartes in the early 1600s: how important is visual experience in early development?

Dr. Torsten Wiesel and his long-term collaborator, David Hubel were attracted to that same question of the relative role of nature and nurture in the development of the visual system in the 1960s at Harvard Medical School (Dr. Wiesel in now president of The Rockefeller University). It was to be a central issue in their joint research concerning the brain's strategies for translating the light that hits the retina of the eye into information that the brain interprets as shape, form and movement—research that was to gain the two scientists the 1981 Nobel Prize in Medicine.

To a layman, the sequence of events in vision seems as simple as light and darkness. The lens focuses incoming light and forms an image on the retina at the back of the eye. Cells of the retina translate this image into nerve impulses and the optic nerve conveys these signals to the brain. That is what we are all taught in school. But how does the brain actually deal with the signals and translate the image? That is where the questions reach Nobel Prize magnitude. The process is exceedingly complicated. It has taken scientists more than a century to sort it all out. The main visual area of the human brain lies at the back in what is known as the occipital region. That is the seat of the primary visual cortex, which anatomists call the striate cortex, because it appears to have stripes. Although adjacent areas of the cortex are also involved in vision, a person is essentially blind without the striate cortex. For all the primates, including humans, vision is a particularly crucial matter. In humans and monkeys about half of the entire cerebral cortex is involved in processing visual signals. The optic nerves, the great trunk cables that connect the retinas to the brain, are each made up of about a million nerve cells.

But none of these hard-won facts explains why both eyes need to send signals to the striate cortex in infancy to develop the capacity for normal vision. It had been known since at least the 1930s that children with congenital cataracts required long and intense training to give them any ability to recognize forms and shapes. Entirely normal vision seldom developed at all. Since the rest of the eye seemed completely normal the problem must be somewhere in the brain. Congenital cataracts might be blamed on nature, since they were present at birth. The persistent vision problems were due to nurture, in the broad sense of experience that affected the brain after birth. But the brain wasn't supposed to be affected in that way. Its circuits were laid done in the embryo and fetus. For most of the brain, that was supposed to be the end of the story.

"We were anxious to learn the site and nature of this disruption in the visual pathway," Dr. Hubel noted in a Harvey Society lecture at The Rockefeller University. There were at least two possibilities. Perhaps the infant brain needed the "exercise" of coping with incoming visual signals to establish the nerve circuits it needed to make sense of shapes and forms. From their studies, Drs. Hubel and Wiesel didn't find this idea persuasive. It seemed more plausible to them that the necessary circuits were already in place. In the children who had cataracts, and the animals that had one eye covered, the nerve circuits related to the occluded eyes may simply have suffered from disuse. But the two scientists concluded that this was not the main problem. The alternative mechanism, which their research confirmed, was a sharp surprise. In his lecture, Dr. Hubel put it this way:

"We concluded that a monocular closure produces its effects largely as a result of competition. It is as though the connections from the open eye had somehow taken advantage of their rivals from the closed eye in the competition for space on postsynaptic cells. "

In short, the nerve circuits dealing with signals from each of the two eyes competed for territory on the visual cortex. If one eye was inactive because it was kept in the dark, the region of cortex that handled signals from the other eye expanded at the occluded eye's expense. Through their research, Drs. Wiesel and Hubel also showed that there is a critical period in infancy in which this had to be corrected or the structural disparity would become permanent. Furthermore, the brain's translation of signals from the deprived eye would be distorted. The sooner the eye is closed after birth, the more devastating the result, and the more brief the eye closure had to be to cause the damage. If both eyes were active during early life, a later period in which one eye was unused did not cause much permanent harm to vision. Indeed, it is well known that an adult cataract patient can have a large measure of vision restored almost immediately after the cataracts are removed and corrective glasses are provided.

The concept of competition in the visual system during the early sensitive period was a striking advance. There may be even more global implications in the findings.

"It seems conceivable," said Dr. Hubel, "that early deprivation of social interaction, such as contacts with a mother, may lead to mental disturbances that have their counterpart in actual structural abnormalities in the brain."

Both from research in animals and studies of humans who have suffered deprivation of various kinds, other scientists have added strength to this concept. Dr. Merzenich's work is a notable example. In addition, a scientist who has studied children kept in closets and deprived of normal verbal communications during infancy and childhood found similar effects. The children sometimes developed good vocabulary, once they were rescued, but they had serious trouble with grammar. They found it hard to form proper sentences. It is reasonable to guess that they have other problems too. When the brain is taken hostage there is a ransom to be paid. The cost is probably highest, and certainly most tragic, when deprivation comes in childhood.

The long saga of joint research by Drs. Hubel and Wiesel went far beyond the studies of what happens to the brain when one eye is deprived of use. Over the years they worked out in great detail the functional anatomy of the visual cortex, determining just where and to what cells the optic nerve delivered its impulses and how the cortex responded. Professors of the Karolinska Institutet in Stockholm summarized it this way in announcing the Nobel Prize award:

"By following the visual impulses along their path to the various cell layers of the optical cortex, Hubel and Wiesel were able to demonstrate that the message about the image falling upon the eye's retina undergoes a step-wise analysis in a system of nerve cells stored in columns. In this system each cell has its specific function and is responsible for a specific detail in the pattern of the visual image."

One system of nerve cell columns are called ocular dominance columns, which lie in a series of alternating bands across the the primary visual cortex. The nerve signals that originate in the right and left eye are sorted out in these alternating ocular dominance bands. Before the work of Drs. Wiesel and Hubel, nobody knew that such an intricate arrangement existed to help the brain understand the signals it was getting from the eyes. There was nothing in the gross anatomy of the brain that hinted at this structural organization of the vision system. The research by the two scientists illuminated a feature of brain function in a way that few people in the field had even thought possible.

While many of the chemical and structural details of the brain's plasticity must be studied in other species, human experience can cast light on important issues that cannot be resolved in animals. Studies of identical twins have put the glare of reality on many theoretical concepts of nature vs nurture. Consider, for example, schizophrenia, one of the most serious and devastating of mental disorders. Is it genetic, is it environmental, or is it both? If it was purely genetic, the disorder would be expected to arise always in both identical twins of a pair, while among fraternal twins it would not. If the causes were all to be found in environment and life experience, the risk of schizophrenia would differ even between two identical twins, and particularly so if they were reared apart from one another.

In fact, studies have shown that schizophrenia does not always strike both identical twins in a pair. If one develops the disorder, the risk is much higher for the other than would be true of nontwin brothers and sisters even if the twins were raised apart as children. But it is far from an all-or-nothing genetic risk. Heredity appears to be a part of the story, but it cannot be the whole. If one of a pair of identical twins develops schizophrenia, the odds are higher than random chance that the other will be affected too. But the concordance is not total. There are some pairs of identical twins in which one does develop schizophrenia, but the other does not.

Yet the brains of schizophrenics are physically different in some respects from normals. Whether these differences—in the size of the interior spaces called ventricles, for example—are part of the cause or the effects is still not certain. But the brains of schizophrenia patients have clearly become hostage to some process related to the disease. It is not all heredity, but perhaps a hereditary tilt in a direction that allows some environmental stress to tip the balance of normalcy too far.

A similar mix of hereditary influence and some aspects of environment

188

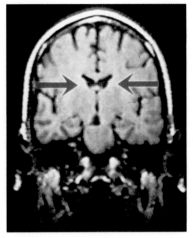

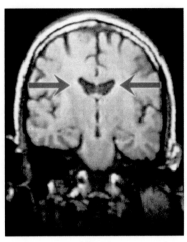

Unaffected

Affected

Some genetic traits for disease are not always expressed to the same extent even in identical twins, which have the same genetic material. Here, one twin with schizophrenia shows enlargement of the cerebral ventricles indicating that there are abnormalities in brain structure and function; the other twin does not have the disorder and does not show the brain abnormality. Images from laboratory of Daniel Weinberger of NIMH. *Courtesy of the Society for Neuroscience.*

also appear to be at work in various kinds of depression. The most serious kind, called bipolar disorder and formerly known as manic depressive illness, seems to be predominantly hereditary. This conclusion arises from a study of 110 pairs of twins cited in a report to Congress by its Office of Technology Assessment. The concordance rate is 0.80. That means that if one of a pair of identical twins develops the illness, the betting odds are about 8 in 10 that the other will be affected also. Among fraternal twins the concordance rate is only 0.16—only a 16% risk. In severe depression that does not involve the violent swings in mood that characterize bipolar depression, the link to heredity seems to be about 59% in identical twins as contrasted with 30% in fraternal twins. For depression of lesser magnitude, the link to genetic factors is still weaker.

It is not necessary to consider such grim disorders as schizophrenia and serious depressive illness to see the extent to which nature and nurture percolate together to produce effects that are unique in each individual. A recent study shows that even the cigarette habit is influenced by both. It has been documented time and time again that peer pressure and the example of family members are important in deciding who will become a smoker. But some people find it relatively easy to quit the habit once they are convinced of its dangers. Others know it is dangerous and destructive to health and yet they can't stop. Is that too a consequence of social environment? A study from the

National Heart, Lung and Blood Institute suggests heredity plays an important role here too. The study dealt with 4,775 pairs of twins, some of whom were identical while others were fraternal. The twins were all born between 1917 and 1927 and had all served in the military during at least part of World War II. That was a time and circumstance in which cigarette smoking was probably far more common than total abstention among young men. The habit was certainly not discouraged. The research team found no evidence that family environment influenced the number of cigarettes a day a man smoked or the extent to which he became addicted to the habit. Genes evidently did. The men were surveyed twice, from 1967 to 1969 and a second time between 1983 and 1985. The prevalence of smoking dropped to nearly half its original level during the sixteen year interval, evidently reflecting society's changed attitude toward smoking in the light of all the data on its dangers. A surprising point in the findings indicated that one of the strongest genetic influences was not on heavy smoking, but on light smoking. The research team sees this as a hint that the habit of light smoking may be influenced by a different gene, or different genes, than is true of heavy smoking.

That surprising conclusion should serve as a warning to anyone who thinks it should be easy to sort out the contributions of nature and nurture to anything as rich in complexities as the functions of the human brain. If a trait as simple as the cigarette habit is forged from a mix of opportunity, peer pressure, the need to cope with stress and, in addition to all of those, a multiplicity of genes, how can one possibly solve a real enigma such as the nature and genetic determinants of intelligence?

In animal research, the first step in a search for genetic influences on behavior would be to make sure that the environment was kept rigorously equal in two groups. Given this environmentally "level playing field," differences between the two groups could logically be ascribed to heredity. One of the grave problems of many such studies of nature and nurture in humans is that the playing field is hardly ever level. Could it ever be possible, for example, to find a pure genetic determinant for violent crime, when many criminals spend their childhood in conditions of poverty with broken homes and peer pressure that pushes toward crime rather than good citizenship? Crimes involving stock fraud or a savings and loan swindle, on the other hand, are seldom committed by the same people who commit armed robberies. Is one to conclude that there are different genes for the two different kinds of crime?

Or, is it more reasonable to judge that environment plays the main role? The opportunity for stock fraud is available to some people, but not to others, and that is certainly a matter of environment, or nurture.

Is it ever possible to dissect such complexities into separate components of nature and nurture? In theory, yes, but in fact it is a prodigious task, except in pairs of twins. A baby's nurture, after all, starts with the health and personal habits of the pregnant woman. After the child is born, nurture continues through such diverse elements as childhood nutrition, family milieu and expectations, if there is a functioning family. Experience in school, job opportunities, personal self-esteem, and the individual's sense of hope for the future all mix into the equation too.

There are genetic disorders, such as Huntington's and Lesch-Nyhan, in which nature is the whole story and no amount of nurture will cancel the patient's tragic fate. That is a common circumstance in diseases caused by single specific gene defects. The cause of Alzheimer's disease is still a mystery, but in this malady also there appears to be nothing much that can be done after the destruction of mind and memory has commenced. What mix of nature and nurture is responsible for Alzheimer's disease is still an open question and it is by no means certain that the causative process is the same in all patients. Familial Alzheimer's disease is different in several respects from the more sporadic disease. The significance of that difference is also mostly unknown.

Nevertheless, nurture includes all of the highest achievements of human ingenuity: one of the brain's strongest suits. There are some cases in which the brain can use that ingenuity to rewrite happy endings into some of the tragedies that are inscribed so indelibly by nature. One example can be found in the devastating genetic disorder phenylketonuria (PKU) and more such victories are almost certain to be scored in the future.

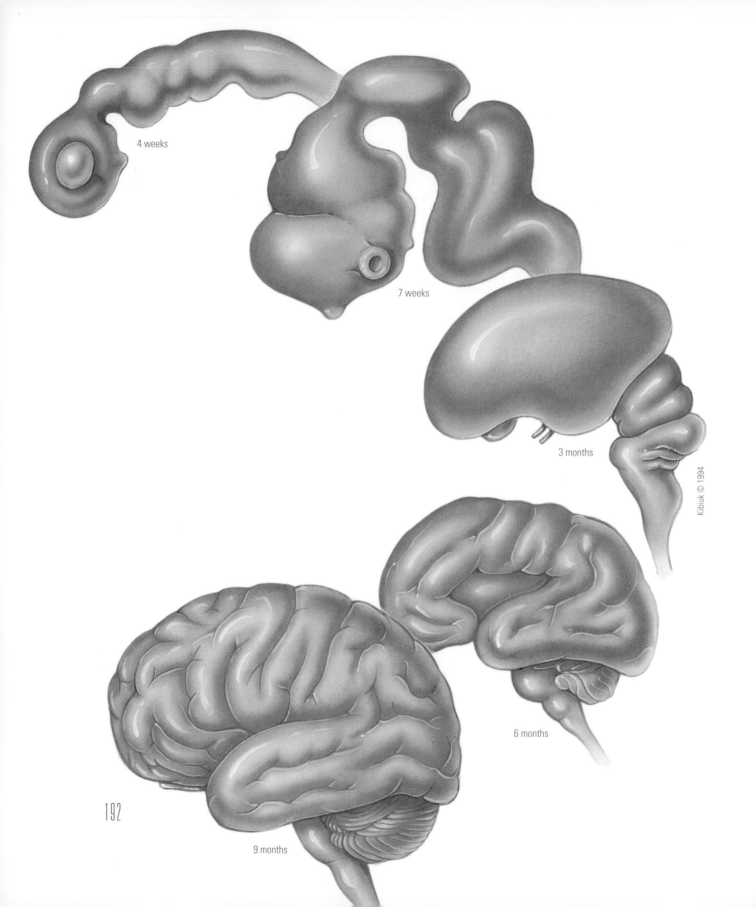

4 weeks

7 weeks

3 months

Kibiuk © 1994

6 months

9 months

THE GOOD NEWS 11

t takes only a few drops of blood, a needle prick to the heel will do it, to fulfill one of the most dramatic triumphs nurture has ever won over nature. The blood comes from infants a few days old. The mission is to find those few who may be at risk of brain damage from phenylketonuria. Unhappily, PKU is a large enough health concern so that many people know it by its initials. It is among the large category of inborn problems that result from seemingly minor errors in the body's intricate chemistry. In PKU, a tiny genetic flaw deprives the body of the enzyme action needed to break down a common food ingredient, phenylalanine. The accumulating chemical debris from this failure kills brain cells. The result is severe mental retardation that occurs within the first few years of childhood. The loss is permanent.

Clearly, PKU is rooted solidly in nature. It stems from the malfunction of one gene which ruins the function of one enzyme. Problems of nurture have nothing to do with it. Because of the genetic error, the liver lacks help from the enzyme phenylalanine hydroxylase to dispose of phenylalanine. This substance is an amino acid present in all food protein. In the normal person, the enzyme converts phenylalanine to another amino acid, tyrosine. When that normal conversion fails, phenylalanine and its by-products accumulate in the body and there is too little tyrosine. If a baby is born with that single flaw in enzyme function, severe mental retardation results. Nature has dealt the newcomer a tragically losing hand.

The human brain develops from a tube-like structure at one end of the embryo. The "neural tube" thickens and folds upon itself and forms the brainstem and cerebellum and the forebrain, which includes the cerebral cortex.

Although the metabolic error is uncommon, phenylketonuria used to be one of the main causes of serious mental retardation. Today, in the United States, it is rare. PKU is a classic case of good news that nurture can wring from the tragic bad news of genetic error. Most, if not all, of the potential damage to the brain can be avoided by a strict diet begun within the first month of life. It keeps the child free of excess phenylalanine. In the U.S., and most of Europe and other developed countries, virtually all babies are tested soon after birth to find those few cases in which the PKU defect exists. Babies who fail the initial test have to be studied in greater detail to make sure that they really do have the problem, but the testing is well worth the effort. It can rescue the hostage brain.

The protective diet must be started early and it is onerous. The natural proteins that we use as food are made up of some twenty amino acids in varying amounts. Phenylalanine makes up about 4% of the total. A PKU child's diet consists mostly of an artificial mixture of amino acids that excludes phenylalanine. It is Spartan and difficult. Most of the appealing foods in our normal diet, including milk, contain more phenylalanine than the affected child can risk. But the diet works and many adults today owe their mental competence to the PKU test in infancy. The fact that corrective measures can be taken to prevent such a tragic condition is one of the great triumphs of modern medicine. It is also heartening evidence that the human brain can be rescued from hostage states imposed, not only by hazards of environment, but also by grave mistakes in biology.

In that sense, the diet to prevent PKU is a triumph of nurture over nature, but even in this clear-cut case the two forces are intertwined. Before doctors understood the disease, it was an indisputable case of heredity ruining a life despite everything good care could do in defense. Today the disease almost never occurs unless nurture fails to provide the protective diet.

Actually, the intelligent use of nurture to rescue human well-being from the frailties of nature is among the most triumphant themes of medicine over the centuries. The use of iodized salt to prevent the mental destruction of cretinism is one of the old triumphs that involve the brain. It might even be argued that, long before the dawn of history, the first uses of beer and opium to give the mind a lift from pains, terrors, and troubles were the first such nature-nurture aids to the besieged brain. These two drugs may also have given humans their first lessons in a grim truth: miracle cures are never as harmless as they seem.

But PKU was among the first cases in which nurture came intelligently to the rescue of the brain through real knowledge of the problem, not some combination of fortunate chances based on a shrewd observation of cause and effect. It was the first inherited metabolic disease in which damage was forestalled by dealing with the accumulating dangerous by-products. Nonetheless, by the standards of the 1990s, the PKU story is a triumph of yesterday's science and primitive, albeit sensible, countermeasures. The nature of the disorder was discovered almost sixty years ago. The widespread use of a detection test came decades later. The testing went through a stage of controversy because its early use was far from infallible and resulted in some children being put on the diet when they really didn't need it. Critics argued that the universal testing was exposing too many normal babies to the rigors of an unnecessary diet that could, itself, be damaging to health and an agreeable life.

Improvements in the scheme of testing and verification have largely stilled these arguments. The PKU testing is so successful that infant blood tests for several other rare disorders have been added. But the preventive treatment is no trivial discomfort and it is still not entirely clear how long the PKU diet has to be continued to prevent brain damage; certainly through the age of six and probably, with some relaxation, through most of the teenage years. Experts still differ on this. In recent years another problem has arisen as young women whose brains were saved from PKU have grown up, married, and become pregnant. They still suffer from the flawed disposal of phenylalanine. This puts the unborn babies at grave risk even when they are free of the genetic flaw. It has been estimated that over 90% of pregnancies in mothers who have the enzyme defect result in mental retardation and physical problems in the infant. Probably the prospective mother should return to a low phenylalanine diet even before pregnancy, but experience is still being accumulated to define how early the diet should be used and how well this strategy works.

Given all the problems of PKU prevention, it would seem there must be a better way to deal with it. Perhaps there is. In today's world, the near-miracles of molecular biology seem to make almost anything possible, including some incredible rescues of the hostage brain. The enzyme that is missing from the PKU patient's liver has been known for decades and the gene that is its blueprint has been cloned and grown in laboratories. Scientists are becoming adept at manipulating and transferring genes. All this raises a real question that would have been just pie in the sky a decade ago: why not transplant the gene for the needed enzyme into the patient's own liver cells and correct the PKU defect instead of simply holding the figurative thumb in the dike to prevent brain damage?

Many puzzles and unsolved roadblocks lie between this thought and its practical use, but medical scientists are making extraordinary progress. The

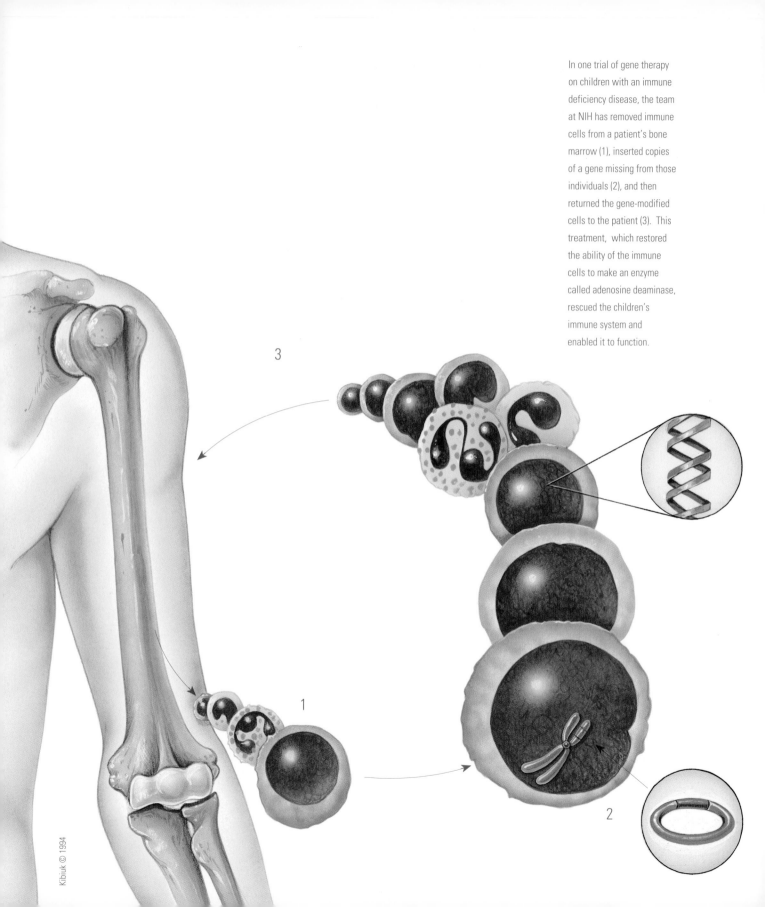

In one trial of gene therapy on children with an immune deficiency disease, the team at NIH has removed immune cells from a patient's bone marrow (1), inserted copies of a gene missing from those individuals (2), and then returned the gene-modified cells to the patient (3). This treatment, which restored the ability of the immune cells to make an enzyme called adenosine deaminase, rescued the children's immune system and enabled it to function.

3

1

2

Kibiuk © 1994

name of this new game is gene therapy. Although still experimental, it is no longer only theory in search of reality. After years of bitter debate and blighted hopes, gene therapy is entering the real world of medicine.

In 1990, at the National Heart, Lung and Blood Institute, Dr. W. French Anderson and a large team of colleagues from his own and other units of the NIH pioneered the first successful use of human gene therapy. They treated two young children who suffered from life-threatening lack of immune defenses. These children too suffered from the failure of one specific gene that was the blueprint for one enzyme. In this case, the enzyme was adenosine deaminase. Its lack throws the immune defenses into failure. The medical team took some of the patients' white blood cells, treated them in the laboratory to add copies of the needed gene, and then returned the gene-modified cells to the patients. The added normal gene allowed those cells to make the crucial enzyme and rescued the children's immunity. The success of those cases has prompted many other recent attempts with different diseases. By Dr. Anderson's tally late in 1992, some forty new gene therapy protocols had been approved by the federal government. Sixty-one patients around the world had received transplanted genes either as therapy or for using the genes as markers to identify cells. Most of the patients had various kinds of cancer. It is not yet clear how useful the new attempts have been, but the catalogue of different diseases being assaulted is growing rapidly.

Dr. Thomas Friedmann of University of California, San Diego, another pioneer in this new field, says the first early exploratory phase of human gene therapy is now ended.

"We are now in an explosive second phase—one of technical implementation," he wrote in a recent review. At least one of the new planned attempts has to do with the brain. It is a proposal to treat brain tumors by gene transfers designed to make the tumor cells genetically susceptible to a drug that normal body cells can resist.

But gene therapy for yet another disease has used a strategy that required putting the new gene into the patient's liver cells, the same target that would be the aim in PKU. This gene transfer was done to combat a disease that causes rampant excess of fats in the blood. The problem is a rare hereditary disorder that sometimes causes heart attacks in childhood. The gene treatment required liver surgery and other drastic measures that would rule out the same tactics for widespread medical use, but the doctors at University of Michigan who treated the first patient of this kind reported that some of her liver cells did take up the foreign gene and put it to proper use. In 1994, the team, now at University of Pennsylvania, reported a substantial reduction in the level of the most dangerous form of cholesterol in their patient's blood. She seemed to be doing well. The doctors have given several other patients the same treatment. While an assault on PKU would involve an entirely different gene, a logical goal would be to put it into liver cells. In PKU, it is also possible that cells other than those of liver could be used to supply enough of the missing enzyme to fill the body's needs. Among gene therapy experts, PKU is already on the list of promising future targets. When and if the treatment is accomplished in PKU, the results could herald a revolution in mankind's ability to deal with this serious hazard to the brain.

As revolutionary in its way as gene therapy, and perhaps a little farther along in development is the actual transplantation of fetal brain cells to treat disease. Specialists call it neural grafting. Like gene therapy, this treatment has had a long frustrating history, but now is beginning to show real grounds for hope.

An important chapter in the story began in the early 1980s in a way no one could have predicted, much less desired. The problem first came to light in 1982 when a patient arrived at a California hospital, stooped, slow of movement, afflicted with muscular tremors and episodes of rigidity. His movements were painfully slow. From the symptoms alone, any doctor would have guessed it was long-term Parkinson's disease. Victims of the disorder often get that way in their sixties or seventies. The problem was that this patient was only twenty-four years old.

In relatively short order at least five such patients came to California hospitals, all relatively young and all suffering from what appeared to be the final stages of Parkinson's disease.

The victims of these bizarre tragedies all had one additional feature in common: drug abuse. That fact soon solved the mystery. In those days, the demand for illicit "recreational drugs" spawned a short-lived cottage industry in manufacturing new ones. One such drug, sold on the West Coast, was touted as homemade heroin. In fact it was a deadly concoction that killed brain cells. It is known as MPTP, shorthand for 1-methyl-4-phenyl-1,2,3,6-tetrahydropyridine. In people who took it, the drug produced, almost overnight, the symptoms of advanced Parkinson's disease including the tendency to freeze into postures of statuelike rigidity. Two patients who took the drug said they woke up the morning after and were terrified when they found they could hardly move. The terror was justified. The effects were devastating and the condition turned out to be permanent. Brain cells had been killed. There was a strange feature to this cell killing that raised the specter of Parkinson's disease; the damage was amazingly exclusive to one tiny region deep in the brain, the substantia nigra. Little else seemed to be harmed.

Scientists quickly discovered that the prime agent of these disasters was MPTP. It was so efficient in killing cells in that particular part of the brain that it soon came into research use. It could produce in animals a disorder that closely mimicked Parkinson's disease in humans. The chemical has produced the best animal model of the disorder, an important achievement for research.

Most of Parkinson's disease is classed as idiopathic, a fancy word meaning simply that no one knows the cause. But the mechanism of the disease is reasonably well known; degeneration of the nerve pathway between the substantia nigra and a much larger central structure called the striatum. What is still unknown is the cause of that degeneration. Natural Parkinson's disease does not ordinarily destroy neurons of the striatum, but loss of cells in the substantia nigra has the effect of starving the striatum of an important neurotransmitter, dopamine. In consequence, patients suffer the typical symptoms of rigidity, tremor, difficulties in standing and walking, and slowness of movement that are typical of the disease. The drug L-dopa, which delivers dopamine to brain cells, is the standard treatment for Parkinson's disease. Unfortunately, its effectiveness for many patients diminishes after a few years. Medical scientists have long sought better answers to the disorder. It is an important quest because Parkinson's disease is a major public health problem. Nobody knows the exact number of current cases in the U.S., but estimates run at least as high as one million.

Because a key problem is a shortage of dopamine in the brain, one tempting strategy has been the transplantation of cells that produce dopamine. Various different cells and various ways of installing them have been tried over many years, but with only questionable benefit. There have been repeated claims of dramatic success followed by general deep discouragement when the treatments finally failed. In recent years, the quest has focused more and more on the use of fetal brain cells obtained after abortions. The tissue contains brain cells capable of growing after transfer and some of these cells are called dopaminergic because they produce the neurotransmitter dopamine, needed by the Parkinson's patient.

"Cautious optimism concerning future success with fetal tissue implantation persisted because there is logic to the idea of dopamine replacement therapy," said Dr. Stanley Fahn of Columbia University's College of Physicians and Surgeons in a recent commentary, "and fetal dopaminergic cells could be the source."

Fetal tissue is desirable for another reason: it is less likely than adult tissue to evoke destructive immune reactions. Altogether, doctors hoped that the fetal cells could be used safely and that they would not only supply Parkinson's disease patients with dopamine, but might, themselves, also grow and help produce new components for the networks of brain cells in the region where Parkinson's patients suffer loss. Fetal brain cells are a potential large-scale source because many abortions are done each year in the United States.

The animal mimics of human Parkinson's disease produced by using MPTP were important in developing the use of fetal brain cells in humans. Experiments in monkeys showed that the transplanted fetal cells could survive, grow, and even help restore the animals' brain functions that the chemical had ruined. Research with other animals had already shown that fetal brain tissue, unlike cells from the adult central nervous system, would often develop and integrate into the recipient's native brain tissue.

What may prove an important turning point came late in 1992 with a series of reports from Sweden and the United States. Doctors of three research teams used fetal brain tissue to treat either natural Parkinson's disease or its equivalent that resulted from illicit use of drugs containing MPTP. Three reports were published in the Nov. 26, 1992 issue of the *New England Journal of Medicine* with accompanying editorials and commentary by other specialists.

The most successful cases were two Americans treated in Sweden. The two had been seriously damaged by MPTP nearly a decade before. Conventional treatments had failed and the patients were almost totally incapacitated. They needed help in eating, dressing, and personal hygiene. They couldn't walk unaided. After the fetal tissue transplants were performed by Dr. Anders Björklund and colleagues at the University of Lund, both patients improved remarkably. The improvements came gradually over a period of almost two years. One of the two patients, a forty-three-year-old man, was able to dress and feed himself and visit the bathroom without help. He even made trips outside his home. The other patient, a thirty-year-old woman, had seldom been able to get out of a chair without help. Once up, she fell frequently. Twenty-two months after her fetal transplant operations, she could get out of a chair unaided and walked with a long, normal stride. She had gone six months without falling.

The other studies were done at Yale by a team led by Dr. Eugene Redmond and at the University of Colorado by Dr. Curt R. Freed. The two groups did a total of ten patients.

As Dr. Redmond described the procedure, it was astonishing in its sophistication, yet apparent simplicity. His team used magnetic resonance imaging to pinpoint the minute target area in the patient's striatum. They plotted paths to the target to avoid hitting any of the brain's major blood vessels. Then they gave the patient a mild sedative and local anesthetic and the surgeons drilled a hole in the skull. Meanwhile, the fetal brain tissue, which had been frozen in liquid nitrogen to preserve it, was thawed to room temperature. The material was fed into the brain through a hollow tube less than 1/200th of an inch in diameter and the fetal brain cells were extruded into the patient's brain along a tract a few hundredths of an inch long.

"Twenty-seven to sixty minutes elapsed between the removal of the tissue from liquid nitrogen and implantation," Dr. Redmond's report said, "during which time the tissue was kept in an oxygenated medium. The patients were discharged on the third postoperative day."

Unlike the two patients in Sweden, all those treated in the United States had natural Parkinson's disease. Almost all of the patients improved after the transplantations, but there is an implicit question that can't yet be entirely answered. The parkinsonian condition produced by MPTP is a one-time injury. It presumably won't get worse with time. But natural Parkinson's disease is different. The cause is unknown and there is no guarantee that the same process that killed the patient's neurons originally might not continue. If it does, that still-mysterious process could destroy the implanted neurons too. In short, the doctors must continue to study the patients over periods of many years to see how well the improvements persist.

Dr. Björklund, a leading pioneer in the fetal transplant field, said improvement in the MPTP patients was greater than in many, if not all, of fifty-five patients in Sweden and elsewhere who received fetal transplants in recent years. He said it seems possible that victims of natural Parkinson's disease have an underlying brain disorder that may continue and nullify some of the improvement

THE GOOD NEWS

Parkinson's disease specifically attacks the substantia nigra and destroys nerve cells that make the neurotransmitter, dopamine. The dopamine-producing neurons send axons to the rest of the brain, where dopamine is released as a neurotransmitter. Lacking dopamine cells, the Parkinson's disease patient cannot control normal movement and suffers other deficits of awareness and ability to think. The "designer drug" MPTP also attacks and destroys these same neurons and causes a disease very much like parkinson's disease. *Modified from* Pathology, *by E. Rubin and J. Farber. Published by J. B. Lippincott Co.*

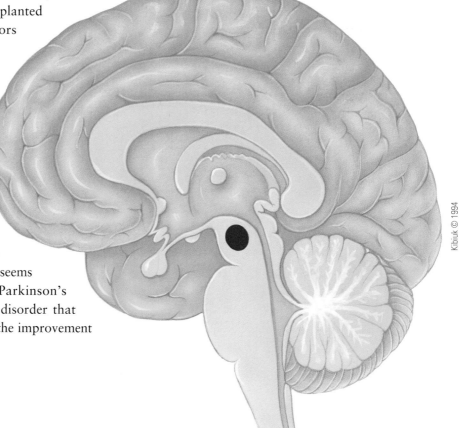

Kibiuk © 1994

achieved by the transplants.

In the lead editorial accompanying the three reports, Dr. Stanley Fahn of Columbia said the results of all three treatment projects were encouraging, but he raised a swarm of questions that still need answers: Do the foreign neurons actually make new synaptic connections in the brain? What are the best target sites for installing the foreign neurons? Will the brain properly control the release of dopamine by the transplanted neurons? And, of course, how long will the benefits persist?

Despite all the questions, he ended on an optimistic note: "We can expect to see further research that will identify the best approach to treating Parkinson's disease by the implantation of fetal tissue into the brain."

That encouraging statement, however, also raises another issue. In the United States, this important research has raised political and religious questions as well as those of medicine. There is a major debate on the use of fetal tissues no matter how useful they may be. In this case, the divisions have nothing to do with brain research itself. The use of fetal tissue has been transplanted into the bitter national controversy over abortion. That long dispute has divided the nation on fiercely contested specifics that range from appointments to the Supreme Court of the United States to the right of individual women to obtain abortions unmolested in their home communities. During

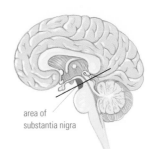

area of substantia nigra

The substantia nigra ("black substance" because of its dark appearance under the microscope) consists of nerve cells of the pars compacta that make dopamine and of the pars reticulata that do not. Attempts to treat Parkinson's or MPTP patients with transplanted cells involve surgical insertion into the brain of nerve cells that produce dopamine to replace those of the pars compacta that have been destroyed.

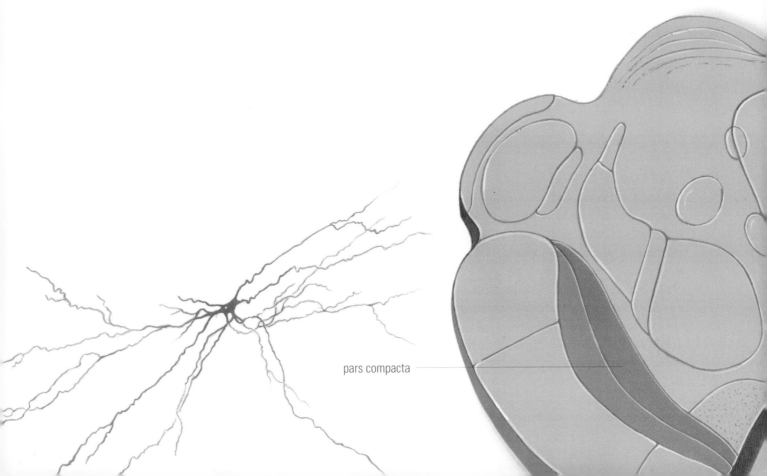

pars compacta

the Administrations of Presidents Ronald Reagan and George Bush the federal government made concerted efforts to discourage abortion. Both Administrations banned use of fetal tissues for brain implants on the assertion that these procedures would encourage women to have abortions.

Major studies sponsored by the government during those Administrations and earlier had concluded that fetal research was valuable to medicine and science, was an issue separate from the abortion debate, and should be continued. The federal ban was kept in force anyway. It had been established by the Reagan Administration. Dr. James Wyngaarden, then director of the National Institutes of Health, asked for guidance on funding from Dr. Robert Windom, assistant secretary of health in the Department of Health and Human Services. The NIH is a part of that department. Dr. Wyngaarden noted that the research "may be characterized in the press as an indication that the Department is encouraging abortions."

Dr. Windom placed a moratorium on funding such studies and appointed a panel of outside experts to review the issues. Just before the end of 1988, the panel decided, by a large majority, that the research was acceptable and could be funded. The Bush Administration kept the ban in place anyway.

In fact, the federal government can't ban such research outright, but it can, and did, rule that the work could not be done with any help from federal

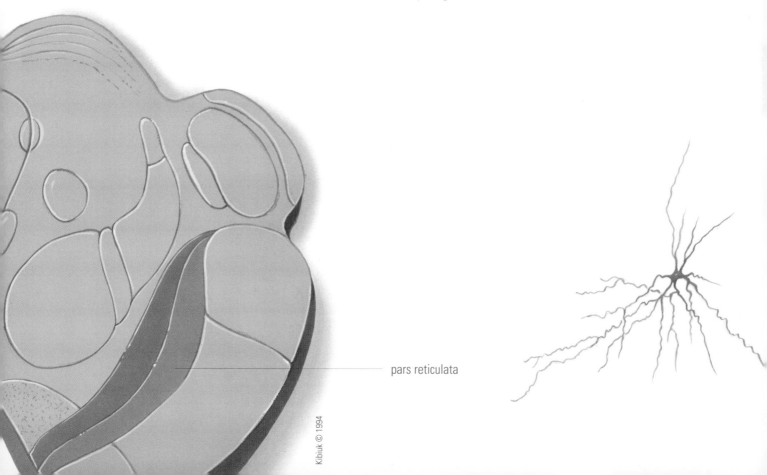

pars reticulata

Kibiuk © 1994

funds. Since most medical research depends heavily on federal grants, the ban choked off most American studies on the uses of fetal brain tissue. The studies at Yale and the University of Colorado avoided the ban because private funding was available to them. They did the work entirely without federal money. In the transplants, they generally used material from only one fetal brain per patient. In Sweden, where the government does not try to hamper such research, the surgeons used tissue from several brains in each operation to get the maximum beneficial effects.

Reflecting the explosive atmosphere of the debate, the *New England Journal*'s reports on the brain tissue transplants were accompanied by a separate editorial and a special commentary specifically on the use of fetal tissue itself. The editorial, by Dr. Jerome P. Kassirer, the journal's editor in chief, and Dr. Marcia Angell, executive editor, called the research promising and urged the new Clinton Administration to lift the ban. In their comments, the editors of the *New England Journal* said the objection to research on fetal tissue transplantation has arisen precisely because it shows promise of being useful immediately in the treatment of patients.

In fact, an executive order lifting the ban was among President Clinton's first acts on assuming office in January, 1993. He signed five memoranda related to abortion on the twentieth anniversary of the Supreme Court Roe vs Wade decision that established a constitutional right to choose abortion. In addition to lifting the fetal research ban he ended the so-called gag rule on abortion counseling at clinics that receive federal financial support; eased the restrictions on abortion at military hospitals, reversed a Reagan Administration ban on aid to international family planning programs that involve abortion or counseling on the subject. He also called for a review of the policy against importation of RU-486, the French drug that can induce very early abortions.

Opponents of abortion have argued that the potential good from use of fetal tissues might induce some women to have abortions even though they had been ambivalent about the procedure at the start. The ban on federal support for medical research that involved fetal cells transplants was justified by the Administrations of Presidents Reagan and Bush on the grounds that the research would be an impetus for more abortions. Commenting on this idea, the medical editors said the use of fetal tissue to treat anonymous patients with Parkinson's disease "is very unlikely to be the principal factor in a woman's decision to have an abortion," but if it is one consideration to some women, the editors asked, why is that a cause for governmental action?

"We find it problematic to focus on the question of a woman's motives for having an abortion," they wrote. "It implies that evaluating the motives of citizens is a legitimate activity of government."

Those who argue that abortion at any stage of fetal development is murder want abortion outlawed and the use of aborted tissues halted. They say it makes no moral sense to argue that use of aborted tissues is justifiable because this may help relieve pain and suffering. One does not commit murder just because it may help someone else.

But this kind of argument is hotly disputed by those on the other side of the debate. Many Americans, probably a majority, do not believe it is murder to abort an eight-week-old embryo. Even the 1992 Supreme Court, with its relatively conservative majority, never agreed to a total ban on abortions. Moreover, surgeons do not throw away a transplantable human heart just because they disapprove of the drunk driving that caused the accident that made the donor available.

Another commentary in the same issue of the medical journal found totally impractical the Bush Administration's alternative proposal that tissue banks be set up to collect material from spontaneous abortions and ectopic pregnancies. The announced intention was to provide a source of nerve tissue that did not require deliberate abortions. The specialists from the University of Minnesota who commented on this proposal said the two alternative sources would yield hardly any usable tissues. In both situations the fetus is usually either damaged or defective and can seldom be retrieved promptly enough to yield nerve tissue suitable for use. In an ectopic pregnancy, the embryo is implanted outside the uterus, usually in the oviduct where it cannot develop properly. Nerve tissue that is alive and capable of continuing to grow can only rarely be recovered from these cases, the authors said. Furthermore, in many spontaneous abortions the cause of the pregnancy failure itself would rule out use of the fetal tissues for transplantation. Major causes of spontaneous abortion include chromosomal errors and other serious defects in the fetus. Infections in the fetus and serious disease in the mother are also important causes. No one would transplant into a patient's brain any tissue that might carry any such lethal hazards.

After the Clinton Administration came to the White House, the main federal bars to neural grafting fell, but the battle over abortion was by no means over. On the day the President signed the executive order ending the ban on fetal tissue transplants, an estimated seventy-five thousand people marched in Washington to protest abortion. Since then there have been murders and attempted murders of doctors who perform abortions. Such acts have added another, and frightening, dimension to the concept of the hostage brain. On the other hand, perhaps it was one of the original dimensions. Since the dawn of history, some human brains have taken countless others hostage by playing on ignorance, fear, greed, and all kinds of fanaticism. Such hostage-taking is the dark side of the human imagination.

Parkinson's disease, although itself a large public health problem, is by no means the only gleam on the horizon that impels scientists to test the possibilities of neural grafting. There are also other tragedies such as Huntington's disease, a rare but devastating affliction, and Alzheimer's disease. The victims of that disorder are numbered in the millions.

Huntington's disease is best known to many people because one of its victims was Woody Guthrie, the folk singer who inspired a whole generation with his ballads. Like many other afflictions that attack brain and personality, the root cause of Huntington's disease is the failure of a single gene. In families where one parent carries that particular bad speck of heredity, every child has a 50–50 chance of falling to the disease too. Unlike many disorders that require two copies of a bad gene to cause damage, the Huntington gene holds any man or woman hostage to disaster whenever one copy appears.

The physical and chemical nature of the disorder is known. Several populations of neurons die, most of them in the striatum. Unlike parkinsonism, where a single neurotransmitter is lacking, the brains of Huntington's patients are starved of many of the important ones. But, in theory, neural grafting might help by replenishing neurons of the striatum. Some animal experiments have raised early hopes that transplantation of neurons might benefit at least some Huntington's patients. On the other hand, an early trial in a patient several years ago produced no improvement. To find out whether the hopes of neural grafting in Huntington's disease are justified, research must continue and be broadened.

Alzheimer's disease, the great brain plague of the late twentieth century, has victims far more numerous than Huntington's disease and probably more numerous than those of parkinsonism. As the American population ages, the expected toll from Alzheimer's disease is rising to the level of several million. This deadly enemy of the mind is also being considered as a possible target for neural grafting. The brain cell loss in Alzheimer's disease seems to be more diffuse than in either parkinsonism or Huntington's disease and there are no animal models that mimic the human disease with any fidelity. But some specialists hope that future transplants of fetal tissue might help the brain restore some of its own cell losses or perhaps replenish supplies of vitally needed neurotransmitters. Dr. Redmond of Yale is among the scientists who believe neural grafting has a future that is far larger than Parkinson's disease, provided the research is encouraged.

Some specialists see this kind of tissue transplantation as a future hope in several other conditions that compromise the brain. Among the possibilities are several kinds of motor neuron disease including amyotrophic lateral sclerosis, which ended the career and life of Lou Gehrig of the New York Yankees. Various kinds of injuries to the spinal cord are also being considered as potential targets.

With the possible exception of parkinsonism, all of these are early hopes with distant goals. As in many other health problems that center on the brain, ever-increasing knowledge of that incredible organ is opening new avenues of hope and experiment. The good news, and there is a lot of it, is that feats have been accomplished that would have seemed impossible just a few years ago. Indeed, specialists in gene therapy too are looking at Parkinson's disease as a possible future candidate for treatment. Their roster of conjectured possibilities also includes the most serious forms of arthritis and diabetes and even Alzheimer's disease.

It would be rank foolishness, however, to trumpet the good news, present and future, without mentioning the dark side too. Disorders of the human brain have always been the ultimate bad news because they can destroy the mind and the personality—the very things that make us human. They have always done so and they still do. But today there is even an element of hope in this grim picture because more has been learned about the brain in the past half century than in all of history before our era. Today, as more and more of the brain's biology is coming into focus, doctors and medical scientists see hope of someday confronting even the worst kinds of bad news that brain disease can produce.

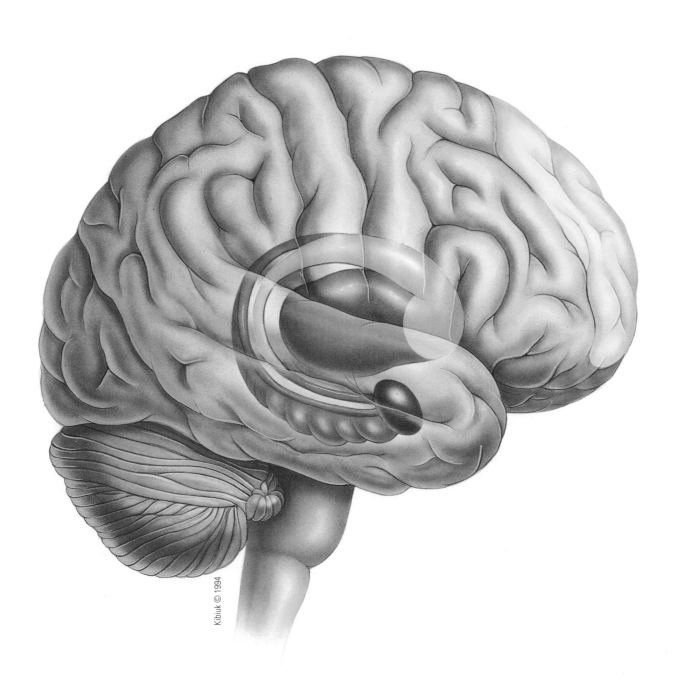

THE BAD NEWS 12

T here is something mercifully dry and academic in the names doctors
assign to human ailments whenever new ones are discovered;
Creutzfeldt-Jakob disease, for example; Huntington's chorea, Lesch-
Nyhan syndrome. Those names honor the discoverers and they sound
scientific, impersonal, and mercifully exotic. The reality behind the
antiseptic labels is heartbreak.

The Lesch-Nyhan disorder was discovered in the 1960s by Dr. William L.
Nyhan, a scientist of University of California, San Diego, and a young
colleague, Michael Lesch, a medical student who worked with him in the
research.

The disorder is one of the many that are caused by errors in single genes.
In medical terms it is an inborn error of metabolism. The enzyme, called
hypoxanthine guanosine phosphoribosyl transferase (HGPRT), is seriously
deficient. To many laymen that fact itself may seem to border on the ludi-
crous. How can anything with so many syllables be important in an age of
shrinking attention spans? Indeed, the effects of this deficiency are complex.
They are also simply disastrous.

To translate the disease into in human terms, see a frail young boy, sitting
in a wheelchair in a sort of disorganized jumble. He looks almost as though
someone had flung him there. His eyes appear huge in a thin face. He talks
about being a firefighter when he gets older, but his visitor knows this will
never happen and so does his mother, standing behind the wheelchair.

Huntington's disease attacks
a different part of the brain
from Parkinson's disease.
The shaded regions show
the caudate-putamen and the
frontal regions of the cerebral
cortex - two brain areas
where degeneration and loss
of neurons takes place in
the victims of this disease.

Whether the boy knows, is hard to say. For the moment he is calm, civil, talks rather well. The hospital nurses all give him a cheery "hello" and call him by name.

But there is also a violent side to the boy's life, because his personality is warped by Lesch-Nyhan disease. His arms are encased in padded splints that hinder his movements. There is nothing at all wrong with his arms. The splints are there to protect him from himself. One of the tragic quirks of his disease is a compulsion to self-mutilation. Lesch-Nyhan victims have outbursts in which they bite their lips and fingertips savagely and even try to stick pencils into their own eyes. The episodes are as terrifying to the patients as to their families. Just why they occur is a mystery.

The gene for the enzyme at fault in this disease was one of the first to be cloned and transplanted into mammalian cells by pioneers in recombinant DNA research. There was early hope of treating Lesch-Nyhan disease by gene therapy. The hope soon faded. Damage to the patient's nervous system seems to occur so early in life that gene therapists would have little time to make the diagnosis and attempt gene transfers. Probably more important, the crucial abnormality is in the brain and it is not clear whether corrective genes would do any good unless many copies could be delivered to cells of the brain itself. Here, the brain might be its own worst enemy. The so-called blood-brain barrier protects against foreign substances, but that barrier also makes it difficult to pass many important medicines and biologicals to the central nerve tissues where the trouble is. The first triumphs of gene therapy have gone to more accessible diseases that threaten life without first damaging the brain.

For Lesch-Nyhan patients there still is not much to be done beyond the old fashioned imperatives of care and compassion. The patients all suffer from gouty arthritis because of excessively high levels of uric acid in their blood. This can be treated, but the treatment has no useful effect on the patient's behavior or other problems of the central nervous system. Dr. Nyhan is a compassionate and determined man. He still hopes the disease will be conquered, but admits cures and treatments are not yet on the horizon. Still, study of the brain and the hormones and enzymes it orchestrates give scientists like him the challenge to transform hope into reality. For the time being, nevertheless, the diagnosis of Lesch-Nyhan disease is unmitigated bad news.

Mercifully, the disorder is rare, as are most of the other single gene disorders. Much more often than not, genetic counselors can bring families good news because even at the worst, the odds are no more than 50-50 that a second child will have the same problem that first brought the family face to face with genetic disease. In most cases, the risk is much less than 50-50.

Nevertheless, there are several thousand different genetic errors that produce incurable diseases. Some affect the brain and central nervous system; others do not. In total, they add up to a massive public health problem. In this universe of fatal errors, none, perhaps, is more loaded with tragedy than the disorder called Huntington's disease. It was originally named Huntington's chorea because of its symptoms. Chorea, coming from a Latin word meaning dance, is a general term for disorders of the nervous system in which patients have irregular, jerking movements because of involuntary muscular contractions. Huntington's disease was named after a physician, Dr. George Huntington, who practiced on Long Island and described the disorder in definitive detail in 1872.

All Huntington's disease patients develop the bizarre jiglike movements, but these are a relatively trivial feature of the disease. The real tragedy is in what the disorder does to the mind and how the destruction unfolds.

In geneticists' terms it is an autosomal dominant disorder, meaning that it involves an error somewhere in one of the nonsex chromosomes and that the existence of the error in just one of the two chromosomes in this pair is enough to bring on the disease. The Huntington's error is in a gene on chromosome 4, one of the larger chromosomes in the human genetic archive. The disease is a genetic time bomb. Most people who develop it have normal childhoods with no behavioral hint that anything is wrong. Then, commonly when the person reaches the thirties or forties, difficulties with memory and physical coordination appear. At first they are just hints, but as time goes on the conditions get worse. Over several decades, the formerly robust and mentally acute person declines into a state of invalidism with brain and body losing the ability to cope with life. The disease has robbed the world of talented and highly effective people who showed no signs of mental abnormality until the Huntington's symptoms began to appear. The most famous case was that of the folk singer Woody Guthrie. Furthermore, the usually late beginning of the disease means that most of its victims are well into or past their childbearing years before the disease becomes apparent.

From the family's point of view one of the worst aspects of the tragedy is its not quite perfect predictability. Every child of a Huntington's patient can see the handwriting on the wall in the decline of father or mother. The son or daughter knows, sometimes from childhood onward, that he or she has a simple yes-or-no chance, like one toss of a coin, of ending the same way and there is no way of escaping that fate. The child of a Huntington's disease patient could avoid having children so the disease would not be perpetuated further, but that is an agonizing decision to make when the odds are 50-50 that any child would be safe anyway.

About ten years ago, scientists at Harvard Medical School and its teaching hospitals discovered which chromosome contained the deadly mistake. Within a few years, tests were developed so that any child of a Huntington's disease patient could learn which way the future would fall: safe from the disease because the gene defect was not present, or destined to go the same way the parent went. The test itself creates another dilemma: take it and you may be freed forever from the dread—or you may know years in advance the grim way in which your life will end. Some people at risk have taken the test. Others have declined.

For years, the research seemed to be frozen just short of the gene's discovery. The faulty gene's location was pinned down, not only to chromosome 4, but even to a small region at one tip of that chromosome. Yet other disease-causing genes were located, identified, and had their genetic messages translated down to the last nucleotide, while the Huntington's disease gene remained maddeningly elusive.

That was the situation up to the spring of 1993. Then scientists of The Huntington's Disease Collaborative Research Group, six laboratories from the United States and Britain, reported that they had at last identified the gene itself and the type of genetic mistake it represented. The fault was an error in the genetic script a little like stuttering—one gene sequence was repeated several times; almost like saying "disease-ease-ease," to put it crudely. In fact, the mistake was excessive repetition of the three nucleotide bases C, A, G. The normal equivalent of the Huntington's gene would have between eleven and about thirty-four of these so-called C, A, G "triplets." In Huntington's disease the same gene may have as many as 100. In the genetic alphabet, the triplet C, A, G is the code word for constructing the amino acid glycine, but what the spelling errors do to the gene and how that erroneous message translates into brain damage is still unknown. Evidence from autopsies of Huntington's patients shows that their brains have lost large numbers of neurons in a structure called the basal ganglia, but how the mutation in the gene sets the destructive process in motion remains an enigma.

Specialists in the study of Huntington's disease were delighted by the announcement in March 1993. Discovery of the gene must be ranked as the most important advance in the modern history of the disease. How soon it will make a difference to patients is anyone's guess, but few expect a quick payoff. One or two other gene discoveries have been followed swiftly by further advances in diagnosis or treatment. In others, Lesch-Nyhan disease among them, progress has been painfully slow even with the faulty gene in hand.

The single gene defects that harm the brain are important to science because of the clues they provide to details of disease and to brain function and organization. They are also important to public health for many reasons. But viewed in the context of a nation's overall health, their impact is probably modest. Huntington's disease is thought to affect about thirty thousand Americans. In addition, all of their children are potential victims, but those numbers are relatively small in the whole universe of public health and most of the other three thousand to four thousand single gene diseases are even less common. Unfortunately, the bad news is not limited to the tragedies of rare genetic disorders that affect the brain.

Other kinds of brain-crippling disease are all too common. The two most important, in public health terms, are schizophrenia and mania. Each is thought to affect about 1% of the U.S. population; more than two million people apiece. These are major disorders of the mind that ruin lives and sometimes end them. Major manic depressive illness is an important cause of suicide. Altogether, depression is thought to be responsible for more than half of all the suicides committed in the United States in a year's time. Mania and depression often go together, following each other in quick succession. But the borders of this realm of mental disorder are fuzzy. Most normal people have moments of high enthusiasm when everything seems possible right now and the world just sits there waiting to be conquered. Most people have periods of gloom when life seems to be battering them and nothing works. It is only when the enthusiasm becomes so wild as to put it far beyond sense or reason that it becomes mania. Depression becomes an illness when it seems to be so hopeless as to defeat every action; when the simplest decisions are impossible and nothing can be done about anything. In many patients the moods alternate and the alternations become increasingly rapid over time.

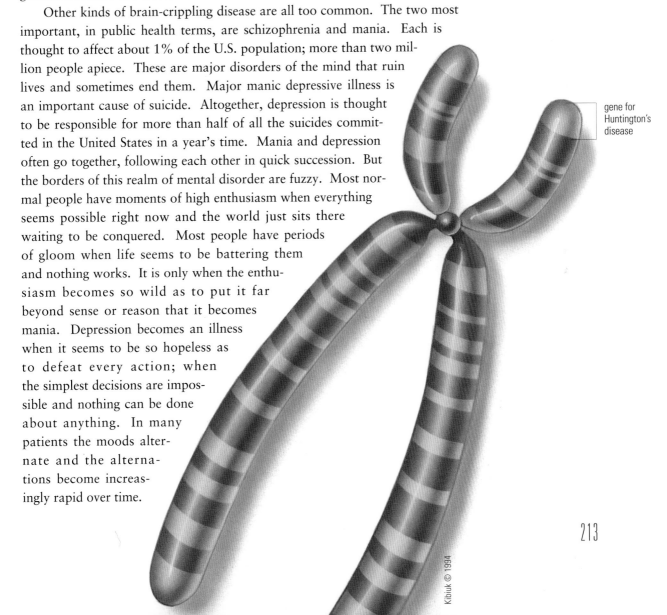

The gene for Huntington's disease has been localized to the end of the short arm of chromosome number 4, as shown in the diagram. The photo inset shows a pair of such chromosomes from a normal human subject.

Courtesy of Dr. Becky Alhadeff and Dr. James German of the New York Blood Center.

gene for Huntington's disease

Kibiuk © 1994

213

Manic and depressive traits have been seen, or imagined, in many famous and highly creative people. Some have weathered the furies at both ends of the spectrum. Others have crashed. Today an arsenal of medications has become available to treat mania or depression, or both. They have almost certainly saved many lives and kept many personalities intact, but some observers of this chemical defense of rationality have begun to wonder how much natural genius the drugs might be squandering to keep some people sane. Others dismiss this idea as foolish nihilism. But the debate is worthwhile even if it never leads to clear answers. The role of devil's advocate is vital to science and to free society as a whole.

The illness that involves mania and depression is often called bipolar to distinguish it from cases in which serious depression is not interrupted by any rebounds into mania. Either disorder can begin gradually or it can erupt with hurricane force at any age, and there seems to be something about the middle and late twentieth century that fosters it. In recent years, public health statisticians have noticed a worrisome upward trend in this category of mental illness. Since the 1940s it appears to have been steadily on the increase in the United States and some of the other highly developed countries of the West. The trend seems to be continuing. It is most marked among people who also have a close relative afflicted with mania or depression or the combination. The cumulative rates increase with age. There is nothing surprising in that, but the increase is substantially steeper for people born after 1940 than for those born earlier. No one knows what has happened, or has been happening, since 1940 to cause that trend.

The other great category of psychotic illness, schizophrenia, is also full of mysteries and unknowns. Typically, schizophrenia begins in late teenage or early adulthood with bizarre feelings that people are watching or talking about you or that something external is controlling your mind. You may blame radio signals from the CIA or outer space and you know absolutely that these malign forces are real. Audible voices talk to each other about you. Thoughts are plucked from your mind. Foreign thoughts and emotions are deliberately inserted. That is the way it seems.

As the disease progresses, hallucinations come, the patient seems to withdraw from reality and normal emotions. Behavior becomes odd and inadequate to whatever occasion is at hand. Most schizophrenics become incapable of managing their own lives and many become permanent patients in mental hospitals. Others make up a portion of the "street people" who live in cardboard boxes, sleep on warmth-giving sidewalk gratings and become constant public reminders that we are neither dealing effectively with mental illness nor caring adequately for its victims.

The label, schizophrenia, has been in use for nearly one hundred years and there has been a seesaw of styles in explaining what it really is and how to cope with it. Early in this century it was blamed on heredity. Studies of the close relatives of schizophrenics and pairs of twins in which one had the disease have confirmed that heredity is a factor. But heredity is by no means the whole story. Environmental influences, in the broadest meaning of that term, must also contribute. Many attempts have been made to find some simple chemical, infectious, or other physical cause. Nothing reliable has been found. Equally unsuccessful have been the attempts to settle the main blame on the trauma of bad childhood upbringing or later personal disasters. These may contribute to the patient's problems, but they are not the cause. Freud tried psychotherapy in treating schizophrenia, but concluded that he was having no significant impact on the disease. Many later psychiatrists have come to the same conclusion. Psychiatric and psychological counseling help some patients cope with their problems through varieties of mental stimulation and occupational therapy. But before the development of modern antipsychotic drugs, the best of treatment had only modest good effects. Sometimes therapy probably did harm.

Today, the causes of schizophrenia are still unproven, but there is ample evidence that there are physical and chemical abnormalities in the schizophrenic brain. Some of the differences from the normal brain are puzzling; others are illuminating. Until recently, these important details could only be studied in dead brains at autopsy. Now, some important features of brain structure and function can be seen while a person is alive, conscious, and thinking. This new way of looking at the mind in action is testimony to the incredible advances of modern technology. For brain study it foreshadows a revolution in understanding because it permits medical scientists to eavesdrop directly on the thinking brain.

Two techniques are particularly important: MRI, which allows pictures of the physical structure of the living brain, and the PET scan, which gives pictures of the brain in the act of thinking and reacting. Both techniques have already given profound new insights into the abnormalities of schizophrenia.

The MRI technique has revealed physical differences between the normal brain and that of the schizophrenic. The most notable difference is in the size of the ventricles, the hollow, fluid-filled spaces within the brain. Using the magnetic resonance imaging technique, Dr. Daniel R. Weinberger and colleagues of the National Institute of Mental Health and St. Elizabeth's Hospital in Washington, DC, as well as others have found that the ventricles are larger in schizophrenics than in normal people. The most dramatic examples are some of Dr. Weinberger's MRI images of the brains of twins. If any two people have a chance of being equipped with closely similar brains, it should be a pair of twins. But the MRI pictures showed that this doesn't apply if one twin has schizophrenia and the other does not. In the twin who is free from the disease, the ventricles are unmistakably smaller than they are in the schizophrenic twin. Whether the overlarge ventricles are a cause of the disease or some kind of effect is still unclear. Perhaps the enlargement reflects a loss of tissue within the brain. The question is being pursued in current research.

While MRI studies have revealed physical differences, the PET scan and other techniques have given new ways of studying the human brain while it is at work; analyzing, making decisions, or calling the body into action. Among the most powerful of these is the PET scan. Without going into the details of how the process works, the end result is that it measures oxygen consumption in tissues. Because oxygen is the universal fuel for metabolic processes, the level of oxygen consumption shows which brain tissues are active and how active they are. PET scans of the human brain in action have been remarkably illuminating. They have shown which areas of the brain are particularly active in various kinds of mental and physical tasks and how the normal brain differs in these patterns from brains afflicted with schizophrenia.

As just one example of the PET scan's sophistication in eavesdropping on the conscious brain, it has shown that distinctly different regions of the brain are active when a person is hearing words, seeing words, or speaking words. Pioneering work of this kind was done by Dr. Marcus Raichle, of the Washington University Medical School in St. Louis. One series of his PET scans showed the normal brain's response to seeing a line of printed meaningless symbols, a line of printed letters that did not spell any word and printed letters that did spell a real word in English. We are all so accustomed to seeing and interpreting such printed symbols that it might seem reasonable that the same brain region should handle all of these seemingly similar tasks. In fact, that is not true at all. Substantially different parts of the brain light up when a person views each of those different lines of symbols.

Those variations might seem to be just a curiosity, but they reveal some of the dynamic details of brain function and some PET scan studies show significant differences in the working of normal and schizophrenic brains.

For example, PET scans taken when a normal adult is doing a contrived psychological task called the Wisconsin Card Sort Test show the prefrontal cortex of the brain lighting up as that region burns oxygen. The test measures the individual's performance in making analyses and choices that lead to

216

immediate action—the physical sorting of cards into various categories. The prefrontal cortex is important in doing that kind of mental gymnastics.

Dr. Weinberger's group used the PET scan technique to find what may have been the first known concrete difference in function between the normal and the schizophrenic brain. While the prefrontal cortex of a normal brain becomes active in the card sorting task, the schizophrenic brain appeared to be overwhelmed. The PET scan shows the patient's prefrontal cortex reducing its activity as though it was overloaded. These PET scan studies showed, not just a defect in the schizophrenic's brain, but a defect in its mental performance. Brain specialists consider that remarkable and significant. The prefrontal cortex is crucial to perception, memory, and judgement. Its circuits function in short-term "working" memory and in dealing with symbolic information. All of these qualities are badly distorted in schizophrenia.

In addition, the prefrontal cortex is the last region of the brain to develop fully. It doesn't achieve maturity until adolescence and early adulthood. Perhaps because of that, children and early adolescents find the Wisconsin card sorting test difficult while normal adults do not. It may be significant that schizophrenia rarely develops before the age of fifteen. Could the disease take the patient's brain hostage during the crucial transition from childhood to adult status? Perhaps, but that possibility still leaves unanswered the crucial question of why it happens in some people, but spares most of us.

Researchers who try to tease out truth from the multiple puzzles of schizophrenia are obsessed with questions such as that. If there are differences in function, there must be differences in chemistry and these have indeed been found. Most of the new insights have been dividends from the use of modern antipsychotic drugs. The era of modern drug treatment for mental illness began in the 1950s with the surprising discovery that chlorpromazine, a compound discarded as an antihistamine because it caused too much sleepiness, had strong beneficial effects on symptoms of both schizophrenia and mania. Doctors who prescribed it soon found that its influence on schizophrenia and mania were not just sedation; it also had direct effects on some of the disabling symptoms of the disorders. The drug proved immensely valuable in reducing the force of patients' episodes of wild agitation. It also helped with schizophrenics' delusions and hallucinations. It seemed to help these patients communicate better and it reduced the catatonic physical rigidity and stupor that afflicted some. After decades of research, scientists today believe chlorpromazine, and others like it, work by blocking the action of the neurotransmitter dopamine at receptor sites in certain populations of neurons. The schizophrenic brain appears to suffer either from too much dopamine activity in

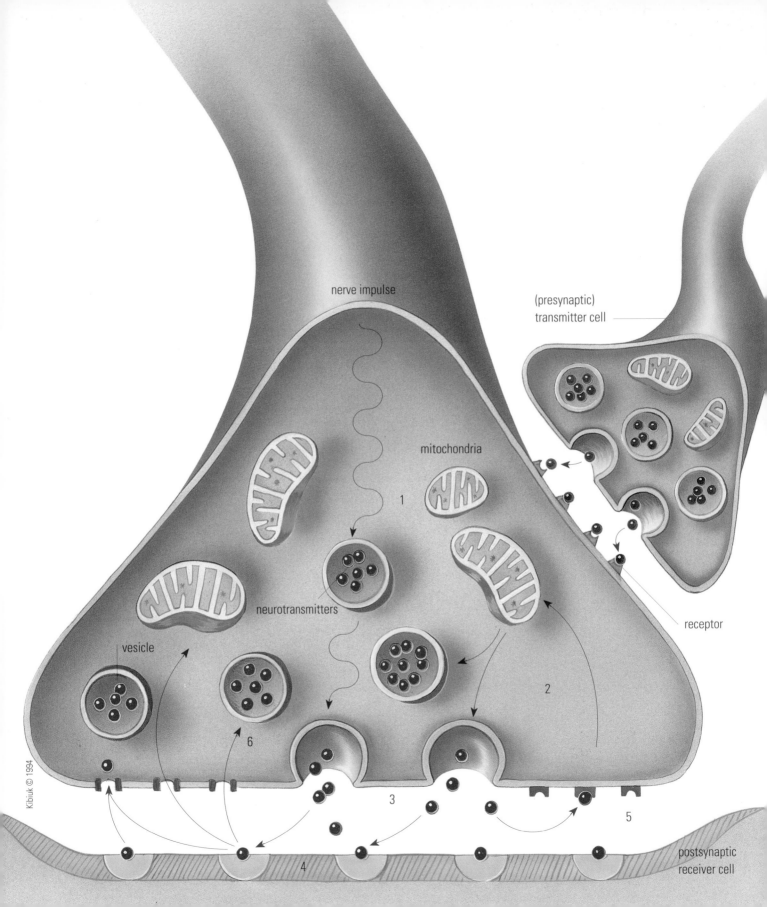

nerve impulse

(presynaptic)
transmitter cell

mitochondria

1

neurotransmitters

receptor

vesicle

2

6

3

5

4

postsynaptic
receiver cell

Kibiuk © 1994

crucial brain regions, or from an imbalance between dopamine-using neurons that originate in the midbrain and others of the cerebral cortex that use glutamate as a neurotransmitter.

Discoveries that some compounds could relieve disordered and despondent minds often came by chance. What followed was not only a new era in the development of drugs to aid the mentally incapacitated, but some spectacular advances in understanding the chemistry, the organization, and the functioning of the brain as well.

Imipramine, first viewed as an alternative to chlorpromazine, soon showed greater promise in treating major depression. The two drugs affected the actions of certain neurotransmitters in the brain. Powerful effects on patients' mental states and detailed knowledge of the drugs' chemical action helped launch a fruitful search for additional medicines to treat mental disorders. One of the most famous drugs to emerge from the search is fluoxetine hydrochloride. It is sold by Eli Lilly and Company under a trade name that has virtually become a part of our common language: Prozac. Its effectiveness against depression, together with a reportedly low risk of unpleasant side effects, has prompted doctors to prescribe Prozac for many emotional problems. The list includes patients who suffer from excessive fear of rejection, those who are deficient in self esteem, or seem excessively sensitive to criticism. In some, the complaint is a low capacity to experience pleasure.

In a commentary on the drug, Dr. Samuel H. Barondes of University of California, San Francisco, said it is being used today for some symptoms that American psychiatrists used to consider the exclusive province of psychotherapy and that the new psychopharmacologic drugs altogether have "stimulated a rethinking of fundamental assumptions in psychiatry."

But he also noted that today's advances in drug design are based more on chance discovery and fragmentary information than on any deep knowledge of how human behavior arises from the elements of brain function. Prozac, for example, is known to act at the synapses, the complex nerve cell connections where one neuron fires its signal to an adjoining cell. The drug blocks a process called reuptake for one specific neurotransmitter, serotonin. When a neuron fires its signal across a synapse a neurotransmitter is released into the cleft between the two cells and affects the receiving cell. Reuptake is a process by which some of that nerve signaling chemical is taken up again quickly by the cell that fired it. This takes it out of action and diminishes the signal to the receiving cell. By blocking reuptake of serotonin, Prozac presumably augments the action of that nerve signal chemical in the neurons that use it. But serotonin is only one of many neurotransmitters that function in the brain,

In the synaptic terminal, neurotransmitters are made (1) and stored in small packets or vesicles (2) using energy generated by the mitochondria, the power house of the cell. Synapses release the packets of neurotransmitters (3), and these transmitters bind to receptors (4) and cause a response in the receiving cell that may increase or decrease the excitability of that cell. Neurotransmitters also bind to receptors on the synaptic terminal itself (5) and stimulate or inhibit further neurotransmitter release. Then, the released neurotransmitters are inactivated (6) either by enzymes which break them down or by being taken up by the synaptic terminal or by a glial cell, so that they are no longer available to act on the receptors. Some synaptic terminals have other terminals on them, which produce and release neurotransmitters that act upon and regulate the activity of the other synaptic terminal (7). Neuropharmacologists, who design drugs for treating nervous and mental disorders, take advantage of all of these features of the synapse in their efforts. For example, reserpine is a drug that disrupts storage of certain neurotransmitters (step 1), whereas fluoxetine (Prozac) is a drug that blocks the reuptake (step 6) of the neurotransmitter, serotonin.

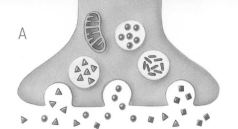

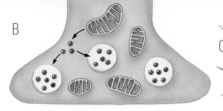

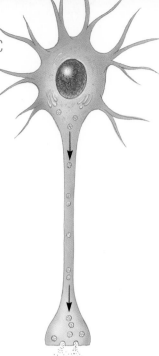

and serotonin itself has many different receptors on which Prozac may act. How could this one specific drug action have such manifold and complex effects on behavior? Why do the therapeutic effects of the drug seem to take weeks to develop? Brain scientists would certainly like to know. Meanwhile, there is much evidence that the drug is useful and knowledge of what it actually does in the brain may help chemists design even better drugs. That is the traditional process, but only with great difficulty can it be made to show how the brain actually orchestrates behavior.

Reserpine, a drug borrowed by modern science from the medicine of ancient India, was one of the first modern treatments for high blood pressure. Some people who used it also got seriously depressed. Some committed suicide. Why? It turned out that reserpine does something to deplete the brain's available stores of certain neurotransmitters such as dopamine, serotonin, and norepinephrine—the class of chemicals called monoamines. Many of the early drugs effective against depression acted in various ways to keep synapses well supplied with their particular neurotransmitters of that class.

In contrast, antianxiety drugs, of which Valium may be the most widely known, bolster the action of another nerve-signaling substance GABA (gamma-amino-butyric acid). Major depressive illness seems to reflect reduced availability at the nerve cell synapses of dopamine and norepinephrine, while mania comes with excess of substances of this same class.

Much recent study has centered on the synapses, the actual connections between the brain's nerve cells. At these connecting sites, the flow and availability of the various neurotransmitters is governed in multiple and complex ways. Typically, the junction will be between the axon of one nerve cell and a dendrite of the other. The signal from one neuron to another starts with an electrical pulse called an action potential, but most of the actual signaling in mammalian brains is done by chemistry. The word synapse comes from the Greek "to clasp." The functioning part of the junction is not as hard a connec-

Synapses come in many types, each of which has certain special features. Many synapses store and release more than one neurotransmitter (A). Some synapses contain neurotransmitters that are made locally by enzymes located in the synaptic nerve terminal itself (B), while other synapses contain neurotransmitters that are made in the cell body because they are actually small proteins; these neuropeptide neurotransmitters are transported in packets down the axon to be stored and released in the synaptic nerve terminal (C). When released from the synaptic terminal, neurotransmitters act on receptors on the receiving cell to transfer a

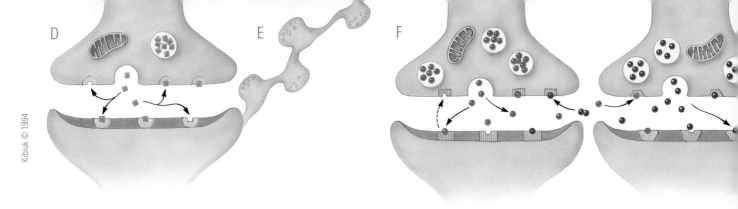

D E F

tion as two wires soldered together. Instead there is the upstream presynaptic side and, on the receiving end, a postsynaptic dendrite. In between is a gap known as the synaptic cleft. When a nerve cell fires, one or another of the neurotransmitters is released from storage vesicles and crosses the synaptic cleft to exert an effect on the other cell. The identity of the particular neurotransmitter depends on the type and location of the nerve cell. There are many ways in which the action can be altered: by breakdown of the key chemicals, by the response of receptors at or near the synapse, and by the process called reuptake, in which supplies of a nerve signaling chemical are restored to their original location. Analyzing this intricate traffic across the synaptic cleft has helped scientists understand the most basic details of brain function. Advances in drug design have also come about as chemists have designed various compounds to act selectively on each and almost every one of the contributors to nerve signal transmission across the synapse.

It should come as no surprise that what happens at these crucial meeting places of the mind is anything but simple. In addition, we can dispense with such adjectives as "tiny" and "minute." All the components come in that category. The cleft between the pre- and postsynaptic sides, for example, is about 20 to 30 nanometers wide. A nanometer is a billionth of a meter, or about 36 billionths of an inch. The vesicles where the signal chemicals are stored in the synapses are about 40 to 50 nanometers in diameter.

It is in the uncountable billions of transactions across synapses, between neurons of many different shapes, sizes, and patterns of connection, that the brain's main information signaling takes place. Even the resting brain is never totally at rest. The signaling goes on continuously in billions of cells and their many billions of connections. That incessant chatter is the individual's passport to a coherent world. It seems incredible that the system works as well as it does so much of the time. When something does go wrong, the effects can be tragically obvious. This is true of major problems such as schizophrenia

signal to that cell; however, in some types of synapses, the released neurotransmitters also act on receptors on the nerve terminal itself to regulate release of more neurotransmitters (D). Some synaptic terminals are not discrete endings but "varicosities" or bulges on a long and winding axon (E); in many cases, these varicosities do not end on a discrete site on a receiving neurons, but rather release there neurotransmitters into the region of another nerve cell, thus producing a rather broad effect on more than one nerve cell. Synaptic terminals often "talk" to each other by responding to the neurotransmitter or neurotransmitters that are released by another, nearby terminal (F); the receptors for these other neurotransmitters are usually on the synaptic terminal itself and control the release of the neurotransmitter produced by that nerve cell.

and manic depressive illness in which the causes are mysterious. It is also true of some other diseases in which the cause is all too well known. Notable among these is AIDS, an infectious disease caused by a known and much studied virus—HIV, the human immunodeficiency virus. From the start of the AIDS epidemic, doctors noticed that some patients also developed mental symptoms; loss of memory and all the other classic features of dementia. It was easy enough to explain these symptoms simply as reflecting the shock of the AIDS diagnosis. It was a death sentence and the worst kind of death sentence at that. It carried the threat of lost friends, lost job, feelings of guilt over the possibility that the infection has been passed on to others, and gradual, painful loss of health and independence with a final stage of agony and weakness ending in death.

Almost any mental symptom; fear, anxiety, despair, feelings of rage and unjust persecution must be rated normal, or at least understandable, as the reality of AIDS sinks in. But the effects of AIDS on the mind are by no means only psychological. The disease often degrades the brain as seriously as it damages the rest of the body.

AIDS' damage to the immune defenses is its best known effect. This loss of immunity often leads to what are called opportunistic infections. These are infections from sources that the normal immune defense system would squelch easily and as a matter of course. Some of the opportunistic infections invade the brain and can cause varieties of potentially fatal meningitis and encephalitis.

But in many AIDS cases, the patient loses memory and mental resilience, and sinks into dementia through damage to the brain and central nervous system long before the immunological disease brings death. Estimates have varied widely on the question of how often this happens. Some studies have found neurological signs and symptoms in 30% of patients, while others have more than doubled that figure. Still other research has found direct evidence of the AIDS virus in the brain tissue of patients. In addition, the brains of some AIDS patients have been found to be shrunken, their interior spaces, the ventricles, are enlarged, and parts of the cerebral cortex have a shriveled look. One study of AIDS patients' brains at autopsy showed that some feature of the infection seemed to break down the protective blood-brain barrier and that this probably hastens and aggravates HIV's attack on the brain. The same study also showed that AIDS patients often had abnormally leaky blood vessels in the white matter of their brains.

New information on the brain damage caused by the AIDS infection has also led to some new strategies to treat the disease and to evidence that conventional treatment is indeed doing some good. AZT (azidothymidine), the best known AIDS drug, seems to have a beneficial effect on the brain function of some patients. A dramatic series of PET scan images produced by scientists of the National Cancer Institute showed this clearly. A scan of the brain of a patient who had AIDS-related dementia showed that brain activity within the occipital region and parts of the temporal lobes is much less than normal. After thirteen weeks of treatment with AZT, the same patient showed a return to almost normal brain activity. Unfortunately, AZT has never yet been proved capable of curing AIDS. For the present, the disease is as much bad news as any other disease. It is far worse than most.

The fact that infection can cripple and kill the brain is not really a surprise. Infectious meningitis, encephalitis, and damage to the fetus that can be caused by maternal infection with the rubella virus are all old and familiar tragedies. A high and prolonged fever, or a lapse of more than a very few minutes in oxygen supply to the brain can cause grave brain damage too. The human brain is incredibly tough and resilient, but it is an organ, like any other, made of living tissue fed by an intricate web of blood vessels. It can be harmed. All this is familiar, but infection that causes dementia seems less commonplace to most people. Originally, dementia meant insanity or madness and it still has that aura. Dementia praecox was an old term for schizophrenia. In today's psychiatric parlance, dementia carries much broader implications. It means loss or impairment of mental powers from any cause. Infection is certainly among the causes of dementia. This too is an old story, but it has had some remarkable new twists. One important new chapter involves Creutzfeldt-Jakob disease, a disorder known for almost a century, that is keeping the concept of infectious dementia at the forefront of health research today.

The damage and loss of neurons in a dementing illness such as AIDS can be visualized by PET studies that show both reduced blood flow and glucose metabolism. Left hand panel shows a normal brain, while right hand panel shows devastation in a degenerating brain of an AIDS patient.

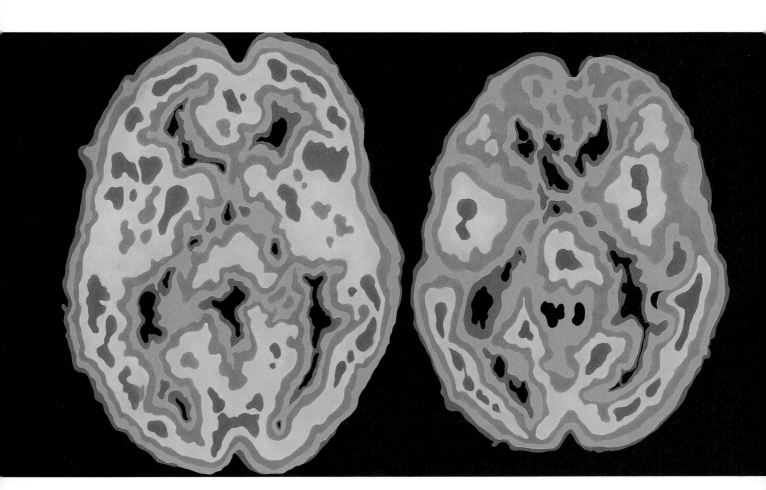

BREAKING AND ENTERING: INFECTIOUS DEMENTIA 13

On March 21, 1974, the *New England Journal of Medicine* published a strange letter to the editor. It was only four paragraphs long and it appeared on one of the back pages of the journal, not a place likely to attract much notice. But it did attract international notice among brain specialists because it was downright frightening. The letter reported a case in which a deadly degenerative disease of the human brain must have been transmitted from a man who had died to a woman who received a cornea from one of his eyes to restore her eyesight. It was the first known case in which that rare, catastrophic brain disorder called Creutzfeldt-Jakob disease, was ever transmitted from one human to another. It was a chain of events that most experts would have dismissed as either flatly impossible or, at the very least, comfortably remote. The letter erased that complacency. The writers were pathologists at Columbia University's College of Physicians and Surgeons in New York. They told this story:

A fifty-five-year-old man died of pneumonia about two months after he began to have memory problems and some difficulties with physical movements and coordination. Immediately after he died, his eyes were taken for use in corneal transplants. Soon after that, an autopsy showed that he had suffered from Creutzfeldt-Jakob disease. By that time, a fifty-five-year-old woman had received a corneal transplant using the man's tissues. The cornea is not a part of the brain even though the optic nerve of the eye is intimately connected to the brain. Transmission of the fatal disease seemed most unlikely, but the corneal transplant had already been done. There was no way to annul that fact. The doctors could only wait and hope.

Unfortunately their wait was brief. About eighteen months after the transplant, the woman began to develop neurologic symptoms. She died eight months later in an advanced state of dementia and brain degeneration. Her autopsy showed all the specific kinds of damage found in the man's brain, but her deterioration was even more severe than his. The letter to the medical journal noted that the brain disease is extremely rare. Coincidence could not explain the woman's fatal illness. The doctors concluded:

" ... the present cases may be the first evidence for the transmission of this disease from one human being to another. Aside from the importance of this report to the transmission of Creutzfeldt-Jakob disease, there are wide implications to be considered in all transplantation programs with relation to the transmission of slow-virus diseases."

That was twenty years ago and there has never been another report of human transmission of a slow-virus infection by corneal transplant, but there have been many cases in which the disease has been passed from human to human in other accidental ways. Such transmissions are still occurring today. They are called iatrogenic cases. The word comes from the Greek "iatros," meaning physician. Doctors use iatrogenic to admit that it's their fault. They keep the admission in Greek, one supposes, in the hope that most laymen won't know what they are talking about.

Creutzfeldt-Jakob disease is one of a handful of mysterious afflictions of the brain that were called slow-virus infections because they developed unusually slowly, but met the accepted criteria for virus infection—they were caused by agents so small that they could pass through filters fine enough to keep out bacteria and all other known sources of infection. When that classical definition first came into use no one had ever "seen" a virus or had any idea what it might really be. The name bespoke an unknown, but demonstrably real, infectious entity. Today viruses are all too well known. The varieties, reproductive cycles, and widely various infectious strategies of innumerable viruses have been documented. They have been studied under the electron microscope and analyzed chemically and genetically down to the last subunit of nucleic acid and protein.

But still, no conventional virus has ever been linked to any of the slow-virus disorders. In the mid-1970s, scientists were just coming to grips with the reality that certain puzzling human brain diseases could actually be passed from person to person by some mysterious, almost unimaginable, agent of infection. The same symptoms could be produced in animals by inoculations

226

with tissue extracts from the brains of humans who died of the diseases. The laboratory transmissions were extremely difficult to achieve. Commonly, the animals did not develop the brain degenerations until years after the inoculations and the transmissions had to be virtually direct from brain to brain. Blood transfusion would not do it. In addition, unlike all known viruses, the slow infections never produced any hint of immune reaction in the victims. There were no antibodies, no inflammation; nothing. Furthermore, no one could detect viruses in the samples of infectious brain tissue.

To make matters worse, virus-killing sterilization treatments such as formaldehyde, boiling heat or exposure to severe doses of ultraviolet light left brain extracts still infectious. Other treatments known to inactivate DNA and RNA did not halt these infections, and yet the infectious life of every virus known to science depends on either of those two nucleic acids. A virus in which the nucleic acid has been destroyed is dead.

Yet, these infections must be virus-caused even though there was not the slightest hint that any conventional viruses were present. It was an enigma and it posed serious dangers to human health. Anti-infection procedures had to be changed in autopsy work and surgery throughout the world. Extra precautions had to be used for handling elderly and demented patients.

The transmission of Creutzfeldt-Jakob disease from one person to another was a shock. But scientists were at least somewhat prepared for it by a story that had begun soon after World War II in the one of the most remote places on earth, the highlands of New Guinea. Among the villages of former cannibals called the Fore people, a devastating epidemic was in progress and whole families were being wiped out.

The Fore people (pronounced FOR-AY) live in two main groups, north and south, occupying highland territories of scarcely a hundred square miles. At its height, the epidemic was their leading cause of death. In the decade from 1957 to 1968 more than 1,100 deaths from the epidemic occurred among the South Fore people in a total population of only about 8,000 and it seemed, among the South Fore in particular, that the entire population was doomed. The people called their illness kuru. The word meant trembling and fear. The illness produced a lot of both. It had three distinct stages and the victims usually knew they were going to die as soon as the first symptoms appeared. The new victim became unsteady in walking or standing, had a tendency to tremble, sometimes developed crossed eyes, and often began to slur speech. The problems all worsened in the second stage. In the last stage, the kuru victims lost command of their muscles, including facial muscles. They staggered and trembled uncontrollably and sometimes broke into sudden, bizarre fits of laughter.

Press reports from Australia called it "the laughing death," but the victims were not really laughing. The sounds and grimaces were involuntary and they meant doom. By the time death actually came, the victim of kuru was likely to be totally helpless, mentally and physically.

The natives were sure kuru was the result of sorcery. Visiting doctors and scientists at first diagnosed the cases as a strange form of hysteria. Later they decided it was probably an hereditary disease that passed mainly from mother to daughter. The illness attacked both sexes, but it occurred with particular grim frequency among women. The fatal illness was so common that it appeared the Fore people were fast nearing extinction. But the appearances were misleading. Kuru was neither hysteria nor a disease of heredity. Furthermore, it was not continuing to gain momentum as Western observers first thought. In fact the disease was waning slowly, continuing to kill the elderly and the middle-aged, but beginning to spare the youngest.

The most surprising thing, perhaps, was that modern public health measures had nothing to do with this hopeful trend. The Fore people's salvation appeared to lie somehow in the fact that missionaries had persuaded them to give up cannibalism by the mid-1950s. The effect could be seen clearly in the age profile of the deaths. Gradually, the fatal illness stopped attacking children and teenagers to concentrate on older and older victims. Plotting the trends backward in time, it became clear that new infections stopped occurring about 1955. That was when cannibalism finally ended among the Fore people. For decades, kuru had been their main cause of death with fatalities as high as 1% of the population per year. But in 1977 only thirty-one people died of the disease. They were all adults and most of them were old. The infections have incubation periods that can be decades long, so it is uncertain just when kuru will end totally, if it has not already done so.

Cannibalism seems to have existed in many forms in New Guinea. Some people reportedly ate the bodies of their fallen enemies. In some it may have been ritual magic, a way to capture the strength and potency of the departed person. The Fore people were not cannibals who feasted on captured enemies. They ate their own newly deceased relatives. Many reports have described their style of cannibalism as a ritual matter in which the family ate portions of the dead person as a mark of respect and to gain that person's innate magic. Shirley Lindenbaum, an anthropologist who spent a long time living among the Fore to study them, said that idea is more a reflection of Western misconceptions than the ideas of the Fore people. She said they took up cannibalism because animal food was scarce and the people found human flesh tasty and nutritious. The dietary habit was also fairly recent. In her book, *Kuru Sorcery*, she quotes one Fore man as describing the reaction to the first human meal:

"What is the matter with us, are we mad? Here is good food and we have neglected to eat it."

Dr. Lindenbaum said the circumstances long ago pointed to the cannibalism itself as the key to the spread of kuru. In the social hierarchy of Fore life, the men kept valuable pig meat for themselves. Women and young children were the most likely consumers of human flesh. A key point in the transmission of kuru, obvious after the fact, is that custom assigned the brains of kuru victims to women. As Fore people described the rules, a man's brain could be eaten by his sister, or his son's wife; a woman's brain went to her son's wife or her brother's wife. Brain tissue that harbors slow virus is by far the most infectious tissue when transplanted.

The true nature of those infections was teased out of the mystery by scientists led by an American, Dr. D. Carleton Gajdusek of the National Institutes of Health, who won a Nobel Prize for his work. He spent several seasons with the Fore people and continued to visit them for many years. In painstaking research, he took samples of brain tissue from people who had died of the disease and injected samples into animals. He had the patience and skill to keep these experiments going long enough to prove the case. Most animal experiments in transmitting a virus disease are completed in a week or less. The transmission of kuru to chimpanzees took years before symptoms appeared. In one animal there was a lapse of more than four years before the animal developed the disease. When it did appear, the symptoms and physical effects were remarkably similar to human kuru. The experiments proved that kuru was actually a slow infection that could be transmitted by something in a victim's brain tissue.

The transmission is still not easy to achieve. To this day, there has been no proven instance of this transmission of kuru, or any other human slow-virus infection by transfusion of blood. Transfer of brain or pituitary tissue seems to be most effective. Among the Fore people who practiced cannibalism it wasn't difficult to see how this could occur, not only from eating the brains, but just from handling them. Repeated hand washing is

Creutzfeld-Jakob disease affects initially posterior regions of the cerebral cortex and the cerebellum.
Modified from Pathology, *by E. Rubin and J. Farber. Published by J. B. Lippincott Co*

BREAKING AND ENTERING: INFECTIOUS DEMENTIA

Kibiuk © 1994

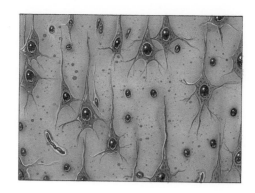

Normal brain tissue is contrasted with the "moth-eaten," spongiform appearance of tissue from brain infected by the slow-virus agent in Creutzfeld-Jakob disease.

seldom one of the virtues of a primitive society and people who had handled a dead kuru victim's brain were likely to rub their eyes and scratch cuts and abrasions on their own bodies. In addition, the women who removed the brains from the dead bodies used bamboo slivers as dissecting tools and often pricked these against their own arms to test sharpness. With these habits, transfer of the infections was all too likely.

In the light of the kuru experience, the transmission of Creutzfeldt-Jakob disease by transplantation of a human cornea was understandable, even though shocking.

Today, the kuru story has essentially ended. The only possibility of new cases would seem to be any Fore people still surviving who were infected as young children. In some known cases, the disease symptoms have taken as long as twenty-three years to appear. There could be longer periods of latency, but just how long is guesswork.

The kuru story shares some ironies with the case of the woman described in Chapter 7 whose systemic lupus was apparently cured by sorcery. Anyone educated in the United States would say immediately that the "cure," if it was real, must have resulted from the brain's effects on the immune system in a person who believed she would be cured. But the witch doctor in the Philippines probably never heard of immunology and might have considered that explanation a trivial quibble about body mechanics. To the sorcerer and his client, the real answer to the illness was sorcery.

The Fore people in New Guinea were always sure their disease was a result of sorcery and the remedy was to deal sternly with the magic-makers. The Christian missionaries who came to convert the Fore could pardonably argue that their faith and the strength of morality really conquered kuru. Certainly the epidemic faded after the end of cannibalism and, just as

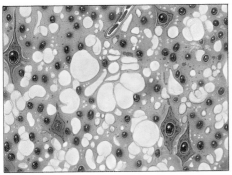

Kibiuk © 1994

certainly, modern science still has no tools to cure kuru or any other slow virus infection.

But in the "civilized" West, kuru is history. The other slow infections that resemble it still exist. They are all called spongiform encephalopathies for the effects they have in killing neurons and leaving the brain with a spongy, hole-riddled look. In terms of human health, Creutzfeldt-Jakob disease is the most important known disease of this kind. After the case of the woman who received the corneal transplant, surgeons and pathologists were alert for repetitions of that disaster, but no more corneal transmissions occurred. What did come to light after that episode were two cases of Creutzfeldt-Jakob disease evidently transmitted by use of metal electrodes that were inserted for diagnostic purposes into the brains of patients who had neurologic symptoms.

In retrospect, the facts are chillingly obvious: patients in whom the electrodes were used came to doctors because of epileptic disorders, but left the diagnostic laboratories infected with fatal Creutzfeldt-Jakob disease. The electrodes were always sterilized carefully between uses, but procedures that kill bacteria and ordinary viruses did not always destroy the agents of the slow infections. It took new and more rigorous sterilization routines to eliminate the risk.

The hazard is apparently not limited to patients. A neurosurgeon, a neuropathologist and two pathology laboratory technicians are known to have died of the rare brain disease. Again, coincidence seems most unlikely to be the explanation.

The Creutzfeldt-Jakob cases and the story of kuru were an energizing challenge to science, but a horror to public health. Fortunately, there seemed to be a respite in new kinds of transmission of the mysterious slow infections. The apparently free period lasted several years, but it was only a respite.

The issue came to light again early in 1985. A twenty-year-old man who had received human growth hormone as a child developed puzzling neurological symptoms, gradually became demented, and finally died. Then there was another case like his and still others. Some medical detective work showed that the common denominator in all the cases was the human growth hormone. All of the victims had received that hormone years earlier when they were children. They were all people who had deficiencies in pituitary gland function. As children, they had not grown at the normal rate. Without the hormone, they would have grown up seriously stunted in stature. The medical label is pituitary dwarfism.

There was only one treatment. The children had to have human growth hormone. Animal growth hormones would not suffice.

Supplies of the scarce human product were obtained by taking the pituitary glands from people who had died (usually accident victims) and harvesting the growth hormone from those glands. This work was done by a government-supported research unit called the National Pituitary Agency. The agency distributed the hormone to doctors for use in children at serious risk of pituitary dwarfism. The program existed for years. It accomplished a great deal of good without doing any harm, until the first cases of Creutzfeldt-Jakob disease appeared.

There is no way of testing a sample of tissue directly for presence of the slow-virus infection that causes Creutzfeldt-Jakob disease. And the disease is so rare that the odds must be something like a million to one against any person, chosen at random, having the infection. Nevertheless, one or two people whose pituitary glands came to the agency must have had it. Probably it was in the early stage of their brain disorders, before any symptoms could be noticed.

As soon as the first cases appeared in growth hormone recipients, the distribution program halted in the United States. It has never resumed. Altogether there have been twelve cases in the U.S. of Creutzfeldt-Jakob disease in people who received human growth hormone in childhood and early adolescence. Thousands of other patients received the hormone without harm and are enjoying the gift of normal stature as a result.

But what happened to the many children who needed growth hormone after the supply program shut down? That is a footnote to the story that illustrates the effects of politics and public perceptions on medical science. The early 1980s were perhaps the last smoldering of the era in which a few "activists" were able to tie medical research in knots by denouncing all recombinant DNA research as the work of the devil. It was the heyday of the "worst case scenario" in which any potential disaster the human brain could imagine could be used as an argument for halting all gene-splicing research and genetic engineering, regardless of how improbable that scenario might be. There never was such a research halt, but at times it seemed imminent.

Only about eight years before the handful of pituitary disasters occurred, a mysterious infection called Legionnaires' disease had erupted among American Legion members who attended a convention in Philadelphia. One of the first responses of the director of the National Institutes of Health was to check all of that agency's records to see what, if any, genetic engineering research was in progress there. He didn't believe there was any connection at all between such research and the disease. He just wanted to be forearmed in case someone raised the charge that it was all the fault of gene-splicing run amok. The cause of Legionnaires' disease turned out to be a previously undiscovered, but quite conventional bacterium.

After the cases of pituitary transmission of Creutzfeldt-Jakob disease, it was the much-denounced genetic engineering that actually came to the rescue. A proposal to license human growth hormone produced by gene-splicing and biotechnology methods had been before the Food and Drug Administration for many months and seemed to be permanently "on hold." Spokesmen for the drug agency denied, of course, that the delays were anything but routine. Many observers were convinced that the politically touchy issue of gene splicing was responsible. In any case, exactly six months after the first public disclosure of the Creutzfeldt-Jakob cases, the biosynthetic human growth hormone was approved by the FDA. Today, children all over the world are receiving the biotechnology product with no fear of infection.

The pituitary story of the 1980s was not the end of iatrogenic transmission of Creutzfeldt-Jakob disease.

Dr. Paul Brown, of the National Institutes of Health, who keeps track of these cases, says the total of pituitary transmissions in the United States stood at twelve at the end of March 1994. There has also been one in Brazil and one in New Zealand, both from growth hormone supplied from the U.S. In addition, there have been four cases of Creutzfeldt-Jakob disease in Australian patients who received another hormone, pituitary-derived gonadotropin, and experts fear that other cases may develop from that source.

Growth hormone supplied in Europe has produced ten cases in Britain and over twenty-five cases in France, where they continued to occur even in the early 1990s. Dr. Brown said almost a third of the pituitary glands used for growth hormone extraction in France came from brains removed from neurology patients who had died.

It hardly takes medical expertise to guess that this source of supply would raise the risk of transmitting Creutzfeldt-Jakob disease. In July, 1993, when the toll in France had risen to twenty-four confirmed cases, two doctors became the target of a judicial inquiry into the circumstances that produced the infections. Doctors in the United States and Britain had halted the use of pituitary glands from cadavers in 1985. In France they continued to use pituitary glands, but subjected the material to an additional purification step.

In addition to the pituitary growth hormone cases, Dr. Brown said there have been fourteen or more cases that arose because surgeons used pieces of dura mater more or less like tire patches in various kinds of surgical repair. The dura mater is the outermost and toughest of three protective envelopes that cover the brain and spinal cord. Four of the fourteen cases occurred in a single hospital in Spain. Most of the dura mater samples implicated in these transmissions came from material produced by one commercial processor in Germany in the early 1980s, but the cases evidently arose from more than one source of contamination.

Like kuru a few decades ago, it is difficult to guess when these cases of Creutzfeldt-Jakob disease will stop altogether because the disease can take so long to appear. Dr. Brown has estimated that incubation periods may be as long as thirty-five years. Meanwhile, scientists have never given up hope of understanding just what infectious material it is that causes these deadly brain disorders. They are making progress, but it is slow work. The apparently total lack of nucleic acid in the kuru agent was one of the early puzzles of the field. That lack seemed to rule out viruses, but it was abundantly obvious that larger agents of infection like bacteria, rickettsia, and parasites of any known kind were not the cause of infection. Dr. Gajdusek and others in the field had no suspects left except some kind of "infectious protein," yet, so far as anyone knew, there was no such thing.

One of the scientists fascinated by the protein aspect of the puzzle was Dr. Stanley B. Prusiner of the University of California, San Francisco. If the cause really was some exotic foreign protein, he vowed to capture it. That meant a difficult and ambitious program of purification; keep removing substances from the infectious mixture of brain materials and continue that extraction process until only one pure, but still infectious, chemical was left. Part of the way through the years of research he coined a name for this mysterious substance: prion. He concocted the name from the phrase proteinaceous infectious particle, which seemed to describe what the infectious substance must be. Many experts continued to scoff at the idea of an infectious protein, but there was a need for a name, and this one has endured.

A fresh surprise of major magnitude came when Dr. Prusiner and his colleagues succeeded in purifying, quite completely, the still hypothetical prion. Most scientists knowledgeable in this field found it hard to envisage some exotic foreign protein that had the ability to infect the human or animal brain, but what Dr. Prusiner actually discovered was even more surprising. It was not a foreign protein at all. It was a "host" protein native to the brain itself. Small mutations in that protein apparently confer upon it an abnormal ability to get itself replicated and multiplied in the brain with somehow disastrous effects.

"Everybody was looking for an infectious agent," said Dr. Brown. "By definition, until now at least, infectious agents come (ultimately) from the outside. Now we are sort of shifting gears and looking for the enemy within."

As of early 1994, the best evidence seemed to show this protein modulating the brain's receptors for the nerve signal transmission substance acetylcholine. The mysterious protein also seems to be a surface protein that affects calcium transport to and from cells. A different protein that has been found in Alzheimer's disease also affects calcium transport and some specialists think this kills neurons. The idea is still unproven.

But the biggest question about the infectious protein of slow-virus infections still remains to be answered.

"The crucial matter in our group of diseases is what makes it multiply," Dr. Brown remarked, "and that is a question no one has answered yet."

A great deal has been learned about this mysterious protein in recent years, but what triggers the initial molecular change is still a mystery.

Dr. Gajdusek still prefers the name virus to identify the agents of infection in all the transmissible amyloid diseases, from scrapie, a disorder of animals, to Creutzfeldt-Jakob.

"The potent abstract concept of a virus as a self-specifying transmissible entity requiring the machinery of the host for its replication did not specify any specific structure," he wrote a few years ago. In other words, a virus could be anything that invaded a living organism and subverted its internal machinery into making new copies of the invader. The virus did not have to take the familiar form of a package of DNA or RNA wrapped in a protein coat. Indeed, that broad portrait of a virus goes back to the old definition used before anyone had actually seen or identified what are now viruses. They used to be called filterable viruses, meaning simply that there was something infectious there that was small enough in size to flow through a filter so fine that it kept out all known microbes such as bacteria.

In any case, the recent identification of the protein that may be the "smoking gun" in Creutzfeldt-Jakob disease means that the gene for making it is also available. This leads to novel strategies that are becoming possible in the new age of molecular biology. Dr. Charles Weissmann, one of Switzerland's leading molecular biologists, did a key experiment. He produced a strain of laboratory mice in which the equivalent mouse gene, and that gene only, was deliberately erased. These are called knockout experiments in the new language of biology. The scientist uses the skills of molecular genetics to extirpate a single target gene. If the gene was absolutely vital to the animal's life, that should be quickly apparent and the nature of that vital function would also be identified.

In fact, the mice got along just fine without the erased gene. At first this seems to fly in the face of logic, but some other knockout experiments with totally different genes have had the same outcome. The results are not quite so surprising as they seem. There is a great deal of life-preserving redundancy in the genetic system. If one metabolic pathway fails, there is often another that can take its place. If one gene fails, another can sometimes fill the gap. That is certainly not true of all genes, but it seems to be the case in at least a few.

That redundancy is probably the answer to the puzzling good health of the mice in the knockout experiments. But a related finding was more signifi-

Knocking out the Creutzfeld-Jakob gene in a mouse starts with preparing embryonic stem cells from a normal mouse embryo and inserting a piece of DNA that disrupts the normal gene. The stem cells containing the defective gene are then inserted into a blastocyst of another normal animal, and a chimeric mouse is produced that contains the abnormal gene in many of its cells. By inbreeding offspring of this chimeric mouse, a few mice are obtained which are homozygous for the defective gene. These are the mice that Dr. Weissman showed are resistant to the slow virus protein and do not develop the Creutzfeld-Jakob disease.

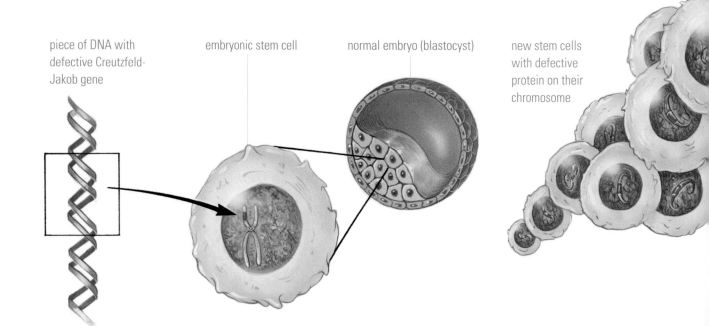

piece of DNA with defective Creutzfeld-Jakob gene

embryonic stem cell

normal embryo (blastocyst)

new stem cells with defective protein on their chromosome

cant for the study of these mysterious brain disorders: lack of the gene seems to give the animals resistance to infection with Creutzfeldt-Jakob disease.

If scientists can capitalize, somehow, on that kind of resistance, the findings may offer the first plausible strategies for treating this fatal and inexorable disease of humans. It might become possible, for example, to stop cells from making so much of the protein that seems to be the key to the disease. If this could be done, it might halt the destructive process. Dr. Brown, who is a member of Dr. Gajdusek's group at the NIH, has been doing some early work on concepts of this sort and others have probably been doing so too in the light of Dr. Weissmann's knockout mice experiments. But the work is difficult and, so far, the whole concept is mostly a gleam of future hope in scientists' eyes.

The slow-virus specialists at the NIH have also studied the protein in detail, including the mutations that have been found in its gene in those few families that seem to carry excessive risk of the brain disorder. The known mutations are not found in the truly sporadic cases that have no family history. But they seem to be a clue to special characteristics of familial cases. Whether the disease mainly destroys the mind and memory, or, instead, is more ruinous to deep-seated cerebellar functions of the brain seems to depend

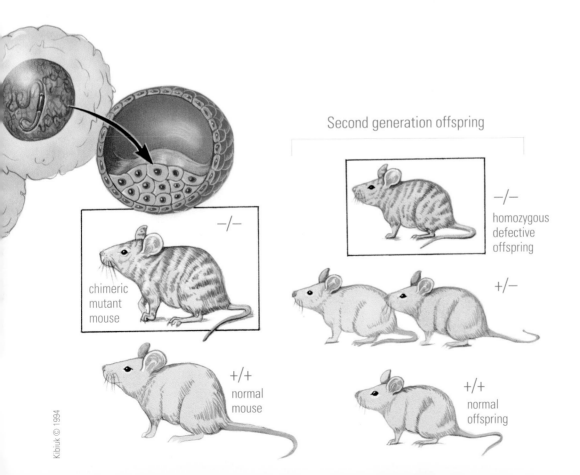

Second generation offspring

−/−
chimeric
mutant
mouse

−/−
homozygous
defective
offspring

+/−

+/+
normal
mouse

+/+
normal
offspring

237

on which particular mutation is involved.

The slow infections are among the most puzzling diseases that afflict animals and humans. They came to the notice of human and veterinary medicine over many years and in widely diverse ways. Kuru was actually a late entrant in the field. The first step in the identification of Creutzfeldt-Jakob disease began in 1920 in the neuropsychiatric clinic of Alois Alzheimer in Breslau, Germany. Hans Creutzfeldt, a doctor there, reported a "new and unusual type of neurological disease" in a young woman. She died a year after her illness became noticeable. In 1921, Alfons Jakob, at the University of Hamburg, published a report of four cases that seemed to him much like Creutzfeldt's case. He and his students pursued the strange illness and gradually attained a strong picture of the disease that today bears the two names. A variant of the disorder is named for three Austrian doctors: Josef Gerstmann, Ernst Straussler, and Isaak Scheinker. None of these gentlemen had any idea what biological process was behind the effects they observed so shrewdly. Meanwhile, sheepherders in Scotland have become all too familiar with a fatal disease that they call scrapie because the animals itch uncontrollably and scrape themselves against trees, fence posts, and anything else available. These animals begin to stagger in the late stages of their illness as their brains degenerate. The scrapie agent, whether it be called a prion or something else, is also transmissible from one animal to another. This disease too is classified as a slow-virus infection. The fact that scrapie could be transmitted was proved experimentally in 1936 when scientists injected healthy sheep with brain and spinal cord of other sheep known to have the disease. A famous mishap of animal vaccine drove home the finding with tragic emphasis a few years later. A batch of vaccine against another serious disease of sheep called louping ill was contaminated with material from scapie-infected sheep and more than 1,200 vaccinated animals developed the slow-virus disease. The vaccine had been inactivated with heavy and prolonged doses of formalin as part of the manufacturing process. Thus, transmission of the deadly disease also proved that the scrapie agent could survive treatment that inactivated all conventional viruses. Transmissible mink encephalopathy is a fatal disease of mink that arose in this way. A more recent killer of animals called mad cow disease, or bovine spongiform encephalopathy, also came from contaminated bone meal.

All of these diseases of humans and animals are now called spongiform encephalopathies and all are caused by slow infections. Kuru was the first human disease in which this bizarre kind of infection was proved. Now there is a new variant called fatal familial insomnia. It got that name because some victims suffered brain damage that seemed to make sleep impossible. The patients die of this and other neurological problems.

In the light of the man-made transmissions of Creutzfeldt-Jakob disease and the slow infections of animals, it is tempting to speculate that most of these tragedies might result from human error. But almost certainly this is not the case. There is a deeper mystery of biology at work.

Most cases of Creutzfeldt-Jakob disease occur sporadically without any slightest hint of direct transmission from person to person. Some other cases seem to run in families. It is those families that have mutations in the gene responsible for the protein that runs riot in the brain disease. Even kuru, although it was spread by cannibalism, must have started somewhere in some individual as a spontaneous event. The mystery is still unsolved.

Almost from its beginnings, this field of medical and veterinary research has been haunted by the specter of another illness that dwarfs all the others in importance. This is Alzheimer's disease. The effects on the mind are strikingly similar to those of Creutzfeldt-Jakob disease. There are important points of similarity in the pathology, too, including the buildup of amyloid, although it takes different forms in Alzheimer's and Creutzfeldt-Jakob diseases. The genes for the two proteins are on different chromosomes. It is chromosome 20 in Creutzfeldt-Jakob disease and chromosome 21 in Alzheimer's disease.

Could Alzheimer's disease be a slow-virus infection? Most of the scientists who have pursued these brain disorders have been struck by that thought. Some specialists, notably Dr. Gajdusek's group at the NIH, have pursued the question in the most decisive way. They have tried to transmit into animals some disease-producing extract from the brains of Alzheimer's victims. Several years ago, the NIH group thought they had succeeded in two cases, but they have since concluded that this was laboratory error.

"Considering the fact that we have inoculated thousands and thousands of monkeys one or two errors can be expected and these clearly were errors," Dr. Brown said. He estimates that close to one hundred Alzheimer's disease brains were used as inoculation sources in their research. A team of scientists at Yale University has also reported transmission of Alzheimer's disease, but this too is yet to be confirmed and is widely thought to be incorrect.

The idea that some kind of infection might explain Alzheimer's disease is difficult to abandon, but some scientists now doubt that it will ever be proved. Yet, on other fronts, much progress is being made in understanding this all too common and devastating human disease. Progress is urgently needed, because Alzheimer's disease must rank as one of the most devastating plagues of the late twentieth century. Only recently has it become clear just how common it is.

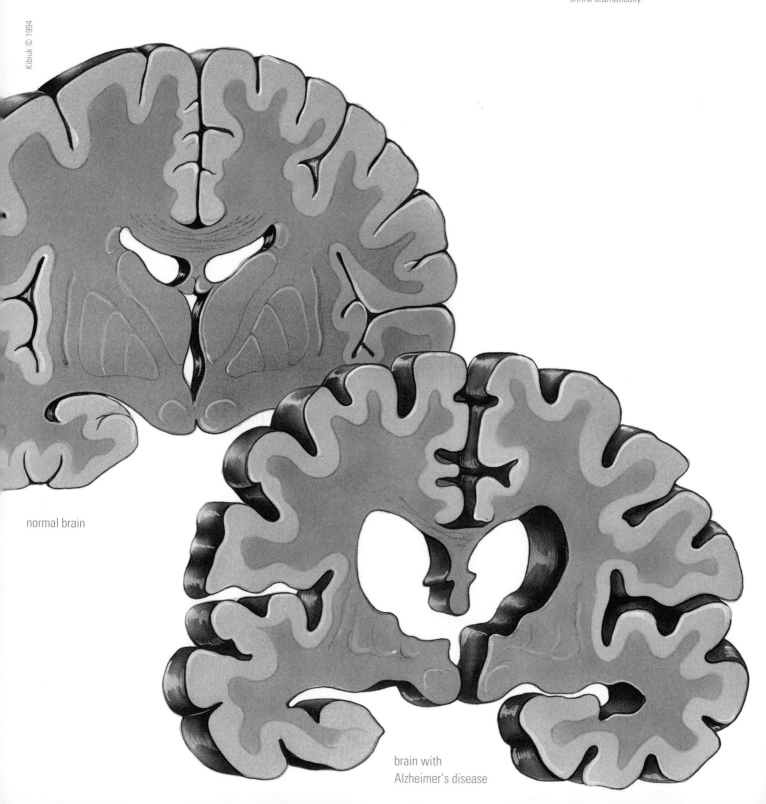

Kibiuk © 1994

Alzheimer's disease causes the brain to lose neurons and shrink dramatically.

normal brain

brain with
Alzheimer's disease

THE THIEF OF REASON: ALZHEIMER'S DISEASE 14

Alzheimer's disease, the great thief of human minds, is full of puzzles and paradoxes. The main cause of senility, it begins with little quirks of forgetfulness, but expands gradually to wholesale loss of memories that took a lifetime to collect. First you forget where you put the car keys and later can't remember your way home from the supermarket. The disease degrades personality, destroys mental reference points, and warps the perception of time and identity. It brings confusion and erases most of the mental skills essential to independent life.

In some ways, the disorder suggests a slow-virus infection, but it has resisted all efforts to transmit it or to find any infection as its cause. In some families, the disorder attacks early and seems to be hereditary. Yet the great majority of cases appear sporadically in old age, not linked to any known family history.

Now, one surprising quirk of chemistry seems to set these sporadic cases apart from people who escape dementia altogether. Some Alzheimer's patients have an excess of a particular blood protein that helps carry cholesterol in and out of cells. It would seem a more likely contributor to heart problems than brain disease. Yet strong evidence links it to Alzheimer's.

Still another paradox: while it finally causes degeneration in the brain, the disorder seems to start with a spurt of restorative growth.

In the final analysis, is it really a disease at all, or is it just the final volley of slings and arrows in the outrageous fortune of growing old?

Medical professionals must cope with all the puzzles of Alzheimer's disease because it is one of the great public health concerns of the 1990s. Senility has captured millions of today's elderly Americans and the toll seems certain to rise further in the new century. Our population is growing older as the old are living longer. Dementia in the elderly will surely keep pace. In this unhappy equation, scientists' interest in the disease is of high importance because understanding is the best hope of doing something about it. At present, little can be done to slow the inexorable destruction of the Alzheimer-stricken mind. The cause is a mystery and there is no cure. A few other diseases have been largely conquered before their true nature was understood, but this is unlikely to happen with Alzheimer's disease. Better knowledge is the main chance.

Until approximately the 1970s, senile dementia was usually blamed on hardening of the arteries of the brain. This process was thought to leave vital populations of nerve cells bereft of oxygen. Cells died and the mind died with them. In recent years, this concept has lost credibility and the focus of research has shifted.

Many scientists today believe Alzheimer's disease is not just evidence that human brains wear out, but a disorder separate and distinct from the aging process. More likely, it is several disorders that have somewhat different causes but the same end effect. This is a more hopeful view than the older idea that senility is simply a consequence of living too long. If it is a disease, some kind of treatment should become possible. Many strategies are being explored today with growing enthusiasm. Most of the research is quite recent. Only within the past ten years or so has any impact on the disease seemed possible. Indeed, general familiarity with the name Alzheimer is scarcely a decade old.

Ever since it was first described in 1906 by the German psychiatrist and neuropathologist, Alois Alzheimer, it had been viewed as an uncommon kind of dementia that appeared in middle age. It was also known as presenile dementia to contrast it with the more "normal" dementia of the aged. The patient whose brain led Alzheimer to define the disease had been severely demented. She died at the age of fifty-six.

In the 1970s and 1980s, study of many brains made it clear that there was no biological difference between dementia of the Alzheimer's type and the main kind that afflicted the elderly. The same signs, symptoms, and physical characteristics appeared, regardless of the patient's age.

The possibility still cannot be ruled out that everyone who lives long enough will eventually become demented. If that is the case, it might be considered an inevitable consequence of aging. But that is a nearly meaningless

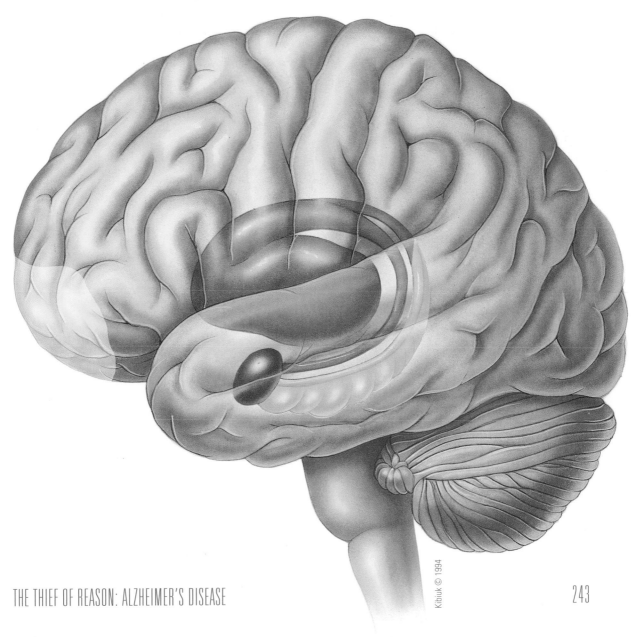

Alzheimer's disease attacks the temporal lobe region including the entorhinal cortex and hippocampus and the frontal regions of the cerebral cortex, as well as many other brain regions not shown in the diagram.

Modified from Pathology, *by E. Rubin and J. Farber. Published by J. B. Lippincott Co.*

Kibiuk © 1994

THE THIEF OF REASON: ALZHEIMER'S DISEASE

243

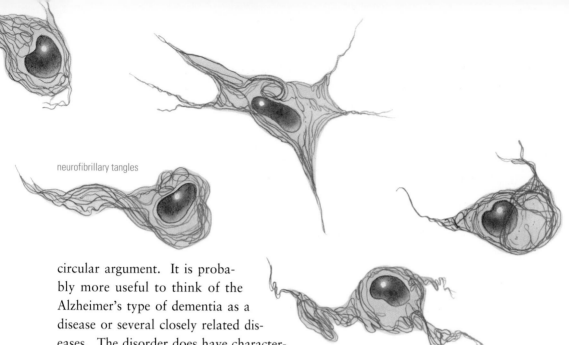

neurofibrillary tangles

circular argument. It is probably more useful to think of the
Alzheimer's type of dementia as a
disease or several closely related diseases. The disorder does have characteristics that suggest disease. While elderly people
who are not demented also lose neurons and have changes in the dendrite
arbors of many surviving brain cells, the changes seen in dementia are more
selective and more drastic. Deposits in the brain of the protein called beta
amyloid are part of the signature of Alzheimer's disease. Normal brains collect beta amyloid too, but the changes in dementia are more severe. The evidence suggests there is something going on in Alzheimer's disease beyond a
gradual decline that could be blamed entirely on the aging process.
Furthermore, there are some people who do live to great age and finally die
without ever becoming demented.

So the questions become: what causes Alzheimer's disease and what can
be done about it? There are increasingly many ideas, but no solid answers yet
to either question.

Regardless of cause, there is no doubt that Alzheimer's disease is closely
related to age. Fewer than 1% of Americans under sixty-five have it, but the
toll rises to at least one person in four among those over eighty and the percentage seems to keep rising with increasing age. According to one estimate,
40% of Americans over the age of eighty-four suffer from senile dementia.
Altogether it has been estimated that about 4.4 million elderly Americans are
demented, the majority of them Alzheimer's cases. Most of the rest suffer
from brain damage caused by repeated strokes.

The picture that Alois Alzheimer saw almost ninety years ago was dementia in the patient and some particular changes in the brain: the senile plaques

In Alzheimer's disease, the
brain tissue contains neurofibrillary tangles and shows
granulovacuolar degeneration.
These sites of abnormal accumulation of cellular debris
cause damage to nerve cells.
Modified from The Early Story
of Alzheimer's Disease,
by A. Alzheimer, O. Fischer,
F. Bonfiglio, E. Kraepelin,
and G. Perusini. Published
by the Liviana Press.

and neurofibrillary tangles that have since become all too well known. Research since his day has added much to the picture. The typical plaque has a core of the beta amyloid protein surrounded by what looks almost like a halo of damaged axons, dendrites, and their fragments. The neurofibrillary tangles contain pieces of protein from tubular fibers common to nerve cells. It all looks like debris from some degenerative process, but the significance of the plaques and tangles is still fuel for debate. Are they just the rubbish of wounded brains or are they, themselves, part of the process of destruction?

Attributing the disorder to some infection is still tempting, but remains speculative. If any disease is infectious, it has to be proved so by showing that it can be transmitted from one individual to another. Research to prove transmissibility in animals has been tried repeatedly and with great diligence. There has been at least one false alarm, but no proven case. Perhaps brain damage from some long-departed infection is part of the cause, but that too remains unproven. There are hints that physical injury to the head, particularly if it occurs late in life, may heighten the risk of dementia. All such fragments of knowledge point toward a still hidden truth, but the cause is still unknown.

When stymied by lack of a definable cause, scientists often look for gene mutations that go with a disease. In Alzheimer's cases there has always been some ambiguity in the evidence for and against heredity as the cause. Some families have many cases and patients are likely to develop dementia before their 70s. Today it is widely believed that something in the genes heightens the risk in these so-called familial cases. Chromosome 21 is a logical place to look because that is where the problem of Down's syndrome has its focus and all Down's patients do develop typical Alzheimer's disease if they live into middle age. Also, a gene for a chemical close relative of the beta amyloid protein is on that chromosome.

Accordingly, Alzheimer's disease specialists were delighted in 1991 when a research team at St. Mary's Hospital Medical School in London discovered a mutation in a gene on chromosome 21 that was linked with the disease in families that had many cases. This was crucial evidence of heredity at work. The mutation changed the gene's blueprint just enough to cause cells to build the precursor to beta amyloid with one wrong amino acid, an isoleucine where a valine should be. How could this single change in a complex process of protein building bring disaster? No one knows.

A quick profusion of follow-up experiments showed that the mutation is extraordinarily rare; too rare to account even for the bulk of other familial cases of Alzheimer's dementia. In addition, the large majority of cases are sporadic and the mutation on chromosome 21 has nothing at all to say about them. Defects in chromosome 21 appear to a be part of the answer, but they do not solve more than a small fraction of the whole riddle of this destroyer of minds. Alois Alzheimer's brainchild is a stubborn foe.

neuronal loss
and lipofuscin

Not long after the chromosome 21 discovery, scientists of the University of Washington in Seattle added another important clue to the genetic puzzle. Using some of the research dividends of the Human Genome Project, they found a genetic defect on chromosome 14. The team did not identify the faulty gene itself, but other groups have confirmed that something abnormal on that chromosome does go with the disease in more than a dozen families. Among their members, dementia is an all too common calamity. It usually develops around the age of forty-five.

Still another gene defect, this one on chromosome 19, has been linked to other familial Alzheimer's families in which the disease usually appears in somewhat older people: men and women in their 60s. It appears now that there are probably other genes that heighten susceptibility to the disorder in still other families as well. All of this new evidence appears to strengthen the case for Alzheimer's disease being a cluster of several closely related diseases all converging on a common type of dementia.

A surprising discovery made in 1992 has drawn some researchers in a sharply new direction. Scientists at Duke University found a link between Alzheimer's disease and a blood substance, called apolipoprotein E, that was previously known only as a suspect in the causes of heart disease. The new evidence is the first that makes a persuasive link between genetic factors and the great bulk of Alzheimer's cases that begin after the age of sixty-five. More than three-quarters of all the patients are in this group.

Apolipoprotein E is usually called ApoE. It was known previously as a protein that binds itself to cholesterol and helps carry that fatty substance in and out of cells. As such, it was under suspicion as a contributor to the artery clogging that produces heart disease. The scientists at Duke made the surprising discovery that ApoE also binds to beta amyloid, one of the prime suspects in Alzheimer's disease. Adding to the excitement of this discovery, the gene for ApoE is located in a region of chromosome 19 that was already suspected of having some link to the brain disorder. The research group led by Dr. Allen D. Roses of Duke and joined by scientists at other major institutions, launched an intensive follow-up of this new lead. By the summer of 1993 they had evidence that others in the Alzheimer's field called exciting and "an epidemiologist's dream."

ApoE is one of the many chemicals in the body that come in variant forms. This natural variation depends on heredity. There are three major variants, called alleles, of the ApoE gene. The variants are known as ApoE-2, ApoE-3, and ApoE-4. They differ slightly from one another. Every person inherits one of the gene variants from each parent giving the possibility of six slightly different forms of ApoE depending on which combination the person has received from father and mother. People who have the E4/E3 combination are thought to have some heightened risk of heart attack, evidently because they have a form of ApoE that is efficient in carrying cholesterol into cells of blood vessels.

Dr. Roses' team and their collaborators found that people who have two copies of E4 have a particularly great risk of developing Alzheimer's dementia. Fortunately, the Epo-4 gene variant is quite rare. It is estimated that only 3% of the general population have it in a double dose. E3 is thought to be the most common form with 90% of the population having at least one copy and roughly 60% having two copies. In Alzheimer's patients studied by the research group and in members of families in which the disease tends to appear late in life, E4 was much more common.

In the families studied that were prone to late-onset Alzheimer's disease, only one person in five who had no copies of the E4 variant developed the brain disorder by the age of seventy-five. Among those who had one copy, nearly half were afflicted by that age, and in those who had two copies the toll rose to 90%.

senile plaque

The research team's report in *Science* said that, in the forty-two families they studied, "...the double dose was nearly sufficient..." by itself, to bring about Alzheimer's disease by the age of eighty. The scientists said the evidence suggests that ApoE-4 is a "major risk factor" for Alzheimer's disease that appears late in life.

Other scientists have confirmed the status of ApoE-4 as a real, and hitherto unsuspected, risk factor in Alzheimer's disease. The findings have provocative implications including the possibility of a blood test that could predict the disease early in life and a host of new strategies for designing drugs to treat the disorder. But the research team at Duke took care to put their discovery in conservative terms. They noted, among other things, that 64 out of 176 Alzheimer's cases that they identified by autopsy had no copies of E4. In short, E4 could not be the whole story. And they cautioned that application of their results to the general population must await major epidemiologic studies that have not yet been done. A study was being organized in 1993 to follow fifteen hundred elderly people for the rest of their lives to see how well the ApoE profile can predict the risk of developing Alzheimer's disease.

Late in 1993, at the annual meeting of the Society for Neuroscience in Washington, DC, Dr. Roses and his colleague at Duke, Warren Strittmatter, added another dimension to their discovery. They offered a theory to explain the precise damage the patient's ApoE profile does to the brain. In their view, it is not directly the presence of ApoE-4, but the lack of the other variants, ApoE-2 and ApoE-3. In the new theory, these two gene variants exert a protective effect that helps the microtubules inside neurons resist damage. These tubelike structures are necessary to the neuron's proper functions. With the protection absent, the neurons are subject to damage and destruction.

Unlike the original discovery, which was widely accepted, the later theory got a mixed reception at the neuroscience meeting and the resultant label controversial. How this part of the Alzheimer's story will unfold remains to be seen.

In any case, many specialists believe that loss of key neurons and their synapses is probably the direct cause of the dementia in the disease. Like the other signs of damage, the loss of neurons and their connections is not diffused uniformly through the brain but is concentrated in particular regions and groups of brain cells. Among the hardest hit are portions of the cerebral cortex, key organ of human thinking and consciousness, and the hippocampus, the structure deep in the brain that is believed to be crucial to memory. Taken together, the cerebral cortex, the hippocampus, and their web of connections to other parts of the brain are the vital creators of thought, planning, memory, and most of the other attributes that make us human. It is easy to imagine how damage to these areas can ruin the minds of Alzheimer's patients. The geography of cell loss makes it look as though the damage isolates the hippocampus from the cerebral cortex. Dementia would be an all too plausible result of that breach in communications within the brain.

The chemistry of the damaged nerve circuits is persuasive too. The brain accomplishes all of its incredible feats with the help of nearly two dozen different neurotransmitters that are the chemical agents of nerve signaling; the semaphore flags of the brain. Among the earliest studied of these signal chemicals was acetylcholine. It was the first to be identified as a neurotransmitter in the central nervous system. Nerve circuits that use it are so intimately involved in the processes of memory that it was once thought that nerve cell synapses that use acetylcholine might actually be storage sites of memory. Today that concept appears to be too simple. The chemical's relationship to memory is considerably less direct.

Nevertheless, whatever does the actual damage in Alzheimer's disease, it seems to have a special bias toward attacking nerve cells that use acetylcholine, or the enzyme that makes it. Deficiency of acetylcholine has appeared to be the most dramatic and predictable chemical change in the patients' brains, although recent studies have also implicated other neurotransmitter systems too.

The loss of brain cells that make acetylcholine is particularly stark in the cerebral cortex and the hippocampus. This evidence, of course, has sparked a search for drugs that increase the action or availability of that neurotransmitter in the hope of gaining some relief of the symptoms of dementia. In one recent set of laboratory experiments, done at Massachusetts Institute of Technology and Massachusetts General Hospital, scientists found that acetylcholine promoted the proper breakdown of the amyloid precursor protein so that it does not lead to excess accumulation of beta amyloid. A shortage of the neurotransmitter increased beta amyloid production. Whether these findings will lead to an important strategy for treating patients remains to be seen.

Several years previously, doctors had begun experimental use of drugs designed to cope with the presumed shortage of acetylcholine. One such drug works by reining in an enzyme that normally breaks down the neurotransmitter. With the drug circulating in the patient's body, there should be more acetylcholine available to do the brain's work. That is the theory behind the drug, called tacrine, produced by the Warner-Lambert Company and now sold under the trade name Cognex. There were early enthusiastic reports of the drug's effects, most of which had to be tempered in the light of further experience. Two large-scale trials of the drug, reported in 1991 and 1992, showed modest benefit to many, although not all, of the patients who took it. One such report, in the *Journal of the American Medical Association*, said patients who took the drug showed some improvement in certain tests that measured intellectual abilities and memory. There was nothing dramatic in the improve-

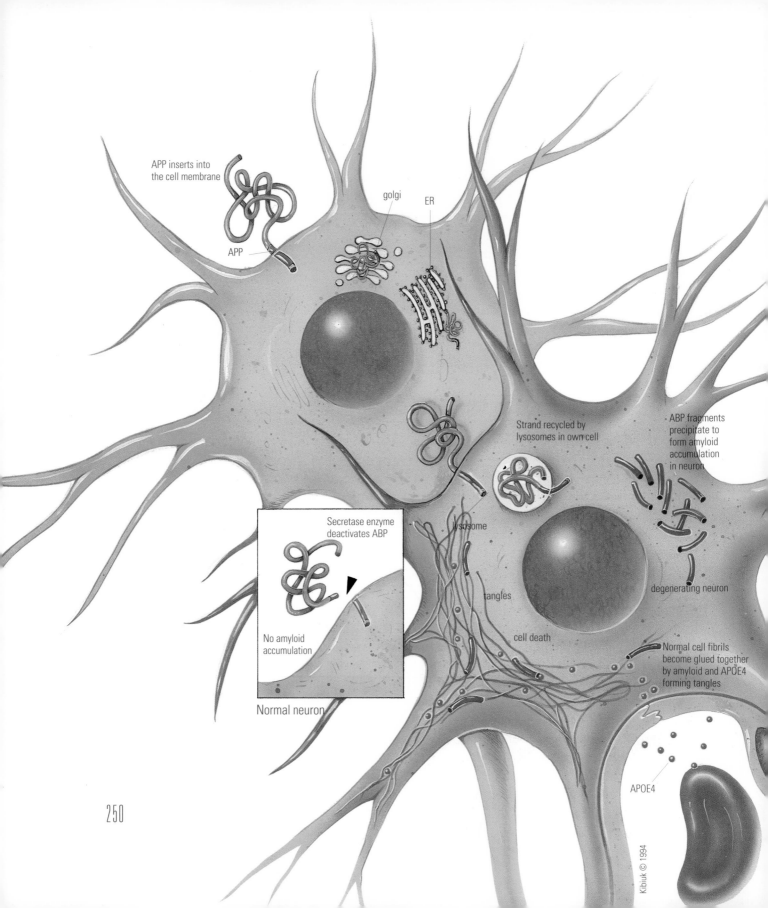

APP inserts into
the cell membrane

APP

golgi

ER

Strand recycled by
lysosomes in own cell

ABP fragments
precipitate to
form amyloid
accumulation
in neuron

Secretase enzyme
deactivates ABP

lysosome

tangles

cell death

degenerating neuron

No amyloid
accumulation

Normal cell fibrils
become glued together
by amyloid and APOE4
forming tangles

Normal neuron

APOE4

250

Kibiuk © 1994

ments, but most patients who have the disease would be expected to decline in ability over time. Any improvement is certainly encouraging. An editorial in the medical journal said tacrine does provide modest relief of some dementia symptoms, but suggested that it may be more helpful to a particular category of Alzheimer patients than to the generality of those afflicted with the disorder. This would be expected if the dementia is a group of several closely related disorders, rather than a single one. Indeed, acetylcholine is by no means the only neurotransmitter that seems to be disordered in Alzheimer's disease. That brain chemical came to research workers attention early, but now scientists searching for answers to the disorder have also been pursuing other substances that carry signals in the brain and the cellular receptors that receive their messages. Important among these are two neurotransmitter systems. In the polysyllabic parlance of brain scientists they are called the adrenergic system and the glutamatergic system. The acetylcholine system is called cholinergic.

Adrenergic refers to the steroid hormones produced by the adrenal glands. Glutamatergic has to do with the neurotransmitter glutamate. In both cases, the systems include the receptors through which they influence cells. In Alzheimer's disease, neurotransmission via glutamate is severely disrupted in the cerebral cortex and the hippocampus. The functions of the so-called adrenergic system show losses in the disorder too. A severe loss of neurons occurs in a structure in the brainstem called the locus coeruleus. In plain English, it could be called the sky-blue spot. From this small bit of brain tissue come important nerve circuits that feed into the entire forebrain. On the other hand, glutamate is important to neurotransmission, information processing and storage in the temporal regions at the sides of the brain. Trond Myhrer, a Norwegian scientist, has suggested that more attention be paid to the recently discovered impact of Alzheimer's disease on the glutamate system and that this be explored for possible clues to new drug treatments for the disorder.

But the idea that disruptions of the acetylcholine system are important in Alzheimer's disease has been circulating since the mid-1970s and it takes time to develop drugs to take advantage of new ideas in science. In any case, an advisory committee to the Food and Drug Administration noted that tacrine, the drug developed to bolster the cholinergic system, appeared to be safe and that two studies had shown it to be of some benefit to about 20% of the patients in whom it was tested. Tacrine was approved by the FDA in 1993 for treatment of the disease. Nobody has suggested it is a cure for dementia or even that its beneficial effects are widespread, dramatic, or permanent, but in

Normally, the beta amyloid precursor protein is inserted into the cell membrane where part of it is clipped off on the outside of the cell by a "secretase" enzyme. The precursor molecule is cut off in such a way that the beta amyloid portion of the molecule (portion in red) cannot be produced. However, according to a current hypothesis for the mechanism by which Alzheimer's disease destroys nerve cells, the beta amyloid precusor protein can be abnormally broken down by enzymes in lysozomes, tiny bodies within nerve cells. The abnormal breakdown product binds to neurofilaments and also combines with other proteins to form the neurofibrillary tangles. A protein normally found in blood, called apolipoprotein E4 (green spheres), binds strongly to these tangles, which eventually kill the nerves cells in which they are produced. There is evidence that people who have apolipoprotein E4, as opposed to other forms of the apolipoprotein E family, are particularly susceptible to developing Alzheimer's disease. At this stage, however, the scheme shown in this figure is only a speculation as to how the disease actually damages the brain.

this mind-destroying disease any help is welcome. Other neurotransmitter systems that are seriously affected in Alzheimer brains are also being explored in the search for effective drugs.

A wide variety of other drug strategies have been developed over the years. Substances that cause blood vessels to dilate have been tried in the hope that they might increase the flow of blood to the brain and thus deliver more oxygen to help keep brain cells alive. Chelating agents, chemicals that grab molecules of metal and remove them from body tissues, have been tried. Their use was suggested by the much-debated idea that excessive aluminum is present in the patients' brains and that this metal may have something to do with the disease process. If that is so and chelating agents can reduce the amount of aluminum, so the argument goes, the effect might be helpful. The hypothesis on aluminum still has some proponents, but it seems to be fading from the forefront of strategies against Alzheimer's disease.

Research has suggested many possible ideas for drug treatment of Alzheimer's disease. There have been a few hopeful reports, but little success, so far, in developing any specific medicines that are useful in slowing the pace of dementia. Nothing has been found that helps all Alzheimer sufferers and there have been no known cures. A handbook, *Understanding Alzheimer's Disease*, published for the Alzheimer's Disease and Related Disorders Association, lists several classes of experimental drugs that have been tested as possible treatments for the brain disorder. But dramatic advances against this common cause of dementia have been all too rare.

Nevertheless, research workers are buoyed by the hope that the wealth of new research on Alzheimer's disease is bound to suggest more leads and ideas and that one or another of these will yield major dividends in the future.

Several years ago, the study of identical twins gave the kind of hint that continues to keep the quest alive despite many disappointments. In one pair of twins, the disease developed in both, but one twin became demented thirteen years before the other. What happened to bring on the disease in one twin? Or, perhaps more important, what protected the other twin for more than a decade? The difference in experience hints that there are answers to be found through some scientist's future ingenuity. A profusion of different possibilities is being explored. A few research teams, for example, have begun to suspect that the intricate immunological process called the complement cascade may have a causative role. Complement is the immunologists' term for a multiprotein defense system in which a couple dozen different substances are triggered into action, one after another, in a powerful chain of steps that helps destroy microbes that have invaded the body. Recent evidence has shown that brain cells are capable of making some of the corrosive complement proteins. Some of them have actually been found in the plaques and tangles that are the brain signatures of the condition.

There is no doubt that these powerful substances could damage nerve cells if they somehow turned against their own brain tissues in some kind of autoimmune reaction. But finding complement proteins at the scene of the crime, so to speak, doesn't prove the point. Their presence may be a late effect rather than an early cause. There is another piece of circumstantial evidence that seems to hint at some immune factor as a contributing cause of dementia. There are somewhat fewer than the statistically expected number of cases of Alzheimer's patients among people who suffer from rheumatoid arthritis. Most such arthritis patients are under almost continuous treatment with antiinflammatory drugs. Could those drugs be having a protective effect on the brains of the arthritis patients? It is a tempting hypothesis to some scientists, but there are alternative explanations for all of the clues that seem to support the immunity theory. The suspected relationship may be real and important, or it may prove to be a red herring of no real significance. That has happened many times with other theories of Alzheimer's disease. Only further exploration will tell which of the possibilities is the truth.

There is also some evidence and much speculation linking Alzheimer's disease to disorders that affect energy metabolism. Studies have shown that Alzheimer's brains have unusually low levels of glucose use, one of the body's main means of providing energy.

Scientists' increasing interest in the effects of hormones on brain function has generated studies that show considerable promise for women who have Alzheimer's disease, or who seem to be developing dementia in the years after menopause. The strategy is to give estrogens, the female hormones. Animal studies have shown that estrogen receptors exist in the brain and that these hormones increase the activity of an enzyme important to acetylcholine production in certain key areas of the brain. Studies have also shown that administration of estrogens is sometimes helpful to the memory and other cognitive functions of elderly women. Pursuing these leads, several studies have been launched to test the value of estradiol, a powerful natural estrogen, and other hormones of that group, on the memory, emotional well-being, and cognitive function of elderly women.

An early pioneer in this work was Dr. Howard Fillit, who was at The Rockefeller University in the middle 1980s and was particularly interested in the possibility that Alzheimer's disease might involve an autoimmune reaction in which the body turns destructively against some of its own tissues. He thought this might include tissues that use acetylcholine in nerve signaling. But his studies led him more and more into the hormonal aspects of the situation. It was apparent even then that there was more Alzheimer's disease in elderly women than in men and that these patients often suffered the bone loss of osteoporosis along with mental decline.

Dr. Fillit was particularly struck by a lecture by one of his colleagues, Victoria Luine, on the effects of estrogens on the acetylcholine nerve signaling system in the brains of female rats. The hormones seemed to stimulate an enzyme that promoted the activity of the neurotransmitter in a key region of the brain. The enzyme, choline acetyltransferase, was also known to be much decreased in people who had Alzheimer's disease.

Estrogens were known to help the osteoporosis problem in some elderly women. Perhaps hormone treatment could help both the mental and the physical problems. Dr. Fillit and his colleagues tried treatment with low doses of estradiol in seven elderly women who suffered from Alzheimer's disease and also from osteoporosis. After six weeks of treatment, the women improved significantly in mood, attention, and in their ability to interact socially with others. When the hormone treatment was halted their mental condition slid gradually down hill. It was exactly the pattern that would be expected if the improvement had been produced by a hormone that was gradually depleted in the body.

To the scientists who did this work, the results were breathtaking, but no research funding agency shared their enthusiasm. Dr. Fillit went on to other work with the elderly. Nevertheless, the research did leave echoes and important lasting effects. The full story has as much to do with aging as with Alzheimer's disease, as we shall see in the next chapter.

A different realm of brain research, the nature of stress and its hormonal effects, has also offered its own hints on what may favor the development of Alzheimer's disease. Stress calls forth a burst of reactions as hormones are mobilized to confront danger. Other hormones flow forth quickly to bring the defenders under control before they do damage themselves. Some parts of this hormone cascade might be damaging to nerve cells. Drs. Robert Sapolsky, then at The Rockefeller University, and Philip Landfield, at Bowman Gray Medical School, originated the idea that glucocorticoid hormones acting in reaction to stress may accelerate wear and tear in the hippocampus. They saw certain amino acids that have an excitatory effect on nerve cells as a part of the process. The hippocampus is one of the key brain regions in which this damage is likely to occur during prolonged stress. The hippocampus is also one of the prime targets of Alzheimer's disease. While it seems unlikely that stress is among the root causes of Alzheimer's dementia, it could be a factor that nudges the disease toward faster destruction of the patient's brain. Perhaps some people who are susceptible to the brain disorder for other reasons may fall victim to it faster if their lives have been marred by excessive stress.

In their various ways, both stress and Alzheimer's disease show the human brain's talent for responding to change. The compulsion to adapt is central to the brain's biology, but the adaptation is not always for the good. It can be another way in which the brain can be taken hostage by its own perceptions of the outside world.

The ability to change in confronting the changing world is what scientists call the brain's plasticity. Plasticity is the central fact of learning and memory, development and growth. Only by continuing to change can the brain fit the everchanging universe into its own three-pound cosmos. Plasticity and the power to regenerate are critical needs in coping with a hostile world. They are keys to confronting the facts of growing old. But they may also be keys to the rising tide of Alzheimer's disease in the American population.

For the affected individual, the inexorable downhill slide into dementia is one of the most tragic ways in which the brain can be taken hostage by forces it can neither understand nor control. That is among the important reasons for studying the brain's plasticity and its ability to regenerate.

"The goals of basic regenerative research include identifying key plasticity mechanisms, understanding what regulates them, and applying this information to better understand normal function and eventually treat disease in man," said Dr. Carl W. Cotman, of University of California, Irvine, one of the leaders in this realm of brain study and its relationship to Alzheimer's disease.

His team has paid particular attention to the hippocampus. It is intimately involved in the plasticity of learning and memory and the changes that accompanying both aging and Alzheimer's disease. Experiments in animals have shown that cuts in the hippocampal nerve circuits are followed within days by reactive growth in the housekeeping cells—the glia—and by the development of new synapses to restore neuron connections. Neurons that have lost contact with their original targets degenerate. In humans, some of the equivalent groups of neurons undergo similar losses and regenerations in the course of Alzheimer's disease. Injury, even in degenerative disease, may stimulate growth. In fact, growth and degeneration coexist in that brain disorder, but the defensive new growth seems to become part of the problem.

Research in Dr. Cotman's laboratory has revealed a complex picture of the brain responding to attack by whatever process is basic to Alzheimer's disease. There are cascades of chemical activity involving recently discovered growth factors and other substances that have been known for decades. In trying to restore its circuits, the brain may cause more beta amyloid to be produced and the deposits of this substance may actively increase the damage. For scientists concerned with treatment of the disorder, the picture becomes particularly dicey because substances that are natural a gents of regrowth and repair may also be capable of growth that leads to terrible harm.

The progression of this grim disease as the action of molecular cascades, and not just one but a series of them, in Dr. Cotman's view, arises from the brain's efforts to restore itself. Sometimes restoration is transmuted into ruin. Dr. Cotman and his co-workers argue that identifying the mechanisms that contribute to this ruinous set of events could show ways of slowing their course, particularly if the counterattack could be launched early. This, they say, could help put brakes on the relentless degeneration of the brain.

Many researchers think it is most important to find ways of detecting Alzheimer's disease early or even predicting it in advance. Treating too late is probably worse than treating too little. That is particularly true of brain disorders because the damage, once done, is likely to be irreparable. Doctors need to see the problem coming, but in Alzheimer's dementia the ruined brain is likely to be its own first evidence.

If it does prove valid, even for a fraction of dementia patients, the ApoE hypothesis could give valuable advance warning. That is one of the idea's main attractions. It is also one of the crucial reasons why the scientists who did the work want further studies to test their ideas in a large population.

The same search for early warning signs applies to studies of an entirely different kind by Dr. M. J. de Leon, a psychiatrist and brain specialist at New York University Medical Center. He has used the CAT scan and magnetic resonance imaging techniques to look at the hippocampus in Alzheimer patients in various stages of their disease. He has found that noticeable shrinkage of the hippocampus occurs very early. Indeed, he believes he can find it even before any other signs of brain damage are detectable. It appears to be one of the earliest warning signs presently available and he claims 85% accuracy for it. He thinks that there is, even earlier than that, a derangement of glucose uptake, which Dr. de Leon believes may also be a useful clue in early detection of the dementia-producing brain disorder. In related studies, a colleague at NYU, Dr. James J. Golomb, has found evidence that some shrinkage in the hippocampus in normal elderly people may explain the mild forgetfulness that usually goes with aging. The key question still to be

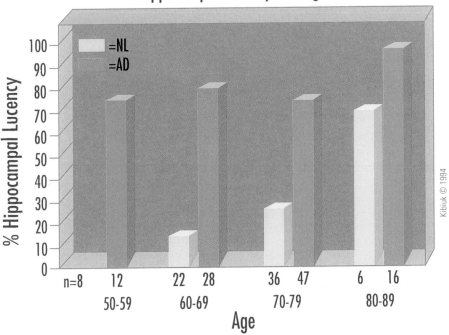

CT Hippocampal Lucency and Age (n=175)

% Hippocampal Lucency

=NL
=AD

Age

n=8 12   22 28   36 47   6 16
50-59   60-69   70-79   80-89

Kibiuk © 1994

According to the research team of Dr. Mony de Leon of New York University Medical Center, shrinkage of the hippocampus ("hippocampal lucency") occurs in normal aging (NL) but only very gradually in the seventh and eighth decades of life. In contrast, people with Alzheimer's disease (AD) show this shrinkage much more dramatically and much earlier in life. *Modified from a figure by Dr. Mony de Leon.*

answered is whether or not these brain changes in "normal" people are really the earliest stages of Alzheimer's disease.

So, progress is being made, slowly, often painfully, but unmistakably on many fronts. Probably many of the ideas that seem promising today will fall away. Hopefully, others not yet conceived, will appear and be tested. The human brain is the most complex thing that has ever arisen since life on Earth began. It should surprise no one that the brain's problems are difficult to understand and solve. Genetics, development, nutrition, infection, physical injury, and harmful personal habits can all affect the brain. All of these have to be considered as the human mind searches for remedies for the condition that robs the mind of itself.

Age always intrudes on the equation. It seems not to be the whole story in Alzheimer's disease, but it could hardly be totally detached. The effects of growing old itself are of intense interest to students of the brain. There are certainly bad ways to treat one's brain during life, but are there any demonstrably good ways? Was Shakespeare right when he saw the final years as a dismal ending? "... second childishness and mere oblivion, sans teeth, sans eyes, sans taste, sans everything."

Was the poet Robert Browning whistling in the dark in his famous exhortation a couple of centuries later?

"Grow old along with me!

The best is yet to be,

The last of life, for which the first was made."

What does science of the late twentieth century have to say about these mutually incompatible visions? The emphasis today is on two other facile turns of phrase that also appear mutually incompatible: use it or lose it, and wear and tear. If wear and tear gradually erodes the brain, perhaps using it means losing it too. That is an unsettling idea much debated today as specialists try to understand everything that growing old does to the human brain and mind.

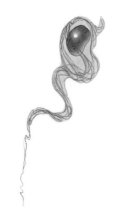

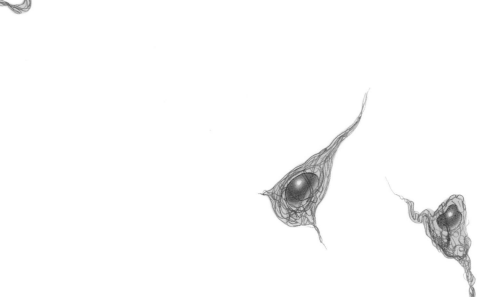

THE THIEF OF REASON: ALZHEIMER'S DISEASE

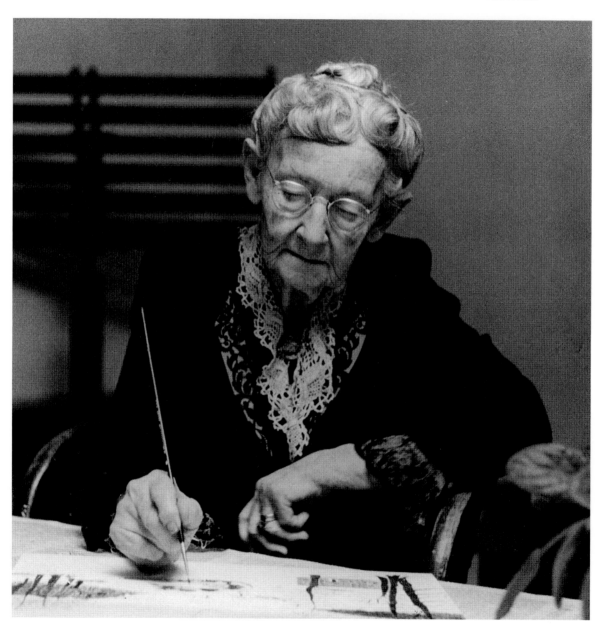

HOW TO GROW OLD? YOU SHOULD LIVE SO LONG   15

Hordes of Americans jog, shun fat in their diets, keep watchful eyes on their weight and blood pressure, and perform a host of personal rituals in hopes of keeping their hearts healthy and their bodies firm. Few take any deliberate steps to make sure their minds live as long as their hearts. Fewer still would have any idea how to go about it.

There are some obvious things that can be done to prevent unnecessary brain damage that compromises the mind. One is to forego professional boxing as a life work. Too much hammering on the head can produce effects much like Alzheimer's disease. The boxers' term is punch drunk. Even more important, brain conservers should avoid addiction to drugs and alcohol. Overuse of amphetamines can produce psychosis. Cocaine, heroin, marijuana, and alcohol all seem capable of damaging the brain if they are used too much, but even here there are ambiguities. It isn't necessarily true that an occasional drink does harm; it may even be good for you. The damage caused by the so-called drugs of abuse is also a matter of debate. Heavy use over a long period of time is certainly harmful, but occasional use, if it can ever be done without addiction, is still very much debatable as a cause of lasting damage.

Of course, some things people do to protect their hearts are good for their brains too. Health habits that reduce the risk of stroke may also prevent dementia from repeated strokes. Avoiding excessive stress in middle and old age is probably good for all of the body's systems and organs. There is solid evidence that it is good for the brain. Physical exercise itself is presumably good for the mind too. The presumption has been part of our heritage since Rome was the center of the western world.

"Mens sana in corpore sano"—a sound mind in a sound body—goes back to the Roman satirist Juvenal and there is no telling what folk saying, ancient even in his day, gave him the idea. On the other hand, it is the style of the late twentieth century to question all unproven presumptions no matter how obvious. At Washington University School of Medicine in St. Louis, psychologists tested the effects of long-term exercise training on mental functions in eighty-seven sedentary older adults. After a year of physical training, the research team documented real improvements in physical condition. They found "little if any effect on improving cognitive function." Physical condition was improved in all the people who tried the experiment, but tests of mental performance showed no significant change. The research team did find improvements in morale among their elderly exercisers and concluded that the training was worthwhile on that ground alone, but actual mental function wasn't raised.

If there is a particular lifestyle that one should follow to keep the brain and the mind in good working order, it is hard to prove. There are all manner of prescriptions, but no solid verdict for any of them.

Most thinking people would opt for keeping their minds active to the end. After all, that is the real purpose of having a mind. The idea also has the lure of being optimistic. If using it to the full helps keep the brain in working order, so much the better. The idea also has common sense logic. Muscles, bones, and virtually everything else in the body deteriorate if unused. Automobiles get rusty if left for months in a parking lot and their batteries are likely to die. Boats left at anchor get barnacles on their hulls and their metal parts corrode. Everywhere in the world there are hints that things need to be used, cleaned, and polished. All this reinforces the intuition that the brain must be active if it is to stay sharp. In any case, keeping the mind in tune with the beauties, grandeurs, and absurdities of the world must rank among the highest pleasures of life. An active mind, almost by definition, is one that continues to be interested in the present and the future. It's worth doing whether it preserves the brain or not. Dr. Trey Sunderland, chief of geriatric psychopharmacology at the National Institute of Mental Health, has defined a healthy older person as "one who has the ability and energy to pursue his or her own interests and who is looking towards the future." All of this implies, indeed requires, an active brain.

In a panel discussion on aging and mental health, Dr. Sanford I. Finkel, of

Northwestern University Medical School, said memory impairment that accompanies aging is common in the decades after the age of fifty. An important contributing factor, he said, may be that virtually no attention is given to maintaining good memory function throughout life and that most people don't really tax their memories after they finish their formal education. In the same panel discussion, Dr. Fredrick T. Sherman, a specialist in internal medicine for middle-aged and older adults, said he tries to keep his patients at the highest level of function that is prudent in their physical condition. "Use it or lose it is my battle cry," he said.

Indeed, conventional wisdom would certainly favor the "use it or lose it" philosophy of life, but conventional wisdom is often wrong. There are some brain specialists who don't think the use it or lose it credo is the whole story. There is also a world of evidence that things wear out when they are used. Tires, cars, and television sets all wear out. Everything grows old. In humans, there is a swarm of changes that seem to be inevitable in the aging process. Some impairment in recent memory and loss in the ability to recall things quickly seem to go with normal aging. Scientists can even estimate just where in the brain the problem probably lies: forgetting where you left the car keys is likely to be the fault of the hippocampus. Being unable to match the right name to a clearly remembered face is more often a problem of the neocortex.

In either case, it is not always a cause for alarm. Some forgetfulness is judged normal in aging. But today any elderly person who can't remember a date, a place, or a face is likely to be terrified over the thought of Alzheimer's disease.

For every human who is growing older, and that means all of us, there is some comfort in modern research on biological clocks. It is likely that more than 60% of adults who are tested for memory skills take their tests in the afternoon. That probably biases the test results in favor of younger adults because most of them tend to be afternoon or evening people, while the large majority of elderly people are more attuned to the morning. Not surprisingly, studies have shown young adults are more adept at many skills of memory than the elderly. But perhaps the results are skewed somewhat by the time of day at which the testing is done.

Research workers at Duke University put this notion to the test with the help of young and old volunteers. The research workers put the two groups to a particularly stiff test: recognizing particular sentences from written passages they had recently read and matching each sentence to the correct passage. When the tests were taken in the afternoon, the younger people scored better by a wide margin. When the tests were taken in the morning, most of that difference evaporated to a point below the level of statistical significance.

Said the authors: "Synchrony between optimal performance periods and the time at which testing is conducted may well be a critical variable in determining group differences in intellectual performance, particularly between older and younger adults."

Data on the effects of aging have been collected over several decades by the Gerontology Research Center in Baltimore. Hand strength and some aspects of visual acuity diminish from early adulthood onward. By the age of seventy, the average human's maximum lung capacity has declined to half of what it was at the age of thirty. Kidney function drops by a comparable amount. The heart's ability to pump blood declines by perhaps a quart a minute and muscular coordination in the seventy-year-old is rated at about 73% of a thirty-year-old's. Facility with short-term memory declines, hearing impairment is common.

Whether these effects result from simple wear and tear is a matter of considerable debate, but they do seem to be inevitable. There is also evidence that the brain diminishes in several important respects, including size, no matter what its owner does. This suggests an unsettling third catch-phrase: "Use it AND lose it." There is a substantial debate among brain scientists over all three of those slogans. Perhaps the everchanging brain is taken hostage finally by the unforgiving arithmetic of the calendar. But it is also possible that there is hope of delaying some of the steps along the way.

Everybody and everything grows old. Shakespeare's seven ages of man reveal a playwright's mind attuned to things happening neatly in distinct acts and scenes. Human biology is not so easily pigeonholed. The process of aging is demonstrably real, but it isn't something that suddenly appears after age twenty-five or thirty or any other milestone. The age at which one certifies its actual beginning is only a matter of convenience. In one sense, aging is everything that happens after conception. Indeed, it is hard to pin down life's calendar in any other way. The human brain seems to start out with far more neurons than it will ever use and loses about half of them before birth. This is certainly a maturing and aging process and it is all completed within the first nine months of life. The thymus gland, vital to development of the immune defenses, is already functioning when the baby is born. It continues to develop up to the time of puberty and then gradually fades. It is one of the earliest glands to show signs of atrophy. This too is a process of aging and it is well advanced before the twentieth birthday even though the gland continues to produce hormones thereafter. A few decades ago, before anyone understood the vital importance of the thymus, its early blooming nature was much mis-

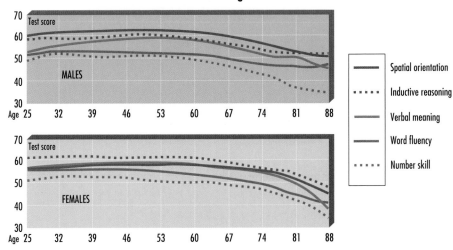

What the Mind Loses as it Ages

MALES

Test score — 70, 60, 50, 40, 30
Age: 25, 32, 39, 46, 53, 60, 67, 74, 81, 88

FEMALES

Test score — 70, 60, 50, 40, 30
Age: 25, 32, 39, 46, 53, 60, 67, 74, 81, 88

——— Spatial orientation

· · · · · Inductive reasoning

——— Verbal meaning

——— Word fluency

· · · · · Number skill

Mental decline in aging is not inevitable, according to a recent study by the MacArthur Foundation Successful Aging Network, headed by Dr. Jack Rowe, President of Mt. Sinai Medical Center in New York. There are individual differences in the skills that change with age. Among the predictors of a sharp-witted old age are the maintenance of keen interests and a flexible attitude, and ongoing mental activity and training may be able to counteract declines in mental functioning in aging people.

Adapted from The New York Times, copyright © 1994.

understood. The adult thymus was widely viewed as unnecessary; almost as dispensable as the appendix. Now it is appreciated as a master gland of the immune defenses, a vital part of life's program even though it plays its main role early.

But where does the adult human brain fit into this complicated flow and ebb of life? Apart from diseases such as Alzheimer's and Parkinson's, aging itself does things to the brain and the mind, but the picture is not as grim as it appeared to be even in recent years.

Americans become "elderly" on their sixty-fifth birthdays, eligible for Social Security, reduced railroad fares, and cheap movie tickets. Today they are given the euphemistic label senior more often than elderly, but either term really means "over the hill." In fact, some sixty-five-year olds are nearing the end of their lives while others are too busy working or playing or both to pay much attention to the milestone. Aging of mind and body varies tremendously from person to person.

It used to be thought that aging and senility marched in lock step together. Yet it was always clear that some people escaped that doom. There were seemingly ordinary men and women who stayed vigorous in mind all the way to the end in their 80s, 90s, and a few even beyond. To drive the point home there are many famous people who have given Shakespeare's prognosis the lie.

George Bernard Shaw was still writing plays in his 90s, and that genius of comic fiction, P.G. Wodehouse, was also still writing in his 90s when he died. Winston Churchill was in his mid-70s when elected to his final term as Prime Minister of Great Britain. Grandma Moses was certainly in the grand-maternal age group when she did the paintings that made her famous. But no one would argue that these remarkable people did their very best work in their last few years. Aging does levy a tax on the brain and it is an ancient truism of politics that the power to tax involves the power to destroy.

There are many theories of aging, but they all fall into either of two large categories: aging is the cumulative effect of a lifetime of errors, accidents, infections, and miscellaneous damage. Or, aging is genetic fate; biological pre-destination, kismet, or karma. For those who prefer less ecclesiastical terms, it is a process of senescence programmed into the body's cells by the genes. Most of the observable facts of aging can be shoe-horned into either type of theory. The biologist Leonard Hayflick found that young skin cells growing in laboratory cultures would divide and reproduce about fifty times and would then quit no matter what anyone did to promote their survival. Their life schedule apparently ran its course. This evidence has long been cited as support for the genetic program theory of aging, but its relevance to the brain has always been a little murky.

In recent decades, one brain finding has been particularly discouraging to people who yearn for mental activity right up to the final curtain. That is the widespread understanding that the adult human brain loses a huge number of neurons as the months and years slide by. In one scientist's estimate, as many as 100,000 neurons are lost every single day. This is the plastic and ever-changing brain with a vengeance. People were somewhat comforted by the knowledge that the brain has billions of nerve cells, but losses on that scale would total over a billion between the decades of the 40s and the 80s and it was hard to believe this could leave the mind totally unaffected. Grow old along with me? It is hard to believe Robert Browning's assurance that "the best is yet to be" if it means giving up a huge number of brain cells to get there.

Fortunately for everyone who plans to live beyond middle age, the upper estimates of neuron loss were based on miscalculations. Dr. Larry R. Squire of the University of California, San Diego calls it "one of the great persisting myths of human neurobiology." The brain does lose some cells, but not on such a prodigious scale. As Dr. Squire explains it, the error arose from the manifest impossibility of actually counting more than a few cells in a small sample of brain tissue. It is necessary to count a few and calculate the many. A starting point was the indisputable fact that the brain does shrink in size as one grows older. The neuron losses were calculated by counting cells in a small sample of youthful brain tissue and calculating how many cells would be lost if a given percentage of the brain mass shrank away. Estimate the number of neurons lost in the shrinkage of a small sample and extrapolate to the whole brain. That should give the answer.

But the answer does not depend totally on the actual loss of brain volume. To an important extent, it also depends on the calculations the scientists put into the estimates and the calculations were often wrong. For one thing, shrinkage during later life is only part of the picture. The brain also shrinks when a pathologist preserves it for study. This loss in the laboratory has to be taken properly into account. A wrong estimate here could throw off the whole end result. There was also another source of error. Recent studies have shown that the brain shrinks with less loss of neurons than had been supposed. The brain cells get smaller in size and they lose dendrites, but they don't all simply vanish.

But what makes the brain give up its tissues to the aging process? There is an accumulation of new evidence that brings the focus back to the role of the hormones that are so influential in earlier stages of life. Take the female hormone estrogen, for example. Normally, it declines after menopause. Many women take hormone supplements today to prevent some of the troubling effects of that decline. Many of them say they feel better. Endocrinologists differ on how good an idea this is, but it is also widely believed that the estrogen supplements help prevent the hip fractures that are so tragically common in elderly women. But, of course, this must be simply a matter of strengthening fragile bones and is totally apart from the aging of the brain. Or is it?

Some scientists think the hip fractures are prevented as much by strengthening the brain as the bones. At first thought this may seem to be nonsense. Epithets about numbskulls and boneheads aside, it would be hard to think of two components of the body that have less to do with each other than brain and bone. But there really is logic to the idea and evidence to support the logic. It all fits into a larger and much more important idea: that a significant part of the mental decline of elderly women is produced by deficiency in the so-called female hormones.

There has been a vast accumulation of evidence in animals testifying to the effects of estrogens on the brain. These effects are by no means limited to brain regions vital to sexual function and sexual differentiation. Estrogen receptors are distributed widely in the brain and central nervous system. That alone suggests the hormone probably has widespread effects and there is a lot of other evidence supporting this idea. Yet the implications for estrogen's widespread effects in the human brain have too often been ignored.

Cutting nerves in a key part of a rat's hypothalamus called the arcuate nucleus produces degeneration of neurons and loss of synapses there. Removing the ovaries from female rats largely eliminates estrogen production. Take an animal that has suffered both of these destructive experiments and give it estrogen; new synapses begin to grow back. In fact, they grow back in remarkably large numbers; up to 75% of the normal number in the same brain regions. How this comes about is still unknown, but the effect suggests strongly that the female hormone must have a growth-promoting effect on nerve cells in the brain. It could be a direct effect or, perhaps more likely, the hormone could be stimulating nerve cells' production of growth substances such as nerve growth factor. Brain studies have shown that estrogen tends to home in on regions of the brain that are also the sites of receptors for nerve growth substances.

Dr. Dominique Toran-Allerand of Columbia University has further illuminated this important subject by showing that estrogens promote growth of nerve cell bodies in embryonic life and probably do so by interacting with

Autopsy studies of brains from people who died at different ages contradict the popular notion that adults lose large numbers of neurons every day as they age. Many areas of the cerebral cortex maintain most of their neurons. However, in brain regions below the cerebral cortex, there is some loss of nerve cells with age that may contribute to loss of motor coordination and mental declines that occur in some elderly individuals.

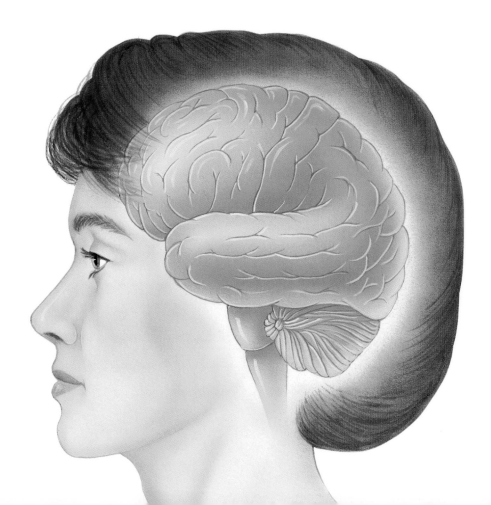

nerve growth factor. The hormones and various growth factors can be found in the same brain localities. The research underlines the importance of estrogens in development.

Molecular biologists have demonstrated that the genes for nerve growth factor and its receptor contain elements that permit the genes to be activated by estrogen in at least some tissues of the body. It wouldn't be surprising if this happens in the brain.

So there are hints that nerve growth factor and similar substances may work closely with estrogen in benefiting the brain. There is ample evidence that the substances that promote nerve growth take part in the brain's attempts to repair itself. When an animal experimenter cuts the axons of nerve cells that project into the basal forebrain, nerve cells die in that part of the brain. Yet, if the animals are given continuous infusions of nerve growth factor into their brains, neurons that use the signal substance acetylcholine are protected. These and other laboratory experiments show that this growth factor and its close chemical relatives are vital to the survival and normal func-

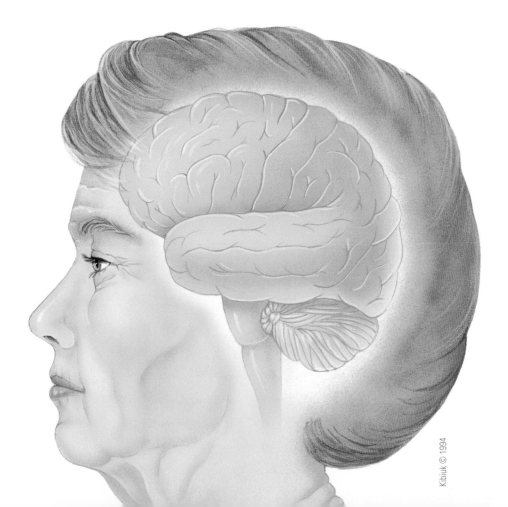

Kibiuk © 1994

tion of nerve cells in the basal forebrain.

The purpose of all this cutting, replacing, and other experimentation, of course, is to learn something of what happens to the human brain in disease and also in the presumably normal process of aging.

The argument goes this way: regions of the basal forebrain are richly endowed with nerve circuits that use the signal substance acetylcholine. These so-called cholinergic circuits project into the hypothalamus, hippocampus, the limbic system and the cerebral cortex. All of these closely related structures of the brain are involved in most of the functions of human memory. Their cells are the earliest to be affected by that destroyer of human memories, Alzheimer's disease. They are also the site of the most severe degeneration that the disease produces in the human brain.

Even though Alzheimer's disease is probably much more than just aging with the accelerator pushed to the floor, it continues to offer important clues to the hazards of growing old. These clues pop up frequently in research on the aging process. The risk of Alzheimer's disease in women rises steeply after the age of sixty-five and that risk is much greater in elderly women than in elderly men. Furthermore, women who have suffered heart attacks are five times more likely to develop Alzheimer's disease than other women of comparable age. Heart disease in elderly women is often blamed on estrogen deficiency and that raises the further possibility that the brain disorder and the heart problems may both be related to estrogen deficiency. There is a hint of that in another seemingly unrelated finding. Fat women are less likely to develop Alzheimer's disease than are their more shipshape peers in age. Fat tissue is rich in an enzyme, aromatase, that converts androgens such as testosterone to estrogens such as estradiol.

But we started down this long trail of chemical clues to brain function through worrying about hip fractures in elderly women. It is time to get back to the point. While obesity seems to help protect elderly women from Alzheimer's disease, statistics show that it also protects against hip fractures. In addition, current estrogen use also reduces the risk of hip fracture and it seems to slow the deterioration of mental processes as well as the sense of balance and related brain responses that help keep a person physically agile.

In a review of research in this provocative field, Dr. Stanley J. Birge, director of the program on aging at the Jewish Hospital of St. Louis and the Washington University School of Medicine in that city, cites another intriguing item:

In elderly women in general, the toll from broken hips and broken wrists rise together up to about the age of seventy, but thereafter, the broken hips become an ever-increasing threat, while broken wrists begin to drop out of sight in the statistics. One of the main reasons for excess stumbling and falling among the elderly is that the brain isn't as nimble as it used to be in helping keep one's balance. One of the first things anybody who is falling is sure to do is reach out with the arms to try to break the fall. As the brain's reactions become slower in the late years of life, the stumbler can't reach out in time. The wrists don't get there fast enough to break the fall or to get broken themselves. Instead, the hips take the fall. So broken hips become a logical consequence of slow reaction time and that lack of quickness has nothing to do with the strength of the bones. It is strictly a problem of the slowing brain. Quod erat demonstrandum, as the logicians used to say: "which was to be proved."

Of course, it isn't quite proved. At present, it is only a tempting hypothesis, but the purpose of making hypotheses in science is to give experimenters something to test in the search for truth. There is evidence that aged female mice do better in tests of mental agility if their body chemistry is manipulated in a way that will increase estrogen. Post-menopausal women who are taking estrogen supplements have also been found to do better on certain brain function tests. Altogether, the evidence suggests it would be worthwhile to test the effects of estrogen replacement on brain function in elderly women. Not much has been done in this until recently. Among the earliest studies was that by Howard Fillit, mentioned in the previous chapter. A Japanese team did similar research shortly after that and confirmed his findings. Several other studies have been done more recently. They have all testified to the usefulness of estrogens in elderly women to sustain mental alertness.

In his report on the subject, Dr. Birge said more careful clinical studies "are desperately needed" to determine whether estrogen replacement therapy can help neurons survive and perhaps even help them regenerate circuits in the human brain. If estrogen was effective, it might help prevent or even arrest the course of senile dementia in women. It may be that estrogen replacement therapy is one of the things women can do to keep their minds vigorous into late old age. It is an idea that merits thorough testing. Men, presumably, will probably have to find some other means.

Dr. Roy Walford, of University of California at Los Angeles, and a colleague, R. H. Weindruch, have made a stir in the lay press as well as the world of science by experiments showing that the lifetime of rats and mice can be substantially lengthened by cutting back on their food supply to about 60% of what they eat normally. In an age when many Americans suffer from obesity anyway, it is tempting to speculate that a stringent lifetime diet could help people live longer without having any ill effects on their natural growth or their mental acuity. This research idea has roots that go back many years. There is no general agreement on its significance. In the current scientific jargon it is still controversial. This is a euphemism meaning that some scientists are persuaded by the evidence while others are hardly even polite about it.

One persistent question is the actual significance of the dietary restriction in human terms. The laboratory rat whose food dish is always available probably gets a lot more food than a rat in the wild and expends a lot less energy. Perhaps these aren't "normal" rats at all, but sedentary, overfed products of laboratory routine that have diminished lifespans because of the way they live.

"In fact," said one research team in a somewhat different context, "most such studies of these animals can only tell us about bored old rats reared with too much food and not enough exercise."

On the other hand, many humans today could be described in the same way.

Much of the emphasis in studies of aging rats, with and without diet restriction, has been on a range of natural effects, including changes in cholesterol in the blood, the ability to make and repair DNA, as well as the function of many vital enzyme systems. Less study has been done on the effects of life-long diet restriction on the aging brain. In the research that has been done, there have been some intriguing findings. Diet restriction was found to prevent some of the loss of dopamine and beta adrenal hormone receptors that ordinarily accompany aging in the brain as well as some of the normal deficits that accrue in the brain's orchestration of physical and mental skills. Since it is not altogether clear what "mental skills" really mean in a rat, the scientists refer to the physical part of the equation as motor skills and the others as cognitive.

In recent studies, investigators have also found that aging rats suffer declines in some of the brain's complex chemistry including production of what are called second messengers. These are chemicals that deliver action orders to a cell after something else, such as a neurotransmitter, has triggered a response in a receptor. A study from Medical College of Pennsylvania, published in 1993, for example, has found that diet restriction prevents some of the loss of one particular second messenger chemical that is important in the brain's widespread use of acetylcholine and dopamine as transmitters of nerve signals. This second messenger chemical is called phosphoinositide. The scientists said it declined with age in rats that had unrestricted access to food, but there was no significant decline in rats up to the ripe old age of two years when they were fed a restricted diet.

As in most topics on the frontiers of science, there is also a conflicting side to the story. The question remains whether the diet-restricted rats are really restricted or simply living on a reasonable diet. Rats are known to be playful and adventuresome when they get the chance. It wouldn't be surprising if the totally boring life of a laboratory cage provoked them into gluttony and that this shortened their lives. As several research scientists have said, the "normal" laboratory rat is not normal at all when compared with animals in the wild.

Male rats apparently don't increase their eating much to compensate for the calories they burn in physical activity. In them, some studies show the results of exercise to be about the same as the results of diet restriction: they live longer on the average. The reason could be the result of fewer calories available for growth and metabolism, whether they expended more in exercise or ate fewer in the first place.

Female rats, in contrast, seem to eat more when they exercise more. So a researcher at Washington University School of Medicine gave some of them as much food as they would eat and access to revolving wheel exercise tracks on which they could run as much as they liked. In fact, they ran a lot and they ate a lot and they lived longer. The scientist concluded that a large increase in food consumption doesn't harm the rats if they balance it by an increase in exercise.

For the moment, the evidence seems to bring things back to the gambler's ancient admonition: "You pays your money and you takes your choice."

That same noncommittal wisdom may apply also to the debate over "wear and tear" versus the "use it or lose it" notion of how best to keep the brain in tune as it grows old. The debate is more than one hundred years old and it is still vigorous.

A case for trying to profit from the "use it or lose it" concept was made by Dr. D. F. Swaab of the Netherlands Institute for Brain Research, Amsterdam, in a review published in *Neurobiology of Aging*. He marshalled the evidence for the brain's ability to repair and restore itself and came up with ten technical reasons for having faith in that restorative capability. A series of companion papers commented on his review, some defending and some disputing his arguments.

In trying to define a principle of successful aging, Dr. Swaab asserted that the brain continues to need stimulation to keep it vital and functioning. But not all stimulation is the same and it is certainly not true that all stimulation is helpful. The glucocorticoid hormones that figure in many aspects of brain function enter the story here too. Dr. Swaab offered the behavior of these hormones as an example of the "use it or lose it" principle. His point was that they reduce the activity of neurons in the hippocampus and also inhibit the uptake of the glucose the nerve cells need as fuel. This could be damaging and it is damage that stems from inactivity.

In fact, however, the glucocorticoids act in concert with excitatory amino acids. These amino acids are released by the activity of neurons, and the chemical processes involved require energy. The glucocorticoids can cause damage by reducing the supply of energy-rich glucose and the whole process is actually a result of neuron activity, not inactivity.

The arguments can go both ways. Excitatory amino acids can kill neurons and yet they are important in excitatory transmission of nerve signals and in the plasticity that goes with what is called long-term potentiation of nerve signals. Long-term potentiation is a durable state of heightened efficiency for the discharge of signals at synaptic junctions. The process is important in many higher brain functions, possibly including learning and memory.

The actions of glucocorticoids can be protective, but can also accelerate the death of neurons. The brain is a complex universe delicately balanced between adaptation and growth on the positive side and wear and tear and destruction on the other. The debate over "wear and tear" versus "use it or lose it" is bound to continue because brain function involves many elements of both.

Indeed, common sense would argue that both sides of the debate are at least partly right. The chemistry of nerve activity must contribute to wear and tear. It also serves to keep nerve tissue vital and promotes its use of growth factors and its life-sustaining plasticity. The brain does lose neurons, synapses, and dendrites as it grows old and the experiences of life seem to add to this destruction. In particular, stress that cannot be controlled seems to have a destructive effect. Robert Sapolsky's studies of stress in monkeys showed this with grim clarity. When the animals died, the subordinate males were the ones who had damage to key parts of the hippocampus. Their brains suffered because of social stresses they could not control. Even without such extra jolts from social injustice, brain activity calls forth the actions of excitatory amino acids and adrenal hormones. Not even the most placid person can avoid this. It is the way the system works and it keeps us alive and conscious. But some of the effects can be destructive. Wear and tear is an inescapable fact of life.

On the other hand, stimulation, within reason, is demonstrably good, particularly if the stimulation starts early in life and continues. Studies in animals have shown that stimulation in infancy and early life increases the web of capillaries that feed the brain with blood and there is evidence that this early growth is helpful in coping with the effects of stress as the animal grows old.

The moral of the story seems to be: Give the child an interesting and constructively exciting childhood and the good effects on the brain will reverberate for a lifetime. All of this seems to argue for using the brain and the mind to the full at every stage of growth and maturity. It is an optimistic view of life where pessimism has nothing constructive to offer.

Indeed, it takes a vivid imagination to picture any doctor telling any patient: "You are growing old, Mr. Jones. Try not to use your brain so much. You'll wear it out."

Much more plausible is what a doctor named P. H. Millard actually did say in the *British Medical Journal*: "Until better evidence is available I think I shall tell my mother to go on doing the crossword: like other organs, may not brains deteriorate with disuse?"

The bottom line, however, harks back to a point made earlier. The process of aging is not something that starts only in old age. Aging begins at the beginning and that is when successful aging should start too. A healthy body can contribute much to a healthy mind even if you can't exercise your way to mental brilliance. Transient oxygen lack can damage nerve cells, and a healthy circulatory system at least reduces the risk of strokes and other problems that can deprive the brain of oxygen. Stress can be too much for the aging brain, unless early experience has honed the tools and shaped the resources for coping with the stresses and excitements of life. In animals, and probably in humans, the skills for coping with the world are best learned early. Stimulation late in life can be destructive, but stimulation and a reasonable amount of excitement early and throughout the lifespan have manifold beneficial effects.

So this glimpse of the natural history of growing old must end with only partial and conditional answers to the questions of aging and the brain. That state of imperfect knowledge is where science stands today.

The issue of youthful preparation for the stresses of old age also offers a partial answer to the question we will pose at the start of the final chapter. But that is by no means the whole answer and it is certainly not the whole message.

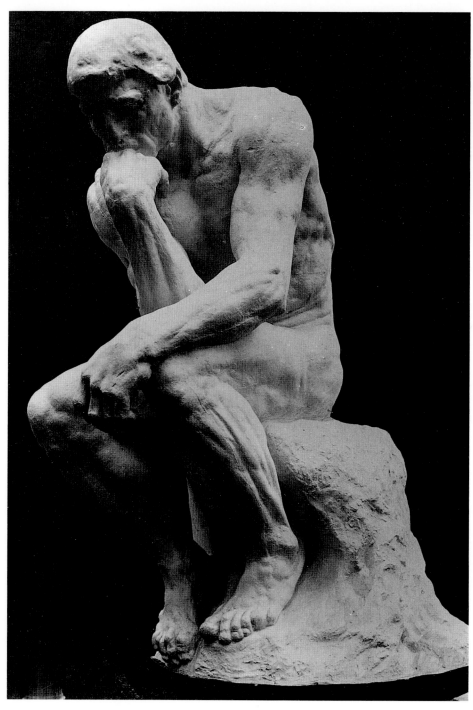

Auguste Rodin, *The Thinker*
Art Resource

Why should anybody care how the brain works? It is a complicated piece of machinery. You can appreciate it and benefit from its incredible talents without really understanding it at all. Like the automobile, it is possible to use a brain without having any idea how it runs. People love art, music, and literature without having any conception of how they are put together or what it is inside the human head that gives those things meaning. Writers and artists can be eloquent in their chosen fields without any knowledge of brain chemistry. The artist Mondrian might be surprised to learn that his abstract paintings appeal particularly to something called the fusiform gyrus. He might even be interested, but it wouldn't change his painting style. Understanding the brain is important to scientists and doctors, but most people can get along perfectly well in perfect ignorance, can't they?

That simple question is where the notion of the hostage brain strikes home. There is such a thing as proper care of the human brain and it can best be exercised through understanding. Failures here can make the brain hostage to all manner of tragedies. Adults reading this book will have noted that they can make a difference for their children, and can hope that their parents have made a difference for them. For adults, an important part of the game has already been played, but all parents have a responsibility to get their children off to a good start. Reasonable care and nurture of the everchanging brain is vital. The proper behavior has been instilled in all of us through generations of precept, example, and cultural lore, but the results are often mixed. With the best of intentions, things can go tragically wrong. There are many ways the brain can be taken hostage by forces beyond its control.

Everybody knows of personal examples. One that was studied in unusual detail was reported from Germany shortly after World War II. Two orphanages were getting shockingly different results in the health and development of the children in their care. The two institutions had equal and adequate supplies of food, but investigators found that the average gain of height and weight in young children in one orphanage was far greater than in the other. Then the supervisors in charge of the two institutions were switched. Before long, the growth rates were reversed too. The curves for children in the orphanage where growth had been good declined sharply, while those in the other institution soared. The investigators who studied this phenomenon sifted the facts. They finally came away convinced that the main difference lay in the emotional atmospheres of the two orphanages. Poor growth and poor social adjustment went with a supervisor who was a "stern and forbidding disciplinarian who ran her institution by instilling fear in the children." She ran it like a prison and the unfortunate children were her prisoners.

A report by the National Institute of Mental Health in the U.S. cited this case as an example of the ill-effects deprivation can have on the young. In this case it was emotional deprivation, affecting the mind and the brain with consequences that penalized the whole body.

This is by no means the only study that has found links between emotional damage and failure of childhood well-being. Not only the brain, but the whole body can be held hostage to some person's malevolent behavior. There are worthwhile reasons for knowing at least a little about the brain and its all-pervading functions.

Poor nutrition by itself can harm the brain and mind. Numerous animal studies have shown that a diet too low in protein can impair learning capacity. Sensory deprivation, a sort of malnutrition of mind and senses, can also lead to retarded biological development with physical ill-effects on the anatomy and physiology of the brain. Some of these changes can be permanent. As noted in Chapter 10, Drs. Torsten N. Wiesel and David H. Hubel found that keeping one of an animal's eyes closed for weeks after birth resulted in reduced responsiveness of the visual cortex to important stimuli after the eye was finally opened. Other studies too have shown that either sensory deprivation or sensory overload can be harmful. Doctors who treat posttraumatic stress syndrome, whether from combat or other causes, have noted that their patients often relate grossly unhappy childhood experiences that occurred long before PTSD developed. This sequence happens often enough to tempt some students of the problem to suspect that early experience may help set the stage for the devastating problems of PTSD that arise after some later crisis. In this and other circumstances, the cost of letting children be abused may well be the existence of many adults with mental problems and defective responses to the stresses of life. These are personal tragedies. They are also expensive in terms of medical care and the waste of human resources.

All of these diverse findings argue for more humanity in treating one's fellow humans to safeguard the heritage of the sometimes too plastic and changeable brain. It shouldn't take brain studies to instill this lesson, but science adds cogent urgency to the message. Injustices can go to the heart of human life, which is not really the heart at all, but the brain.

Beyond that, not only inhumanity, but ignorance concerning the brain can exact real penalties that make the world a worse place. Anyone can see these effects in stories reported by the daily press. Consider the Florida court ruling in 1993 that rejected the modern definition of death based on the absence of brain function. The parents of an infant born anencephalic (almost without a brain) had petitioned the court for permission to donate their doomed baby's healthy organs for transplantation so that other babies would have a chance at life. The court, according to the news stories, denied the petition and ruled that even this infant, born with no chance of ever achieving human consciousness, could only be considered legally dead when its heart stopped beating. It took time for the effects of anencephaly to run their course. During that time, the brain-dead infant's healthy organs decayed too. There is a chronic shortage of organs available for transplantation in this country. Babies often die because no organ transplants are available for them. With organs from the anencephalic baby in Florida it is at least possible that one or more other babies might have been saved to become joys to their families, to lead lives and have futures. That chance for life went to waste. The judges adhered to the medieval, Valentine's Day theory of biology that puts the heart at the core of human life. That probably cost lives even though the court decision could never be held legally responsible.

Consider also the macabre Louisiana prosecutors who wanted to force an insane convicted killer to take an antipsychotic drug to make him sane enough so the state could kill him. Ironically, the murderer was at least sane enough to refuse. After years of legal wrangling that went even to the U. S. Supreme Court in Washington, the Louisiana State Supreme Court ruled against the death-through-sanity idea. The killer, of course, is no model of civic virtue. The Associated Press described him as a schizophrenic who had murdered his mother and father, a nephew, and two cousins. The court said making even such a man take the drug just so he could be executed would be cruel and unusual punishment. The ruling left dangling the possibility that he could be executed some day if his sanity ever returns on its own. The killer is probably sane enough to stay insane.

Beyond the horrifying inhumanity of the original plea to make a deranged killer kill himself, the prosecutor's idea makes no biologic sense. It is as rational as giving a diabetic one shot of insulin and declaring him cured. If the diabetic dies later of the disease, well, too bad. We did cure him. His blood sugar was completely normal the last time we looked at him.

Ignorance does have effects, but these examples are rare cases. They involved only a relatively few people and some of the consequences are problematic anyway.

There is also a larger picture. The brains of its citizens constitute the ultimate, and most important, resource of any nation. Malnutrition, poverty, poor education, and social injustice in all of its forms can erode that resource just as surely as poor land use can erode the vital topsoil from our continent. Most of this crucial truism is often lost on most people, but sometimes not. There is hope in the fact that some politicians, as well as some scientists and other observers of the national scene, do become concerned. Senator Daniel Patrick Moynihan, Democrat of New York, encapsulated part of the message in an Op Ed article in *The New York Times*, quoting Carl Zinsmeister of the American Enterprise Institute:

"There is a mountain of scientific evidence showing that when families disintegrate children often end up with intellectual, physical, and emotional scars that persist for life ... We talk about the drug crisis, the education crisis, and the problems of teen pregnancy and juvenile crime. But all of these ills trace back predominantly to one source: broken families."

Perhaps it can't quite be proved that broken families beget broken minds, but the probability of harm to the mind should never be overlooked. There have been numerous reports, for example, that the victims of child abuse often grow up to be child abusers themselves.

It is also almost certain that some people who kill or maim others, including their own children, are schizophrenics acting out the demented orders of the voices that lacerate their lives.

Again, a glance at the daily newspaper is instructive. June 1993 was an ordinary month, but in one week a Long Island gardener was arrested, charged with murdering at least seventeen women after he paid them for sex. Another person, unknown and unapprehended, sent letter bombs, one of which seriously injured a research professor at the University of California, San Francisco. Federal officials concluded that it was the same person who had sent a series of similarly deadly missives to professors on college campuses in the 1970s and 1980s. By any rational definition, both of these individuals are dangerously insane. Yet science has no solid explanation of why they act the way they do, how they can be identified in time to prevent tragedy, and what, if anything at all, could be done to prevent the mental disorders that have engulfed them and crippled or killed their innocent victims. Psychologists say the Long Island gardener and other notorious serial killers share some traits and quirks. They tend to be loners who live in worlds that are largely fantasy. Neighbors often remember them as quiet, sometimes even as "polite" and "helpful," and express surprise when the grisly crimes are revealed. These killers also tend to be cool in emergencies that might lead to their arrests and they share enough cleverness to perpetrate repeated atrocities before being caught. But these similarities are far too vague to differentiate the killer from a recluse who shares many of those same traits, yet has never harmed a soul.

More to the point, the descriptions and psychological profiles are too vague to allow any such person to be tagged in advance, or even to be certain on any ground save past experience, whether a psychopathic killer is likely to kill again. There is still a huge amount for science to learn about the disordered human brain. It can be held hostage, not only to viruses, poisons, and physical damage, but also to the myriad forms of harm people do to each other through ignorance or spite. Understanding the brain shows the true horror of these effects and shows also how a little care and humanity might make the world better. Still, many of the worst cases remain total mysteries.

To appreciate any of these points, it is not necessary to know which nerve circuits use acetylcholine and which use dopamine, or even to have a definition of the limbic system at one's fingertips. But a modest amount of knowledge, coupled with an appreciation of the brain's plastic and responding nature, helps promote considerate treatment of all human brains; our own and those of everyone else.

The obligation to treat brains and minds with care is particularly heavy on doctors and scientists because it is a plausible guess that they know more about the brain than most other people. From the accounts in this book, it should be obvious that these knowledgeable people are sometimes caught in error themselves. One chilling example is the ignorant mistreatment of the parents of autistic children by specialists who blamed the parents' behavior for the disorder. In those earlier days, autism was widely blamed on "bad parent-

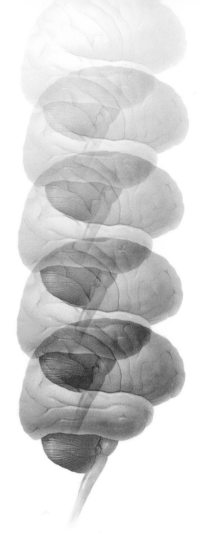

At any age, the brain is an ever-changing and adaptable organ.

CAN WE CHANGE OUR MINDS?

ing" in some elusive Freudian sense. The idea destroyed families without helping the children. Now autism is generally believed to be a physical or chemical disorder of the central nervous system. The specifics are still a mystery, but there is substantial evidence that autism really is a disorder of the brain, not a response to ill-treatment in infancy.

Another controversial idea for coping with brain disorder was the class of surgical procedures called psychosurgery. Essentially, the term connotes surgical operations on the brain to improve, or at least to modify, human behavior. Studies many years ago showed that severing parts of the most frontal portions of the cerebral cortex from the rest of an animal's brain made that animal gentle and manageable even if it had been violent and aggressive before. Today, when much more is appreciated of the integrated functions of the brain than was even imagined a few decades ago, anyone could guess that such an operation would have many effects beyond those that were desired. But in the mid-1930s and later, it was a quick logical jump from the animal studies to the thought that violent and incorrigible humans might be brought back into the civilized fold through similar operations. Thereafter, the procedure was probably grossly overused. During the two decades beginning in 1936, according to one expert's estimate, as many as fifty thousand drastic psychosurgical operations, called lobotomies, were done in the United States.

Most of them were for violent cases of schizophrenia; men and women who were almost impossible to control and whose minds were far too disordered to function normally. But the operations were also recommended for a wide range of other problems, according to Lyle W. Bivens, of the National Institute of Mental Health. On the list were depression, homosexuality, childhood behavioral disorders, and some of the more dangerous aspects of criminal behavior.

In violent patients, many of the operations did produce a gratifying passivity, but unfortunately a lack of normal emotions and a decline in intelligence often went with that change. Critics have charged that the operations destroyed the patients' personalities and turned them into walking vegetables.

Today an impressive range of drugs is available to ameliorate depression and a substantial number can help subdue the most dangerous symptoms of schizophrenia. With such treatments available, it is easy to be shocked by the reckless arrogance of surgeons who tried to cure the mind by carving up the brain.

In fact, the world of the mentally ill was a great deal different before the days of the antipsychotic drugs. Schizophrenia was a hopeless diagnosis, foreshadowing a lifetime locked in the back ward of a mental hospital with long interludes in a padded cell or restraint in a straitjacket. The prospect was that nothing but death would free the patient. Modern brain research has produced a much better future for most victims of mental illness.

As the previous chapters of this book have shown, a vast store of knowledge of the human brain, its ever-evolving functions, chemistry, physiology, and its own internal strategies for making sense of the world have all blossomed within the past few decades. In the 1990s, declared by the U.S. Government to be the Decade of the Brain, the prospect is for even greater advances. But brain scientists today are little more justified in arrogance than the psychotherapists and psychosurgeons of the 1930s and 40s. Those who treat mental illness today are still groping for solutions to intractable problems.

Nevertheless, research on the brain has continued to make clear some of the mysteries of the mind and the truths or untruths of popular perceptions. Nowhere is this more true than in the realm of the steroid hormones, chemicals that are being seen more and more as crucial to the functions and malfunctions of the human brain.

The estrogens are steroid hormones produced by the ovaries. Progesterone is produced in the corpora lutea of the female reproductive tract and the placenta. It is also produced in the adrenal glands in both sexes. The importance of these hormones in the female reproductive system has been beyond doubt for decades. But until recently many people categorized them simply as female hormones, vital to reproduction, but not necessarily to much else. That narrow concept is being shattered by the explosion of research showing that these hormones have much broader effects, influencing the brain in a broad range of functions and governing issues of health and disease in a fashion never before understood or much appreciated, at least by males.

The murky vision of hormone effects is changing for the better. Animal studies are beginning to reveal the specific neurochemical and structural consequences of hormone action on the adult human brain. Two key players in the hormone orchestra are estradiol, the most potent estrogen that occurs naturally in humans, and progesterone. Studies in patients are beginning to show the wide variety of estrogen actions on brain processes of normal life and disease. The hormones influence mental functions and pain sensitivity. They can aggravate the symptoms of Parkinson's disease and epilepsy. Estrogen replacement in elderly post-menopausal women has been shown to improve their mental function. There are indications that women using such hormonal replacement are less likely than others to develop dementia. The hormones even seem to help some female patients who have Alzheimer's disease. Studies are in progress to test that idea further in the hope that dementia can at least be delayed in elderly women, perhaps in some cases, even for the rest of their lives.

The advances of research are never a signal for public complacency. Sometimes, study of the brain suggests conclusions that fly in the face of the dogma of the moment. The brains of men and women do differ from each other physically and chemically. In some specifics, they function differently too. "Unisex" biology is not biology at all. It is nonsense generated for political purposes. On the other hand, it is also pure nonsense to assert that one is "better" than the other. That idea has a much longer and more deplorable history than the recent unisex dogma.

Much current debate on homosexuality boils down to the question of whether it is sin or lifestyle. In fact, there is ample evidence that it is neither, except in the eye of the beholder. The condition appears to be largely a matter of biology: brain chemistry and probably anatomy as well, although the chemistry is likely to be the governing principle.

Those conclusions are probably anathema to the outer fringes of the debating cohorts, but the evidence can be seen in the brain by anyone who cares to look and knows what to look for. So politically charged are the issues, however, that even scientific reports sometimes slip over the edge from research results into pleas for particular brands of social conscience. An example was the report from Dean Hamer's team, at the National Cancer Institute, on the discovery of something on the X chromosome that affects sexual preferences. Their research article in *Science* ended with this paragraph:

"Our work represents an early application of molecular linkage methods to a normal variation in human behavior. As the human genome project proceeds, it is likely that many such correlations will be discovered. We believe that it would be fundamentally unethical to use such information to try to assess or alter a person's current or future sexual orientation, either heterosexual or homosexual, or other normal attributes of human behavior. Rather, scientists, educators, policy makers, and the public should work together to ensure that such research is used to benefit all members of society."

Perhaps because the brain is so central to mind and personality, portions of the public have always viewed brain research and treatment of brain disorders with suspicion. Research and novel ideas in treatment have often sparked controversy. Psychosurgery is a particularly strong example.

Sometimes the controversy is warranted, sometimes it is a waste of time. One relatively recent issue is the use of genetic engineering for purposes that could affect the human brain. Would it be possible, for example, to use the new techniques of molecular biology for mass mind control? Alternatively, could one increase a child's intelligence through manipulations in the fetus or, who knows, maybe in early infancy? Nobody in a free society such as ours should tolerate attempts at mind control or admit to doubts that greater intelligence is a good thing. In fact, both issues evaporate rapidly into fantasy when they are examined. Propaganda and military force have always been tyrants' best weapons of mass mind control. They are likely to remain so. Those methods have often been effective in the past. Fortunately they have never been effective enough to keep people from ridding themselves eventually of the despots. Brain research has little that is practical to offer the world's dictators. Direct intervention in the victims' brains would be impossibly cumbersome even if anyone could figure out how to do it. At present, no one knows how. And history shows that despots prefer brute force.

A more complicated issue is that of efforts to increase human intelligence by direct manipulation of the brain. A federal commission looking into hazards and promises of genetic engineering warned against using tools of genetics in attempts to "improve" the human species. The commission was worried over ill-conceived attempts that did harm rather than the good that was intended. Their focus was mainly on schemes to remodel the human body, rather than the mind. The widespread use of human growth hormone for bodybuilding was a legitimate concern. There was no convincing evidence that brain rebuilding was even plausible for the foreseeable future.

On the purely technical issues, nobody today has any clear idea of what genetic engineering strategy might be used to raise anyone's intelligence. The related fears that some despot might try to generate a real "master race" according to that despot's own blueprint are absurd. It is hard enough to define "intelligence" in any useful sense. What little is known about its biology suggest it is the combined effect of a whole host of genes working in concert in complex ways that can't be fathomed today.

Brain research has shown that proper nutrition and prenatal care of the mother, a nourishing diet and good family life for the child can certainly give the individual a chance to maximize his or her intelligence. These are things that can be done now and need to be done anyway. Everything known today supports the idea that better and more effective human brains can best be developed through the old-fashioned means of good nutrition, environment, and education. That kind of subversion should be welcomed, indeed promoted, on a worldwide scale. If additional ways ever become obvious through future research, they should certainly be used too as widely as possible. The effects would no doubt surprise everyone.

The questions of "mind control" and "super race" are political fantasies.

Scientists have often harbored the illusion that their sphere of life is beyond, even above, politics and that they should be left in peace to do their constructive work with a minimum of interference. The idea has always been naive and self-defeating. The truth of that statement goes back at least as far as 1633. It has thundered down the centuries from what Galileo said, probably in a whisper, after the Inquisition forced him to recant his view of the Earth's motion around the sun:

"But it does move."

All of the history of science is punctuated with similar lessons: the banning of dissection of human corpses during the early Renaissance and the burning of books in every age since Gutenberg.

In our own "enlightened" era there has been a sad profusion of similar atrocities. Potentially promising research with human fetal tissues was held hostage for years by the debate over abortion. Research on contraception stagnated even longer in this country because the NIH was discouraged from doing anything that evoked the politically forbidden words "birth control." Recombinant DNA research was hampered by the debate over the alleged, but totally undocumented, "dangers" of gene splicing. That field of research is still hobbled in some countries.

Another issue that often arises in discussions of brain study, as in most fields of biology, is the use of animals for research. Unfortunately, the totally compassionate use of animals is not possible when the end-point of an experiment must be that of killing the animal to study its brain. Some people consider humans to be just one species among the vast number that exist today on earth. From this egalitarian view, they take the conviction that we humans have no more right to kill a mouse or a monkey than a chimpanzee would have to use humans as experimental subjects. This is a legitimate viewpoint, although a minority one. With people who sincerely hold that view there is no point in arguing and no real possibility of debate. The difference is too profound to be spanned.

Those of us who have sentiments of partiality for our own species take a less absolutist view of animal rights. This is bolstered every time one sees a child who has been cured of some deadly disease that animal research helped conquer. Most of all, it is reinforced by seeing a child waste away in pain and hopelessness because no cure or treatment has yet been devised. No humane person excuses wanton cruelty to any creature, human or any other species. Cruelty is despicable. It is sad, but probably true, that humans have committed more cruelties than any other species. Most of human cruelty has been practiced on other humans.

But the whole panoply of modern medicine and disease prevention rests ultimately on research in which animal experiments have played an indispensable role. One of the crucial reasons for such animal studies is to do away with the terrible cruelties that disease plays on humans of all ages and conditions.

Every chapter of this book has cited case after case in which discovery has been made and error has been dethroned with the aid of animal research. In study after study, there has been no other way. All of the great triumphs over the plagues and diseases of humans—and other species too—have been built on knowledge which could not have been gained without animal research. At multiple points in the search for understanding, animal research has been decisive. It goes all the way back to the first mapping of the circulation of the blood, discovery of the biological uses of oxygen and the existence of nerves. The search for knowledge of life has always depended on the study of animals. Hopes for better treatment for Alzheimer's disease, Huntington's disease, and almost every other disorder of the human mind are sure to need animal research for their achievement.

But the war against diseases of the mind is not, by any means, the only motive for study of the human brain. That three-pound package of tissue, blood vessels, and nerves is the most fascinating puzzle on our infinitely fascinating planet. Probably, humans have been captivated by the puzzles of human behavior and human genius ever since our species first became self-conscious enough to realize that we are a family and inhabit a world. Yet even today, no one knows just what this kind of consciousness is, how the brain achieves it, or how far up the evolutionary ladder one must go before that state appears. Chimpanzees are probably conscious of their own existence. Earthworms are probably not, although they have enough nervous system to react to stimuli. Lovers of dogs and cats certainly hope that these species are "conscious" too, but bees, birds, mice, dolphins, elephants? Everybody can join the argument. None of the "experts" really knows the answer.

Explaining in terms of the chemistry and architecture of the brain some of the intensely human experiences and reactions that people have observed since the dawn of time is another fascinating part of the puzzle. Why do some people come through incredible stress apparently undamaged while others do not? What makes one person go berserk and another go silent? What made Beethoven's universe of music or Einstein's universe of physics?

For that matter, what was the incredible change in our species about forty thousand years ago that generated the breathtaking cave paintings and sculptures of Lascaux and Altimira and continued on to give us the Sistine Chapel and the Pieta? The search for answers to these questions is fascinating and fundamental.

The point has sometimes been made that the brain has as many neurons as the Milky Way has stars. With puzzles of such magnitude it is probable that we shall never reach total understanding, either of the physical universe around us or the internal universe inside the skull.

As machinery, the human body is the envy of engineers and the brain is a marvel to computer experts. But is the human mind nothing more than that? Is it all just quirks of electricity, chemistry, and anatomy that begin with conception and end with death? For science, those are certainly the end-points because science must deal with the palpable, the measurable, and that which can be predicted from the evidence. As a measurable fact of life, the mind does not exist without the brain. That's where the argument ends.

But perhaps just looking at the evidence is too myopic a view. It misses the wonder of it all and scientists have always been enchanted by the wonder. Albert Einstein wrote of "joy and amazement at the beauty and grandeur of this world of which man can just form a faint notion."

"The most beautiful thing we can experience is the mysterious," he wrote on another occasion. "It is the source of all true art and science."

The universe is beautiful. It is incomparably mysterious, but it is not just total chaos. There seem to be rules, and research workers have spent their lives trying to puzzle out parts of them. There would be no point in trying if there were no rules at all. A jigsaw puzzle is nothing but disposable solid waste if there is no picture within it. Brain science would be pointless if each human brain operated by rules that applied to it alone. Astronomy would be nothing but stargazing if no galaxy bore any relationship to any other. But the galaxies do have common themes and all life on earth has just one genetic language. To search for rules requires faith that rules exist and faith is one of the human brain's most awesome talents. It can find order in the midst of chaos. It easily imagines the unimaginable.

Astrophysicists can chronicle to the minute what happened next after the primordial Big Bang. They can estimate how long ago Earth's raw materials coalesced to become a planet. Biologists can judge how many further billions of years elapsed before life began. They can outline the crucial events of life's origin; what the next steps were after the first organism generated another in its own image. Such "hows" and "whens" are the universal questions of science. The fact that we have generated many answers is a source of wonder at the potency of the human brain. But why does the universe exist and why did life arise? That is where the wonders blossom into awe over the fact of the creation itself.

Just as the debate over nature vs nurture became moot as the web of interplay between the two came into focus, so it is with the ancient, bitter war between religion and science. A little humility would be welcome in all the combatants. Unthinking dogma tarnishes both sides. All too often the human brain has been taken hostage by dogma. People who deny the findings of science when these seem at odds with points of their religion are as lacking in true faith as those who see nothing at all in life beyond the chemistry of DNA.

The human brain is the universe of both faith and reason. It has brought fear and desolation to broad reaches of the planet, but it has also brought hope and a rekindling of life. As we have seen, the brain is sometimes its own worst enemy, but more often its best and only friend. The second part of the proposition must be true, else our species would soon have vanished from the planet. The human brain is hostage ultimately to its own great powers, but that hostage state is also our best defense. The three-pound galaxy of cells within the skull has made everything possible that humans have ever done on earth. Some of it has been good; some bad; but it is our only hope for a better world and a better humanity. It is vital that this and future generations insure that each human brain be allowed to develop to its best capacity and be free to explore life and the cosmos without constraint. The brain is what makes us human. Humanity, as we egotistically define such strange traits as intelligence, kindness, and compassion, is our only hope.

CHAPTER 1

The New York Times. Page C-4, March 24, 1993, by Deborah Scoblionkov. Report on a seminar of University Museum of Archeology and Anthropology at University of Pennsylvania: "Historically Drinking: Beers Past and Present."

Plants of the Gods: Origins of Hallucinogenic Use. Richard Evans Schultes and Albert Hofmann. 1979. New York: McGraw Hill Book Company.

Note: The quotation, "Drink this and gods will enter . . . " is sheer imagination. It is the only direct quote in the book that is not derived either from a published source or direct personal communication. There is, however, a whole literature devoted to the importance in early religions of substances that affect the mind when ingested.

Neurobiology of androgen abuse. Richard E. Harlan and Meredith M. Garcia. In *Drugs of Abuse and Neurobiology.* Ronald R. Watson, editor. Boca Raton, FL: CRC Press.

The effects of fat and cholesterol on social behavior in monkeys. Jay R. Kaplan, Stephen B. Manuck, and Carol Shively. 1991. *Psychosomatic Medicine.* 53:634–642.

Social behavior and gender in biomedical investigations using monkeys: studies in atherogenesis. Jay R. Kaplan, Michael R. Adams, Thomas B. Clarkson, Stephen B. Manuck, and Carol A. Shively. 1991. *Laboratory Animal Science.* 41:1–9.

Effects of a low fat diet on brain serotonergic responsivity in cynomolgus monkeys. Matthew F. Muldoon, Jay R. Kaplan, Stephen B. Manuck, and J. John Mann. 1992. *Biological Psychiatry.* 31:739–742.

The brain re-maps its own contours. Research News by Marcia Barinaga. *Science.* Vol. 258, Oct. 9, 1992.

Selected psychological characteristics of anabolic-androgenic steroid users. Letter to the editor. Michael S. Bahrke, James E. Wright, John S. O'Connor, Richard H. Strauss, and Don H. Catlin. 1990. *New England Journal of Medicine.* 323:834–835.

Estimated prevalence of anabolic steroid use among male high school seniors. W. E. Buckley, C. E. Yesalis, K. E. Friedl, et al. 1988. *Journal of the American Medical Association.* 260:3441–3445.
Editorial on anabolic steroids. 1993. *American Journal of Sports Medicine.* 21:337.

"Current Concepts" article on anabolic steroids and growth hormone. Herbert A. Haupt. 1993. *American Journal of Sports Medicine.* 21:468–474.

Viewpoint: Might treatment of hypercholesterolemia increase non-cardiac mortality? Michael F. Oliver. 1991. *Lancet.* 337:1529.

Lowering cholesterol concentrations and mortality: a quantitative review of primary prevention trials. Matthew F. Muldoon, Stephen B. Manuck, and Karen A. Mathews. 1990. *British Medical Journal.* 301:309–314.

The effects of fat and cholesterol on social behavior in monkeys. R. Kaplan, Stephen B. Manuck, and Carol Shively. 1991. *Psychosomatic Medicine.* 53:634–642.

Anabolic-androgenic steroids: effects on social behavior and baseline heart rate. W. Jack Rejeski, Edward Gregg, Jay R. Kaplan, and Stephen B. Manuck. 1990. *Health Psychology.* 1990:774–791.

The New York Times. Letter to editors. Sept. 18, 1992. From Peter R. Breggin, Director, Center for the Study of Psychiatry, Bethesda, and Norman G. Finkelstein, Professor, General Studies Program, New York University. Both letters are on the withdrawal of funding from U. Maryland study of violence conference in 1992.

Differential rearing conditions in rats: effects on neurochemistry in neocortical areas and cognitive behaviors. Trond Myhrer, Laila Utsikt, Jorunn Fjelland, Evy Grini Iverson, and Frode Fonnum. 1992. *Brain Research Bulletin.* 28:427–434.

Current perspectives on anabolic-androgenic steroid abuse. Scott E. Lucas. 1993. *Trends in Pharmacological Sciences.* 14:61–67.

Memory and the brain. M. R. Rosenzweig. 1984. *American Psychologist.* 39:365–376.

Effects of environmental complexity and training on brain chemistry and anatomy. M. R. Rosenzweig, et al. 1962. *Journal of Comparative and Physiological Psychology.* 55:429–437.

How scary things get that way. Research News by Marcia Barinaga. 1992. *Science.* 258:887–888.

Neurobiology of androgen abuse. R. Harlan and M. Garcia. In *Drugs of Abuse and Neurobiology.* R. R. Watson, editor. 1992. Boca Raton, FL: CRC Press. 185–207.

Physical Control of the Mind: Toward a Psychocivilized Society. Jose M.R. Delgado. 1969. New York: Harper Colophon Books.

Violence and the Brain. Vernon H. Mark and Frank R. Ervin. 1972. New York: Harper and Row.

Our changing ideas about steroid effects on an ever-changing brain. Bruce S. McEwen. 1991. *Seminars in Neuroscience.* 3:497–507.

Decade of the Brain. Proclamation 6158, July 17, 1990. By the President of the United States of America, proclaiming the 1990s the Decade of the Brain.

Neuron. Sanford L. Palay and Victoria Chan-Palay. *Encyclopedia of Neuroscience.* Vol. 2. 1987. George Adelman, editor. Basel: Birkhaeuser Verlag. p. 812.

Improvement in symptoms of depression and in an index of life stressors accompany treatment of severe hyper-triglyceridemia. Charles J. Glueck, Murray Tiegar, Robert Kunkel, Trent Tracy, James Speirs, Patricia Streicher, and Ellen Illig. 1993. *Biological Psychiatry.* 34:240–252.

The Social Brain. Michael S. Gazzaniga. 1985. New York: Basic Books, Inc.

Discovering the Brain. Sandra Ackerman. 1992. Washington, DC: Institute of Medicine, National Academy of Sciences.
Scientific American. Sept. 1992. Special issue devoted to the mind and brain.

Differential rearing conditions in rats: effects on neurochemistry in neocortical areas and cognitive behaviors. Trond Myhrer, et al. 1992. *Brain Research Bulletin.* 28:427–434.

He cites M. R. Rosenzweig, Experience, memory and the brain. 1984. *American Psychologist*. 39:365–376; and M. R. Rosenzweig, et al., Effects of environmental complexity and training on brain chemistry and anatomy: a replication and extension. 1962. *Journal of Comparative and Physiological Psychology*. 55:429–437. All this is pursuant to the statement that " . . . environmental factors can modify several aspects of the central nervous system." Rosenzweig and co-workers demonstrated some decades ago that rats housed in enriched environments displayed increased brain weight, higher levels of acetylcholinesterase in neocortex, and an increased number of dendritic spines compared to control rats reared in isolated social environments. The brain measures were found to correlate positively with learning and memory.

CHAPTER 2

AIDS brain research broadens in search of mechanisms. Celia Hooper. *Journal of NIH Research*. Nov. 1991, 17–19. "Hypotheses on homosexuality and the hypothalamus." Celia Hooper. *Journal of NIH Research*. Nov. 1991, 20–21.

Sexual dimorphism in the preoptic area of the rat. Geoffrey Raisman and Pauline M. Field. 1971. *Science*. 173:20.

An enlarged suprachiasmatic nucleus in homosexual men. D. F. Swaab and M. A. Hofman. 1990. *Brain Research*. 537:141.

Is homosexuality biologically determined? *Current Contents*, May 25, 1992. Institute for Scientific Information. *Current Comments*, by Eugene Garfield, based on an article in *Search*, The Rockefeller University magazine, Spring 1992, vol. 2, no.1.

Is homosexuality hard wired? Editorial by John Maddox. 1991. *Nature*. 353:13.

A difference in hypothalamic structure between heterosexual and homosexual men. Simon LeVay. 1991. *Science*. 253:1034–1037.

The five sexes. Anne Fausto-Sterling. *The Sciences*. March/April 1993, 20–24.

Mice can do without male genes. *New Scientist*, Nov. 5, 1981.

Two sexually dimorphic cell groups in the human brain. Laura S. Allen, Melissa Hines, James E. Shryne, and Roger A. Gorski. 1989. *Journal of Neuroscience*. 9:497–506.

Sexual orientation and the size of the anterior commissure in the human brain. Laura S. Allen and Roger A. Gorski. *Proceedings of the National Academy of Sciences USA*. August 1, 1992.

Sexual dimorphism of the anterior commissure and massa intermedia of the human brain. Laura S. Allen and Roger A. Gorski. 1991. *Journal of Comparative Neurology*. 312:97–104.

Sex determination and the generation of sexually dimorphic nervous systems. Jonathan Hodgkin. 1991. *Neuron*. 6:177–185.

Sex determination in marsupials: evidence for a marsupial-eutherian dichotomy. M. B. Renfree and R. V. Short. 1988. *Philosophical Transactions of the Royal Society of London B Biological Sciences*. 322:41–53.

Sex survey of American men finds 1% are gay. Felicity Barringer. *The New York Times*, April 15, 1993. Page A-1, 16. Survey done for the Guttmacher Institute by Battelle.

A gene mapping to the sex-determining region of the mouse Y chromosome is a member of a novel family of embryonically expressed genes. John Gubbay, et al. 1990. *Nature*. 346:245–250.

A gene from the human sex-determining region encodes a protein with homology to a conserved DNA-binding motif. Andrew H. Sinclair, et al. 1990. *Nature*. 346:240–244.

Male development of chromosomally female mice transgenic for Sry. Peter Koopman, John Gubbay, Nigel Vivian, Peter Goodfellow, and Robin Lovell-Badge. 1991. *Nature*. 351:117–121.

The New York Times. Op Ed, Dec. 17, 1991, by Michael Bailey, Assistant Professor of Psychology at Northwestern University, and Richard Pillard, Associate Professor of Psychiatry at Boston University School of Medicine.

A linkage between DNA markers on the X chromosome and male sexual orientation. Dean H. Hamer, Stella Hu, Victoria L. Magnuson, Nan Hu, and Angela M. L. Pattatucci. 1993. *Science*. 261:321–327.

Steroid and thyroid hormones modulate a changing brain. Bruce S. McEwen, et al. 1991. *Journal of Steroid Biochemistry and Molecular Biology*. 40:1–14.

Re-examination of the glucocorticoid hypothesis of stress and aging. Bruce S. McEwen. 1992. *Progress in Brain Research*. 93: 365–383.

Our changing ideas about steroid effects on an ever-changing brain. Bruce S. McEwen. 1991. *Seminars in Neuroscience*. 3:497–507.

News and Views: Developmental biology: insects are constructed piecemeal. Peter A. Lawrence and Gines Morata. 1993. *Nature*. 366:305.

Developmental Anatomy. A Textbook and Laboratory Manual of Embryology. 7th edition. Leslie Brainerd Arey. 1965. Philadelphia: W. B. Saunders Company.

On Development. The Biology of Form. John Tyler Bonner. 1974. Cambridge, MA: Harvard University Press.

Human Structure. Matt Cartmill, William L. Hylander, and James Shaftland. 1987. Cambridge, MA: Harvard University Press.

From Egg to Adult. A Report from the Howard Hughes Medical Institute. Maya Pines, editor.

Behavioral research: sex surveys come out of the closet. 1993. *Science*. 260:615.

CHAPTER 3

Molecular Biology of the Cell. Bruce Alberts, Dennis Bray, Julian Lewis, Martin Raff, Keith Roberts, and James D. Watson. 1983. New York: Garland Publishing, Inc.

Molecular Cell Biology. James Darnell, Harvey Lodish, and David Baltimore. 1986. New York: Scientific American Books.

Cytogenetics and Cell Genetics. Human Gene Mapping 10. New Haven Conference. 10th International Workshop on Human Gene Mapping. 1989. Basel: S. Karger AG.

The sex-determining region of the human Y chromosome encodes a finger protein. D. C. Page, et al. *Cell*. 51:1091–1104.

A gene mapping to the sex-determining region of the mouse Y chromosome is a member of a novel family of embryonically expressed genes. John Gubbay, et al. 1990. *Nature*. 346:245–250.

A gene from the human sex-determining region encodes a protein with homology to a conserved DNA-binding motif. Andrew H. Sinclair, et al. 1990. *Nature*. 346:240–244.

Male development of chromosomally female mice transgenic for Sry. Peter Koopman, John Gubbay, Nigel Vivian, Peter Goodfellow, and Robin Lovell-Badge. 1991. *Nature*. 351:117–121.

Dr. David Thaler, The Rockefeller University, provided valuable suggestions for the design of the figure showing types of mutations.

Gene Expression in the Mammalian Brain. J. Gregor Sutcliffe. *Encyclopedia of Neuroscience*. Vol. 1. 1987. George Adelman, editor. Basel: Birkhaeuser Verlag. pp. 454–455.

Alzheimer's disease: a cell biological perspective. Kenneth S. Kosik. 1992. *Science*. 256:780–783. (The amyloid deposits appear to be important in the disease process, but whether they are part of the ultimate cause or one of the effects of Alzheimer's disease is still unknown.)

Chloroplast DNA sequence from a miocene Magnolia species. E. M. Golenberg, et al. 1990. *Nature*. 344: 656–658. Reference for the magnolia statement in this chapter.

Human CCAAT displacement protein is homologous to the *Drosophila* protein. E. J. Neufeld, D. G. Skalnik, P. M. Lievens, and S. H. Orkin. 1992. *Nature Genetics*. 1:50–55. "An unexpected connection between a human protein linked to white blood cell maturation and a fruit fly protein that directs embryonic neural development may provide general lessons in regulation of developmental genes."

Steroid hormones are multifunctional messengers to the brain. Bruce S. McEwen. 1991. *Trends in Endocrinology and Metabolism*. 2:62–67.

Selfish genes: the phenotype paradigm and genome evolution. W. Ford Doolittle and Carmen Sapienza. 1980. *Nature*. 284: No. 5757.

Recombinant DNA and medical progress. John D. Baxter. *Hospital Practice*. February 1980.

The Transforming Principle. Discovering that Genes Are Made of DNA. Maclyn McCarty. 1985. New York: W.W. Norton & Company.

The Molecular Biology of the Cell. Bruce Alberts, Dennis Bray, Julian Lewis, Martin Raff, Keith Roberts, and James D. Watson. 1983. Garland Publishing, Inc.

Recombinant DNA, A Short Course. James D. Watson, John Tooze, and David T. Kurtz. 1983. W. H. Freeman and Company.

The Morbid Anatomy of the Human Genome. A Review of Gene Mapping in Clinical Medicine. Victor A. McKusick. 1988. Howard Hughes Medical Institute.

The new genetics. Harold M. Schmeck, Jr. *Medical and Health Annual 1981*. Encyclopaedia Britannica, Inc.

A Century of DNA. Franklin S. Portugal and Jack S. Cohen. 1977. Cambridge, MA: MIT Press.

The Biology of Mental Disorders. Fourth in the series *New Developments in Neuroscience*. U.S. Congress. Office of Technology Assessment. Sept. 1992. Twin study notes manic depressive illness shows 80% concordance in identical twins, only 16% for fraternal twins.

CHAPTER 4

Explorers of the Brain. Leonard A. Stevens. 1971. New York: Alfred A. Knopf. Pages 55–59 are on Golgi and Cajal.

The science of nervous systems: a historical sketch. In *Neurophilosophy*. P. S. Churchland. 1986. Cambridge, MA: MIT Press.

Neurobiology of androgen abuse. Richard E. Harlan and Meredith M. Garcia. In *Drugs of Abuse and Neurobiology*. Ronald R. Watson, editor. Boca Raton, FL: CRC Press.

Neuroscience Encyclopedia. 1987. George Adelman, editor. Basel: Birkhaeuser Verlag. Vol. 1, page 470, "The Golgi Method" by Miguel Marin-Padill, says it was developed in 1873 and is still one of the best techniques available for study of the "fibrilloneuronal architecture of the nervous system."

Interactions between hormones and nerve tissue. Bruce S. McEwen. 1976. *Scientific American*. July: 48–58.

The CIBA Collection of Medical Illustrations. Vol. 1, "Nervous System." F. H. Netter. 1957.

The CIBA Collection of Medical Illustrations. Vol. 4, "Endocrine System." F. H. Netter. 1965.

Search. The Rockefeller University Magazine. Annual report. Vol.1, No.4, Winter 1991.

Steroid hormones and the brain: linking nature and nurture. Bruce S. McEwen. *Neurochemical Research*. 13:663–669.

Anabolic-androgenic steroids: effects on social behavior and baseline heart rate. W. Jack Rejeski, Edward Gregg, Jay R. Kaplan, and Stephen B. Manuck. 1990. *Health Psychology*. 9:774–791.

Steroid hormones are multifunctional messengers to the brain. Bruce S. McEwen. 1991. *Trends in Endocrinology and Metabolism.* 2:62–67.

Non-genomic and genomic effects of steroids on neural activity. Bruce S. McEwen. 1991. *Trends in Pharmacological Sciences.* 12:141–147.

Steroid and thyroid hormones modulate a changing brain. Bruce S. McEwen. 1991. *Journal of Steroid Biochemistry and Molecular Biology.* 40:1–14.

Our changing ideas about steroid effects on an ever-changing brain. Bruce S. McEwen. 1991. *Seminars in Neuroscience.* 3:497–507.

Evidence for impaired activation of the hypothalamo-pituitary-adrenal axis in patients with chronic fatigue syndrome. M. A. Demitrack, et al. 1991. *Journal of Clinical Endocrinology and Metabolism.* 73:1224–1234.

Philip W. Gold, et al. *Journal of Clinical Endocrinology and Metabolism.* December 1991. (Hormone deficiencies in chronic fatigue syndrome.)

CHAPTER 5

Anabolic-androgenic steroids: effects on social behavior and baseline heart rate. W. Jack Rejeski, Edward Gregg, Jay R. Kaplan, and Stephen B. Manuck. 1990. *Health Psychology.* 9:774–791. (24 monkeys: the steroids "disrupted the social milieu such that all dominant animals exhibited increases in dominant behavior and subordinates manifested increased submission.") They cite a study by Buckley et al. (1988) estimating that 6.6% of all male sixth graders have had experience with anabolic-androgenic steroids.

Stress and the individual: mechanisms leading to disease. Bruce S. McEwen and Eliot Stellar. *Archives of Internal Medicine.* 153: 2093–2101.

Is this relevant to the human? Chapter 14, *Stress, the Aging Brain, and the Mechanisms of Neuron Death.* Robert M. Sapolsky. 1992. Cambridge, MA: MIT Press.

Depression: the predisposing influence of stress. Hymie Anisman and Robert M. Zacharko. 1982. *Behavioral and Brain Sciences.* 5:89–137.

Steroid hormones are multifunctional messengers to the brain. Bruce S. McEwen. 1991. *Trends in Endocrinology and Metabolism.* 2:62–67.

Steroid and thyroid hormones modulate a changing brain. Bruce S. McEwen, et al. 1991. *Journal of Steroid Biochemistry and Molecular Biology* 40:1–14.

Re-examination of the glucocorticoid hypothesis of stress and aging. Bruce S. McEwen. 1992. *Progress in Brain Research.* 93:365–383.

Stress in the wild. Robert M. Sapolsky. 1990. *Scientific American.* 262:116–123.

The New York Times, Feb. 14, 1993, p. 37.
   Miami. A killer's bid to save his life by claiming that he is a victim of lingering trauma from service in Vietnam has stirred the sympathy of fellow veterans and focused attention on what is known as posttraumatic stress disorder.
   (The Vietnam vet killed a gas station attendant fourteen years ago. At a clemency hearing last year, mental health experts testified that Mr. Johnson, the killer, could have acted without control while reliving a traumatic experience in the war. Gov. Lawton Chiles gave him a stay of execution while reviewing the case.)

Science News, Feb. 13, 1993, Vol. 143, p. 108, says doctors and lawyers have worried that "many criminal defendants might improperly claim" that PTSD "rendered them insane and not accountable for their behavior." But this appears not to have happened according to "the largest study of the insanity defense to date" which covered 8,163 defendants pleading not guilty by reason of insanity. Only twenty-eight had a diagnosis of PTSD. This was published in *American Journal of Psychiatry*, Feb 1993, by Paul S. Applebaum, a psychiatrist at University of Massachusetts Medical Center in Worcester.

The New York Times, May 10, 1993, p. A-20.

Starke, FL. A Vietnam veteran diagnosed with posttraumatic stress disorder was executed Saturday night in the electric chair for the 1979 killing of a gas station attendant. The prisoner, Larry Joe Johnson, had been in a Navy construction unit in Vietnam. Honorably discharged. Served later in Kentucky National Guard where he was injured by a smoke grenade that, the story said, damaged his brain. Supreme Court denied two petitions.

Months earlier, Gov. Lawton Chiles had ordered a review of the case case and afterwards issued another death warrant. Evidently in April he said he recognized the "Vietnam veteran syndrome" but didn't think it applied in this case.

Hypothalamic-pituitary-adrenal dysfunction in posttraumatic stress disorder. Rachel Yehuda, Earl L. Giller, Steven M. Southwick, Martin T. Lowy, and John W. Mason. 1991. *Biological Psychiatry*. 30:1031–1048. This group studied the hypothalamic-pituitary-adrenal axis in PTSD because "the HPA axis is one of the major hormonal systems mediating the stress response."

Paradoxical effects of adrenal steroids on the brain: protection versus degeneration. Bruce S. McEwen, et al. 1992. *Biological Psychiatry*. 31:177–199.

Phenytoin prevents stress- and corticosterone-induced atrophy of CA3 pyramidal neurons. Yoshifumi Watanabe, Elizabeth Gould, Heather A. Cameron, Deborah C. Daniels, and Bruce S. McEwen. 1992. *Hippocampus*. 2:431–435.

Hypothalamic-pituitary-adrenal dysregulation associated with a high fat diet. B. M. Tannenbaum, D. N. Brindley, M. F. Dallman, and M.J . Meaney. 1992. *Society for Neuroscience Abstracts*. 18:643.6.

Altered cortisol response to stress after four months practice of the transcendental meditation program. Kenneth Walton. 1992. *Society for Neuroscience Abstracts*. 18:643.6.

Personal communications from Terence Keane.

Posttraumatic stress disorder. The stressor criterion. Naomi Breslau and Glenn C. Davis. 1987. *Journal of Nervous and Mental Disease*. Vol. 175, No. 5, Serial No. 1254.
Efficacy of treatments for post-traumatic stress disorder. An empirical review. Susan D. Solomon, Ellen T. Gerrity, and Allison M. Muff. 1992. *Journal of the American Medical Association*. 268:633–638.

Elevation of urinary norepinephrine/cortisol ratio in posttraumatic stress disorder. John W. Mason, Earl L. Giller, Thomas R. Kosten, and Laurie Harkness. 1988. *Journal of Nervous and Mental Disease*. 176:498–502. Doctors at Yale University and the West Haven Veterans Adminstration Medical Center in Connecticut found unusually high levels of the stimulant hormone adrenalin, now known as epinephrine and its companion chemical norepinephrine in the urine of PTSD patients.

Nonhuman primate model of alcohol abuse: effects of early experience, personality, and stress on alcohol consumption. J. D. Higley, M. F. Hasert, S. J. Suomi, and M. Linnoila. 1991. *Proceedings of the National Academy of Sciences USA*. 88:7261–7265.

The Swedish childhood diabetes study: indications of severe psychological stress as a risk factor for type 1 (insulin-dependent) diabetes mellitus in childhood. B. Hagglof, L. Blom, G. Dahlquist, G. Lonnberg, and B. Sahlin. 1991. *Diabetologia*. 34:579–583.

Stress and the brain. Joseph Carey. 1991. *Brain Concepts, Society for Neuroscience*.

Science News. Vol. 144, p. 196. Sept. 25, 1993. "Psychological stress linked to cancer." (Citing September 1993 *Epidemiology*, a report by Joseph G. Courtney et al. based on a large Swedish data base on patients in the Stockholm area. "Those who reported a history of workplace problems over the past 10 years faced 5.5 times the colorectal cancer risk of adults who reported no such problems.")

CHAPTER 6

Trauma-related symptoms in veterans of Operation Desert Storm: a preliminary report. Steven M. Southwick, Andrew Morgan, Linda M. Nagy, Douglas Brenner, Andreas L. Nicolaou, David R. Johnson, Robert Rosenheck, and Dennis S. Charney. 1993. *American Journal of Psychiatry*. 150:10.

Survivors of imprisonment in the Pacific Theater during World War II. G. Goldstein, W. van Kammen, C. Shelley, D. J. Miller, and D. P. van Kammen. 1987. *American Journal of Psychiatry*. 144:1210–1213.

Stress and the individual: mechanisms leading to disease. Bruce S. McEwen and Eliot Stellar. *Archives of Internal Medicine*. 153:2093–2101.

Forty-year follow up of United States prisoners of war. J. C. Kluznik, N. Speed, C. Van Valkenburg, and R. Magraw. 1987. *American Journal of Psychiatry*. 144:1210–1213.

Efficacy of treatments for posttraumatic stress disorder. An empirical review. Susan D. Solomon, Ellen T. Gerrity, and Alyson M. Muff. 1992. *Journal of the American Medical Association*. 268:633–638. Source for "One interesting common finding has been that people in the long-term grip of PTSD seldom get much help from placebos."

The cycle of violence. C. S. Widom. 1989. *Science*. 244:160–166.

Personal communications, Terence Keane.

Posttraumatic stress disorder. The stressor criterion. Naomi Breslau and Glenn C. Davis. 1987. *Journal of Nervous and Mental Disease*. Vol. 175, No.5, Serial No. 1254.

Hypothalamic-pituitary-adrenal dysfunction in posttraumatic stress sisorder. Rachel Yehuda, Earl L. Giller, Steven M. Southwick, Martin T. Lowy, and John W. Mason. 1991. *Biological Psychiatry*. 30:1031–1048.

Elevation of urinary norepinephrine/cortisol ratio in posttraumatic stress disorder. John W. Mason, Earl L. Giller, Thomas R. Kosten, and Laurie Harkness. 1988. *Journal of Nervous and Mental Disease*. 176:498–502.

Autonomic responses to stress in Vietnam combat veterans with posttraumatic stress disorder. Miles E. McFall, M. Michele Murburg, Grant N. Ko, and Richard C. Vieth. 1990. *Biological Psychiatry*. 27:1165–1175.

The role of the amygdala in fear and anxiety. Michael Davis. 1992. *Annual Review of Neuroscience*. 15:353–375.

A triune concept of the brain and behavior. Paul D. MacLean. 1973. Hincks Memorial Lectures (1969). T. J. Boag and D. Campbell, editors. Toronto: University of Toronto Press.

How scary things get that way. Research News by Marcia Barinaga. 1992. *Science*. 258:887–888.

CCK in animal and human research on anxiety. Jaanus Harro and Jacques Bradwejn. 1993. *Trends in Pharmacological Sciences*. 14:244–249.

The central amygdala is involved in conditioning but not in retention of active and passive shock avoidance in male rats. B. Roozendaal, J. M. Koolhaas, and B. Bohus. 1993. *Behavioral and Neural Biology*. 59:143–149.

Central amygdaloid involvement in neuroendocrine correlates of conditioned stress responses. B. Roozendaal, J. M. Koolhaas, and B. Bohus. *Journal of Neuroendocrinology*. 4:483–489.

Diferential contribution of amygdala and hippocampus to cued and contextual fear conditioning. R. G. Phillips and J. E. LeDoux. 1992. *Behavioral Neuroscience*. 106:274–285.

Stress and the individual: mechanisms leading to disease. Bruce S. McEwen and Eliot Stellar. 1993. *Archives of Internal Medicine*. 153:2093–2101.

Allostasis: a new paradigm to explain arousal pathology. Handbook of life stress. Peter Sterling and Joseph Eyer. 1988. Chapter 34. *Cognition and Health*. New York: John Wiley & Sons, Inc.

Hippocampal formation volume, memory dysfunction, and cortisol levels in patients with Cushing's syndrome. Monica N. Starkman, Stephen S. Gebarski, Stanley Berent, and David E. Schteingart. 1992. *Biological Psychiatry*. 32:756–765.

Endocrine activity in air controllers at work. I. Characterization of cortisol and growth hormone levels during the day. Robert M. Rose, C. David Jenkins, Michael Hurst, Linda Livingston, and Rogers P. Hall. 1992. *Psychoneuroendocrinology*. 7:101–111.

The Breaking of Bodies and Minds. Torture, Psychiatric Abuse and the Health Professions. Eric Stover and Elena O. Nightinggale, editors. 1985. W. H. Freeman and Company.

A functional anatomical study of unipolar depression. Wayne C. Drevets, Tom O. Videen, Joseph L. Price, Sheldon H. Preskorn, S. Thomas Carmichael, and Marcus E. Raichle. 1992. *Journal of Neuroscience.* 12:3628–3641.

CHAPTER 7

Witchcraft and lupus erythematosus. Case report. Richard A. Kirkpatrick. 1981. *Journal of the American Medical Association.* 245:1937.

Penetrating the mysteries of human immunity. Harold M. Schmeck, Jr. *Medical and Health Annual 1987.* Encyclopaedia Britannica, Inc. pp. 112–127.

Effect of psychosocial treatment on survival of patients with metastatic breast cancer. David Spiegel, Joan R. Bloom, Helena C. Kraemer, and Ellen Gottheil. *Lancet.* October 14, 1989, 888–891.

The Neuro-Immune-Endocrine Connection. Carl W. Cotman, Roberta E. Brinton, Albert Galaburda, Bruce S. McEwen, and Diana M. Schneider, editors. 1987. New York: Raven Press.

Immunology—Basic and Clinical. William E. Paul and Thomas A. Waldmann. In *NIH: An Account of Research in its Laboratories and Clinics.* DeWitt Stetten, Jr., editor, and W. T. Carrigan, associate editor. 1984. New York: Academic Press, Inc.

Stress and the individual: mechanisms leading to disease. Bruce S. McEwen and Eliot Stellar. *Archives of Internal Medicine.* 153: 2093–2101.

Neuroanatomy of lymphoid tissue. K. Bulloch. 1985. In *Neural Modulation of Immunity.* R. Guillemin et al., editors. New York: Raven Press.

Life, death and the immune system. *Scientific American.* Sept. 1993. How the immune system develops. Irving L. Weissman and Max D. Cooper, pp. 65–71. Autoimmune disease. Lawrence Steinman, pp. 107–114. *A History of Immunology.* Arthur M. Silverstein. 1989. New York: Academic Press, Inc. 160 pp.

Sickness behavior. Stephen Kent, Rose-Marie Bluthé, Robert Danzer, and Keith W. Kelley. 1992. *Trends in Pharmacological Sciences.* 13:24–28.

Human CCAT displacement protein is homologous to the drosophila. E. J. Neufeld, D. G. Skalnik, P. M. Lievens, and S. H. Orkin. 1992. *Nature Genetics.* 1:50–55. Cites "An unexpected connection between a human protein linked to white blood cell maturation and a fruit fly protein that directs embryonic neural development may provide general lessons in regulation of developmental genes."

Medical intelligence. Current Concepts: Regulation of the immune response—role of the macrophage. Alan S. Rosenthal. 1980. *New England Journal of Medicine.* 303:1153–1156.

Immunology: The Many-Edged Sword. Harold M. Schmeck, Jr. 1974. George Braziller, Inc.

HLA and Disease Associations. Jawahar L. Tiwari and Paul I. Terasaki. 1985. Berlin: Springer-Verlag.

Genetic Control of Immune Responsiveness: Relationship to Disease Susceptibility. Hugh O. McDevitt and Maurice Landy, editors. 1972. New York: Academic Press, Inc.

First International Workshop on Neuroimmunomodulation, National Institutes of Health, December, 1984. Reports via Dr. Novera Herbert Spector of National Institute of Neurological and Communicative Disorders and Stroke, NIH.

Discovering the Individual. Jean Hamburger. 1978. New York: W.W. Norton, Inc.

Immunology: basic and clinical. William E. Paul and Thomas A. Waldmann. In *NIH: An Account of Research in Its Laboratories and Clinics.* DeWitt Stetten, Jr., editor, and W. T. Carrigan, associate editor. 1984. New York: Academic Press, Inc.

CHAPTER 8

The Clocks That Time Us. Physiology of the Circadian Timing System. Martin C. Moore-Ede, Frank M. Sulzman, and Charles A. Fuller. 1982. Cambridge, MA: Harvard University Press.

Biological Rhythms: Implications for the Worker. Third in the series *New Developments in Neuroscience.* U. S. Congress, Office of Technology Assessment, Sept. 1991.

Brief Report: Traveler's Amnesia—Transient Global Amnesia Secondary to Triazolam. Harold H. Morris and Melinda L. Estes. 1987. *Journal of the American Medical Association.* 258:945–946.

Phase shift in circadian rhythms produces retrograde amnesia. Walter N. Tapp and Frank A. Holloway. 1981. *Science.* 211:1056–1058.

Letters commenting on the jet lag-triazolam report in JAMA, Aug. 21, 1987. *Journal of the American Medical Association.* 259:350–352.

Next-day memory impairment with triazolam use. Edward O. Bixler, Anthony Kales, Rocco L. Manfredi, Alexandros N. Vgontzas, Kathy L. Tyson, and Joyce D. Kales. 1991. *Lancet.* 337:827–831.

Sex differences in cognitive function vary with the season. D. Kimura and C. Toussaint. 1991. *Society for Neurosciences Abstracts.* 17: 340-13.

American Journal of Cardiology. Nov. 6, 1990. A symposium issue which "provides the first compilation of reports in the emerging field of study of triggering and circadian variation of onset of acute cardiovascular disease." Introduction by James E. Muller and Geoffrey H. Tofler.

Clinical Progress Series. Circadian variation and triggers of onset of acute cardiovascular disease. James E. Muller, Geoffrey H. Tofler, and Peter H. Stone. *Circulation.* Vol. 79, No. 4, April 1989.

Transplanted suprachiasmatic nucleus determines circadian period. Martin R. Ralph, Russel G. Foster, Fred C. Davis, and Michael Menaker. 1990. *Science.* 247:975–978.

Timing of breast cancer excision during the menstrual cycle influences duration of disease-free survival. Ruby T. Senie, Paul Peter Rosen, Philip Rhodes, and Martin L. Lesser. 1991. *Annals of Internal Medicine.* 115:337–342.

Menstrual cycle timing stirs debate. Robert Carlson. *Oncology Times*, February 1991.

Jet lag and depression. Letters to editor. Letter by Leon Tec. 1981. *American Journal of Psychiatry.* 138:6.

Circadian rhythms and patterns of performance before and after simulated jet lag. Walter N. Tapp and Benjamin H. Natelson. 1989. *American Journal of Physiology.* 257:R796–R803.

Social zeitgebers and biological rhythms. A unified approach to understanding the etiology of depression. Cindy L. Ehlers, Ellen Frank, and David J. Kupfer. 1988. *Archives of General Psychiatry.* 45:948–952.

Effect of melatonin on jet lag after long haul flights. Keith Petrie, John V. Conaglen, Leonard Thompson, and Kerry Chamberlain. 1989. *British Medical Journal.* 298:705–707.

Effects of melatonin on vertebrate circadian systems. Vincent M. Cassone. 1990. *Trends in Neurosciences.* 13:457–464. Followed by an item on: Regulatory sites in the melatonin system of mammals. Diana N. Krause and Margarita L. Dubocovich.

Corticosteroids and hippocampal plasticity. Bruce S. McEwen. 1994. *Annals of the New York Academy of Sciences.* In press.

Human circadian rhythms in continuous darkness: entrainment by social cues. J. Aschoff, et al. 1971. *Science.* 171:213–215.

Effect of shift work on the night-time secretory patterns of melatonin, prolactin, cortisol and testosterone. Y. Touitou, et al. 1990. *European Journal of Applied Physiology.* 60:288–292.

Physiological changes underlying jet lag. Josephine Arendt and Vincent Marks. 1982. *British Medical Journal*. 284:144–146.

Environmental physiology. Sleep after transmeridian flights. A. N. Nicholson, M. B. Spencer, Peta A. Pascoe, Barbara M. Stone, T. Roehers, and T. Roth. *Lancet*, Nov. 22, 1986, 1205–1208.

Estrogen-related variations in human spatial and articulatory-motor skills. Elizabeth Hampson. 1990. *Psychoneuroendocrinology*. 15:97–111.

The relationship between testosterone levels and cognitive ability patterns. Catherine Gouchie and Doreen Kimura. 1991. *Psychoneuroendocrinology*. 6:323–334.

The New York Times. Feb. 5, 1992, page C-12. Cancer Surgeons Debate Timing of Breast Operations. By Elizabeth Rosenthal.

Review: The molecular biology of circadian rhythms. Michael Rosbash and Jeffrey C. Hall. 1989. *Neuron*. 3:387–398.

Intervention on coronary risk factors by adapting a shift work schedule to biologic rhythmicity. Kristina Orth-Gomer. 1983. *Psychosomatic Medicine*. 45:407–415.

Interaction of colocalized neuropeptides: functional significance in the circadian timing system. H. Elliott Albers, Shyh-Yuh Liou, Edward G. Stopa, and R. Thomas Zoeller. 1991. *Journal of Neuroscience*. 11:846–851.

Optimal time of day and the magnitude of age differences in memory. Cynthia P. May, Lynn Hasher, and Ellen R. Stoltzfus. 1993. *Psychological Science*. 4:326–330.

Variations in memory function and sex steroid hormones across the menstrual cycle. Susana M. Phillips and Barbara B. Sherwin. 1992. *Psychoneuroendocrinology*. 17: 497–506.

Diurnal variation in vasopressin and oxytocin messenger RNAs in hypothalamic nuclei of the rat. J. Peter Burbach, et al. 1988. *Molecular Brain Research*. 4:157–160.

Circadian changes in arginine vasopressin level in the suprachiasmatic nuclei in the rat. Keitaro Yamase, et al. 1991. *Neuroscience Letters*. 130:255–258.

Nuclear mechanisms mediate rhythmic changes in vasopressin mRNA expression in the rat suprachiasmatic nucleus. David A. Carter and David Murphy. 1991. *Molecular Brain Research*. 12:315–321.

Anisomycin, an inhibitor of protein synthesis, perturbs the phase of a mammalian circadian pacemaker. Joseph S. Takahashi and Fred W. Turek. 1987. *Brain Research*. 405:199–203.

Light pulses that shift rhythms induce gene expression in the suprachiasmatic nucleus. Benjamin Rusak, et al. 1990. *Science*. 248:1237–1240.

Stimulated activity mediates phase shifts in the hamster circadian clock induced by dark pulses or benzodiasepines. O. Van Reeth and F. W. Turek. 1989. *Nature*. 339:49–50.

A benzodiazepine used in the treatment of insomnia phase-shifts the mammalian circadian clock. Fred W. Turek and Susan Losee-Olson. 1986. *Nature*. 321:167–168.

Effects of diazepam on circadian phase advances and delays. Martin R. Ralph and Michael Menaker. 1986. *Brain Research*. 372:405–408.

Illuminating jet lag. Experiments show that bright light can reset the human internal clock by any desired amount, offering treatment for sleep disorders. Robert Pool. 1989. *Science*. 244:1256–1257.

Bright light induction of strong (type 0) resetting of the human circadian pacemaker. Charles A. Czeisler, et al. 1989. *Science*. 244:1328–1333.

Repeated changes of dendritic morphology in the hippocampus of ground squirrels in the course of hibernation. V. I. Popov, L. S. Bocharova, and A. G. Bragin. 1992. *Neuroscience*. 48:45–51.

Medical progress. Circadian timekeeping in health and disease. Part 1. Basic properties of circadian pacemakers. Martin C. Moore-Ede, Charles A. Czeisler, and Gary S. Richardson. 1983. *New England Journal of Medicine.* 309:469–476.

Medical progress. Circadian timekeeping in health and disease. Part 2. Clinical implications of circadian rhythmicity. Martin C. Moore-Ede, Charles A. Czeisler, and Gary S. Richardson. *New England Journal of Medicine.* 309:530–536.

Regulation of circadian rhythmicity. Joseph S. Takahashi and Martin Zatz. 1982. *Science.* 217:1104–1110.

Circadian in the frequency of onset of acute myocardial infarction. James E. Muller, Peter H. Stone, Zoltan G. Turi, John D. Rutherford, Charles Czeisler, Corette Parker, W. Kenneth Poole, Eugene Passamani, Robert Roberts, Thomas Robertson, Burton E. Sobel, James T. Willerson, Eugene Braunwald, and the MILIS Study Group. *New England Journal of Medicine*, Nov. 21, 1985.

"Dark-active" rat transformed into "light-active" rat by destruction of 24-hr clock: function of 24-hr clock and synchronizers. Curt P. Richter. 1978. *Proceedings of the National Academy of Sciences USA.* 75:6276–6280.

Bright light resets the human circadian pacemaker independent of the timing of the sleep-wake cycle. Charles A. Czeisler, et al. 1986. *Science.* 233:667–671.

Sex differences in cognitive function vary with the season. Doreen Kimura. Dept. of Psychology, University of Western Ontario. Research Bulletin No. 697.

Variations in sex related cognitive abilities across the menstrual cycle. Elizabeth Hampson. 1990. *Brain and Cognition.* 14:26–43.

Estrogen-related variations in human spatial and articulatory-motor skills. Elizabeth Hampson. 1990. *Psychoneuroendocrinology.* 15:97–111.

Reciprocal effects of hormonal fluctuations on human motor and perceptual-spatial skills. Elizabeth Hampson and Doreen Kimura. 1988. *Behavioral Neuroscience.* 102:456–459.

The relation between testosterone levels and cognitive ability patterns. Catherine Gouchie and Doreen Kimura. Dept. of Psychology, University of Western Ontario. Research Bulletin No. 690, May 1990.

Neural and hormonal mechanisms mediating sex differences in cognition. Doreen Kimura and Elizabeth Hampson. Dept. of Psychology, University of Western Ontario. Research Bulletin No. 689, April 1990.

Are men's and women's brains really different? Doreen Kimura. 1987. *Canadian Psychology.* 28:133–147.

CHAPTER 9

Memory and Brain. Larry R. Squire. 1987. Oxford: Oxford University Press.

The Biology of Memory. L. R. Squire and E. Lindenlaub, editors. 1990. Stuttgart: F. K. Schattauer Verlag. Closing remarks by L. R. Squire, pp. 644–650.

The neurobiology of learning and memory. Carl W. Cotman and Gary S. Lymch. 1989. *Cognition.* 33: 201–241.

Human amnesia and the medial temporal region: enduring memory impairment following a bilaterial lesion limited to field CA1 of the hippocampus. Stuart Zola-Morgan, Larry R. Squire, and D. G. Amaral. 1986. *Journal of Neuroscience.* 6:2950–2967.

Experiental modification of the developing brain. William T. Greenough. 1975. *American Scientist.* 63:37–46.

Synaptic reorganization in the hippocampus induced by abnormal functional activity. Thomas Sutula, He Xiao-Xian, Jose Cavazos, and Grayson Scott. 1988. *Science.* 239:1147–1150.

Remodeling of synaptic architecture during hippocampal "kindling." Yuri Geinisman, Frank Morrell, and Leyla deToledo-Morrell. 1988. *Proceedings of the National Academy of Sciences USA.* 85:3260–3264.

Chemical and anatomical plasticity of brain. Edward L. Bennett, Marian C. Diamond, David Krech, and Mark R. Rosenzweig. 1964. *Science.* 146:610–618.

Covert intelligence operations. Georgina Ferry. 1980. *New Scientist.* 31:308–311.

The medial temporal lobe memory system. Larry R. Squire and Stuart Zola-Morgan. 1991. *Science.* 253:1380–1386.

Memory: organization of brain systems and cognition. L. R. Squire, S. Zola-Morgan, C. B. Cave, F. Haist, G. Musen, and W. A. Suzuki. 1990. *Cold Spring Harbor Symposia on Quantitative Biology.* LV:1007–1023.

The malleability of human memory. Elizabeth F. Loftus. 1979. *American Scientist.* 67:312–320.

The brain: mechanics of memory. Shigetada Nakanishi, Elias K. Michaelis, and Mark L. Mayer. *Nature,* Nov. 7, 1991, p. 31.

Activation of the hippocampus in normal humans: a functional anatomical study of memory. Larry R. Squire, J. G. Ojemann, F. M Miezin, S. E. Peterson, T. O. Videen, and M. E. Raichle. 1992. *Proceedings of the National Academy of Sciences USA.* 89:1837–1841.

The New York Times, Dec. 21, 1970, pp. 1 and 34. Depths of brain probed for sources of violence. Harold M. Schmeck, Jr.

The New York Times, Jan. 16, 1992, p. B-9. Study detects brain abnormality in patients with chronic fatigue. Lawerence K. Altman.

A triune concept of the brain and behavior. Paul D. MacLean. 1973. Hincks Memorial Lectures. T. J. Boag and D. Campbell, editors. Toronto: University of Toronto Press.

Neural subsystems for object knowledge. A critical issue in cognitive neuroscience. *Nature*, Sept. 3, 1992, p. 60.

The New York Times, Jan. 28, 1992, p. C-1. A brain cell surprise: genes don't set function. Natalie Angier.

Widespread dispersion of neuronal clones across functional regions in the cerebral cortex. Christopher Walsh and Constance L. Cepko. 1992. *Science.* 255:434–440.

Cell milieu directs cortex development. Research by Constance Cepko and Christopher Walsh. *Harvard Focus*, Jan. 23, 1992.

The role of the amygdala in fear and anxiety. Michael Davis. 1992. *Annual Review of Neuroscience.* 15:353–375.

Nature, Sept. 17, 1992, p. 181. A letter by Dolph Schluter on the brain size debate calls the differences between men and women and between races a statistical artifact.

How scary things get that way. Research News by Marcia Barinaga. *Science,* Vol. 258, Nov. 6, 1992, pp. 887–888.

Hemispheric specialization for skilled perceptual organization by chessmasters. Christopher F. Chabris and Sania E. Hamilton. 1992. *Neuropsychologia.* 30:47–57.

Personal communication, Larry R. Squire, March 3, 1992, at VA Medical Center, San Diego.

Neurotropic factors. Wilfried E. Seifert. 1985. *Endeavor.* 9:183–190.

The Mystery of the Mind. Wilder Penfield. 1975. Princeton: Princeton University Press.

Something Hidden. A Biography of Wilder Penfield. Jefferson Lewis. 1981. New York: Doubleday.

Mapping the Brain and its Functions. Integrating Enabling Technologies into Neuroscience Research. 1991. Constance M. Pechura and Joseph B. Martin, editors. Institute of Medicine. National Academy Press.

CHAPTER 10

David Thaler, The Rockefeller University, kindly provided suggestions regarding the first figure.

Handbook of Autism and Pervasive Developmental Disorders. Donald J. Cohen and Anne M. Donnellan, editors; Rhea Paul, associate editor. 1987. Silver Spring, MD: V. H. Winston & Sons. A Wiley Interscience Publication.

Neuroanatomic imaging in autism. Eric Courchesne. 1991. Supplement, pp. 781–790, on neuroanatomic imaging, from *Pediatrics.* Copyright American Academy of Pediatrics.

Brainstem and cerebellar vermis involvement in autistic children. Toshiaki Hashimoto, Masanobu Tayama, Masahito Miyazaki, Kazuyoshi Murakawa, and Yasuhiro Kuroda. 1993. *Journal of Child Neurology.* 8:149–153.

The Fatal Shore. The Epic of Australia's Founding. Robert Hughes. 1988. New York: Vintage Books, a division of Random House.

Postnatal development of the visual cortex and the influence of environment. Torsten N. Wiesel. 1982. *Nature.* 299:583–592.

The visual cortex of the brain. David H. Hubel. *Scientific American,* Dec. 1963.

Science, technology and man: population and education. Lord Vaizey of Greenwich. In *Science and Future Choice.* Vol. 2, *Technological Challenges for Social Change.* 1979. Philip W. Hemily and M. N. Ozdas, editors. Oxford: Oxford University Press.

Hippocampus and memory for food caches in black-capped chickadees. 1989. David F. Sherry and A.L. Vaccarino. *Behavioral Neuroscience.* 103:308–318.

Repeated changes of dendritic morphology in the hippocampus of ground squirrels in the course of hibernation. V. Popov, L. Bocharova, and A. Bragin. 1992. *Neuroscience.* 48:45–51.

The visual cortex of normal and deprived monkeys. David Hubel. 1979. *American Scientist.* 67:532–543.

Thirty-first Faculty Research Lecture, University of California, San Francisco, April 7, 1988. The lecture was given by Michael M. Merzenich.

The brain remaps its own contours. Research News by Marcia Barinaga. 1992. *Science.* 258: 216–218.

Steroid hormones and the brain: linking nature and nurture. Bruce S. McEwen. *Neurochemical Research.* 13:663–669.

Commentary: Adrenal steroid influences on the survival of hippocampal neurons. Bruce S. McEwen and Elizabeth Gould. 1990. *Biochemical Pharmacology.* 40:2393–2402.

The New York Times, Sept. 5, 1992, p. 1. Agency rejects study linking genes to crime. Philip J. Hilts.

Violence research: NIH told to reconsider crime meeting. 1993. *Science.* 262:23.

The role of inheritance in behavior. Robert Plomin. 1990. *Science.* 248:183–188.

Genetics of alcoholism. Eric J. Devor and C. Robert Cloninger. 1989. *Annual Review of Genetics.* 23:19–36.

Human behavioral genetics. Robert Plomin and Richard Rende. 1991. *Annual Review of Psychology.* 42:161–190.

Perspectives on Human Deprivation: Biological, Psychological and Sociological. National Institute of Child Health and Human Development, NIH, U. S. DHEW. 1968.

Autism. Uta Frith. *Scientific American,* June 1993, p. 108–114.

Trends in behavioral genetics: eugenics revisited. John Horgan. *Scientific American,* June 1993, p. 122–131.

Aging twins offer clues to late-onset diseases. David Ansley. 1993. *Science.* 259:1826–1828.

Why divorce runs in families. From Minnesota Twin Studies. 1992. *Science.* 258:1734.

CHAPTER 11

Inherited disorders of amino acid metabolism. Leon E. Rosenberg. 1988. In *Harrison's Principles of Internal Medicine*, 11th edition. New York: McGraw Hill.

Genetics. Raymond L. Teplitz. 1981. *Journal of the American Medical Association.* 245:2191–2193.

Blood: Bearer of Life and Death. New Ways to Fight Disease Caused by Faults in the Bloodstream. A report from the Howard Hughes Medical Institute. 1993. Maya Pines, editor.

The ultimate therapy for blood disorders: new genes. Harold M. Schmeck, Jr. Presentation by W. French Anderson at a conference on gene therapy held at the National Institutes of Health, Bethesda, MD, October,1992.

Curing Disease through Human Gene Therapy. National Heart, Lung and Blood Institute, National Institutes of Health. NIH Publication No.93-2888. July 1993.

Bilateral fetal mesencephalic grafting in two patients with parkinsonism induced by 1-methyl-4-phenyl-1,2,3,6-tetrahyrdopyridine (MPTP). Hakan Widner, James Tetrud, Stig Rehncrona, Barry Snow, Patrik Brundin, Bjorn Gustavii, Anders Björklund, Olle Lindvall, and J. William Langston. 1992. *New England Journal of Medicine.* 327:1556–1563. MPTP is short for 1-methyl-4-phenyl-1,2,3,6-tetrahydropyridine.

Unilateral transplantation of human fetal mesencephalic tissue into the caudate nucleus of patients with Parkinson's disease. Dennis D. Spencer, Richard J. Robbins, Frederick Naftolin, Kenneth L. Marek, Timothy Vollmer, Csaba Leranth, Robert H. Roth, Lawrence H. Price, Albert Gjedde, Benjamin S. Bunney, Kimberlee J. Sass, John D. Elsworth, E. Leon Kier, Robert Makuch, Paul B. Hoffer, and D. Eugene Redmond, Jr. 1992. *New England Journal of Medicine.* 327:1541–1548.

Survival of implanted fetal dopamine cells and neurologic improvement 12 to 46 months after transplantation for Parkinson's disease. C. R. Freed, et al. 1992. *New England Journal of Medicine.* 327:1549–1555.

Editorials by Stanley Fahn and by Jerome P. Kassirer and Marcia Angell, and a Sounding Board article, "Are there really alternatives to the use of fetal tissue from elective abortions in transplantation research?" by Daniel J. Garry, Arthur L. Caplan, Dorothy E. Vawter, and Warren Kearne. 1992. *New England Journal of Medicine.* 327:1589–1595.

Neural Grafting: Repairing the Brain and Spinal Cord. October 1990. Second in the series *New Developments in Neuroscience.* U. S. Congress, Office of Technology Assessment.

Location of Parkinson's degeneration in brain. In *Pathology.* E. Rubin and J. L. Farber, editors. Philadelphia: J. B. Lippincott Co. p. 1481.

Minireview: Identification of disease genes and somatic gene therapy: an overview and prospects for the aged. Pragna I. Patel. 1993. *Journal of Gerontology: Biological Sciences.* 48:B80–B85. Abstract says "Once the success and reliability of ongoing gene therapy trials for various human diseases is established, it may then be considered in the prevention and treatment of chronic, disabling diseases such as Alzheimer's disease, Parkinson's disease, arthritis, and diabetes as well as intervention of immunosenescence, when the relevant genes have been cloned. Ethical considerations for gene therapy for aging are similar to those for gene therapy in general. In addition, the ethics of gene therapy for treating diseases versus intervention of the normal aging process must be considered."

The New York Times. Jan. 23, 1993, p. 1. Story on Clinton's order reversing abortion restrictions. Also, an editorial on Clinton discarding the Reagan and Bush anti-abortion "gag rule" and related regulations.

Chlorpromazine and mental health. Proceedings of the symposium held under the auspices of Smith, Kline & French Laboratories. 1955. Lea & Febiger.

Promising protein for Parkinson's. Research News by Rick Weiss. 1993. *Science.* 260:1072–1073.

CHAPTER 12

Location of Huntington's disease degeneration in brain. In *Pathology*. E. Rubin and J. L. Farber, editors. Philadelphia: J.B. Lippincott Co. p. 1481.

Diagnosis of dementia and depression. A roundtable discussion: part 2. Panelists include Robert N. Butler, Trey Sunderland, Sanford Finkel, and Frederick Sherman. 1992. *Geriatrics*. 47:49–57.

A functional anatomical study of unipolar depression. Wayne C. Drevets, Tom O. Videen, Joseph L. Price, Sheldon H. Preskorn, S. Thomas Carmichael, and Marcus E. Raichle. 1992. *Journal of Neuroscience*. 12:3628–3641.

Stressful experience, brain and emotions: developmental, genetic and hormonal influences. Bruce S. McEwen. In *The Cognitive Neuroscience*. Michael S. Gazzaniga, editor. 1994. Cambridge, MA: MIT Press. In press.

Stress and the individual: mechanisms leading to disease. Bruce S. McEwen and Eliot Stellar. 1993. *Archives of Internal Medicine*. 153:2093–2101.

The New York Times, Jan. 13, 1993, page C-12. Sandra Blakslee on search for causes of chronic fatigue syndrome.

Letter commenting on the self injurious behavior of Lesch Nyhan patients. By B. H. King and R. E. Poland. 1991. *American Journal of Psychiatry*. 148:1617–1618.

Identification of 17 independent mutations responsible for human hypoxanthine-guanine phosphoribosyltransferase (HPRT) deficiency. B. L. Davidson, et al. 1991. *American Journal of Human Genetics*. 48:951–958.

Characterization of mutations in phenotypic variatiants of hypoxanthine phosphoribosyltransferase deficiency. Karin Serge-Peterson, J. Chambers, T. Page, O. W. Jones, and W. L Nyhan. 1992. *Human Molecular Genetics*. 1:427–432.

Protein metabolism in phenylketonuria and Lesch-Nyhan syndrome. By members of the Nutrition Research Group, Clinical Research Center, Harrow, United Kingdom. 1990. *Pediatric Research*. 28:240–246.

A potential animal model for Lesch-Nyhan syndrome through introduction of HPRT mutations into mice. M. R. Kuehn, A. Bradley, E. J. Robertson, and M. J. Evans. 1987. *Nature*. 326:295–298. Abstract says "How the resulting alterations in urine metabolism lead to the severe symptoms characteristic of Lesch-Nyhan patients is still not understood."

Biochemical evidence of dysfunction of brain neurotransmitters in the Lesch-Nyhan syndrome. Kenneth G. Lloyd, et al. 1981. *New England Journal of Medicine*. 305:1106–1111.

Expression of human HPRT in the central nervous system of transgenic mice. J. Timothy Stout, Howard Y. Chen, John Brennand, C. Thomas Caskey, and Ralph L. Brinster. 1985. *Nature*. 317:250–252.

Lesch-Nyhan disease and HPRT deficiency. Karen Sege-Peterson, William L. Nyhan, and Theodore Page. In *The Molecular and Genetic Basis of Neurological Disease*. 1992. Stoneham, MA: Butterworth and Heinemann. pp. 241–259.

Biochemical Correlates of Auto-Aggressive Behavior. Theodore Page and William L. Nyhan. In *Application of Basic Neuroscience to Child Psychiatry*. Stephen I. Deutsch, Abraham Weizman, and Ronit Weitzman, editors. 1990. New York: Plenum Publishing Corp.

The Lesch-Nyhan disease. William L. Nyhan. In *Destructive Behavior in Developmental Disabilities: Diagnosis and Treatment*. T. Thompson and D. G. Gray, editors. 1994. Newbury Park, CA: Sage Publishing Co. pp. 181–197.

Abnormalities of purine and pyrimidine metabolism. Theodore Page and William L. Nyhan. In *Neurologic Aspects of Pediatrics*. B. Berg, editor. 1992. Stoneham, MA: Butterworth-Heinemann.

Sounding Board: The Frankenstein factor. 1977. *New England Journal of Medicine*. 297:665. A commentary on the debates over psychosurgery and recombinant DNA work.

Causes of schizophrenia: an overview. Kayla F. Bernheim and Richard R. J. Lewine. In *Schizophrenia: Symptoms, Causes, Treatments*. 1979. New York: W. W. Norton & Company.

Hypothesis. Dopamine and schizophrenia: a theory revisited and revised. Fritz A. Henn. *Lancet*, Aug. 5, 1978, pp. 293–295.

Preliminary Communication. Schizophrenia-like psychosis caused by a metabolic disorder. L. Pepplinkhuizen, W. Blom, J. Bruinvels, and P. Moleman. *Lancet*, March 1, 1980.

The New York Times, March 18, 1986. Schizophrenia focus shifts to dramatic changes in brain. Harold M. Schmeck, Jr.

Quantitative cytoarchitectural studies of the cerebral cortex of schizophrenics. Francine M. Benes, Jessica Davidson, and Edward D. Bird. 1986. *Archives of General Psychiatry*. 43:31–35.

Postmortem evidence of structural brain changes in schizophhrenia. Differences in brain weight, temporal horn area, and the hippocampal gyrus compared with affective disorder. Rosemary Brown, Nigel Colter, J. A. Nicholas Corsellis, Timothy J. Crow, Christopher D. Frith, Roger Jagoe, Eve C. Johnstone, and Laura Marsh. 1986. *Archives of General Psychiatry*. 43:36–42.

The New York Times, Oct. 15, 1985. New ravage of AIDS: brain damage. Harold M. Schmeck, Jr.

HIV-1 envelope gp 120 alters astrocytres in human brain cultures. Lynn Pulliam, David West, Nancy Haigwood, and Raymond A. Swanson. 1993. *AIDS Research and Human Retroviruses*. 9:439–444. Their abstract says the majority of AIDS patients will experience some degree of dementia induced by HIV. They hypothesize that AIDS dementia may partially involve a perturbation of astrocyte function by gp120.

AIDS brain research broadens in search of mechanisms. Celia Hooper. 1991. *Journal of NIH Research*, November 1991, pp. 17–19.

Silent HIV infections. Editorial by William A. Haseltine. *New England Journal of Medicine*. 320:1487–1489.

The changing rate of major depression. The Cross National Collaborative Group. 1992. *Journal of the American Medical Association*. 268:3098–3105.

NIMH Media Advisory 11/26/93. "Higher rates of depression observed in women may be linked to differences in biochemistry and childhood socialization that render some women more vulnerable than men to the illness." These findings were developed at a workshop developed as part of the women's health research initiative at the NIMH. Published as a special November issue of the *Journal of Affective Disorders* devoted exclusively to women and depression.

General Review: Steroids and depression. Beverley E. Pearson Murphy. 1991. *Journal of Steroid Biochemistry and Molecular Biology*. 38:537–559.

Neuroanatomical circuits in depression: implications for treatment mechanisms. Wayne C. Drevets and Marcus E. Raichle. 1992. *Psychopharmacology Bulletin*. 28:261–272.

Preferential reduction of binding of 125I-iodopindolol to beta-1 adrenergic receptors in the amygdala of rat after antidepressant treatments. G. A. Ordway, et al. *Journal of Pharmacology and Experimental Therapeutics*. 257:681–690.

The New York Times, Jan. 24, 1993. Homeless, insane and on crack. A danger to themselves and others. Celia W. Dugger.

Harvard Focus, April 1, 1993. Huntington's flaw discovered. James Gusella, et al., as reported in *Cell*. Same issue: Protein critical to brain-muscle communication identified. Gerald Fischbach. They call the protein ARIA for acetylcholine receptor inducing activity. May be the first of a new family of proteins. They say it may have clinical applications including myasthenia gravis and Alzheimer's disease.

Wall Street Journal, Dec. 2, 1993. Michael W. Miller. Dark days: the staggering cost of depression. Chart cites November,1993, *Journal of Clinical Psychiatry*, study by Paul Greenberg et al. putting total cost of depression at $43.7 billion a year and substantially higher than schizophrenia which is put at $33 billion. The story says the study published in *JCP* "includes some disputable estimates and is likely to become a hotly debated political document."

Thinking about Prozac. Samuel H. Barondes. 1994. *Science*. 263:1102–1103.

Molecules and Mental Illness. Samuel H. Barondes. 1993. New York: Scientific American Library.

Postpubertal emergence of hyperresponsiveness to stress and to amphetamine after neonatal excitotoxic hippocampal damage: a potential animal model of schizophrenia. Barbara K. Lipska, George E. Jaskiw, and Daniel R. Weinberger. 1993. *Neuropsychopharmacology*. 9:67–75.

Evidence of dysfunction of a prefrontal-limbic network in schizophrenia: a magnetic resonance imaging and regional cerebral blood flow study of discordant monozygotic twins. Daniel R. Weinberger, Karen Faith Berman, Richard Suddarth, and E. Fuller Torrey. 1992. *American Journal of Psychiatry*. 149:890–897.

Archives of General Psychiatry "News and Views." Cortical maldevelopment, anti-psychotic drugs and schizophrenia: a neuroanatomical reductionism. Daniel R. Weinberger and Barbara K. Lipska.

Schizophrenia. Henry R. Rollin. *British Medical Journal*, June 30, 1979, pp. 1773–1775.

Mapping the Brain and its Functions. Integrating Enabling Technologies into Neuroscience Research. Constance M. Pechura and Joseph B. Martin, editors. 1991. Institute of Medicine. National Academy Press.

CHAPTER 13

Possible person-to-person transmission of Creutzfeldt–Jakob disease. Philip Duffy, John Wolf, George Collins, Arthur G. DeVoe, Barbara Streeten, and David Cowen. 1974. *New England Journal of Medicine*. 290:692.

Location of Creutzfeld–Jakob disease degeneration in brain. In *Pathology*. E. Rubin and J. L. Farber, editors. Philadelphia: J. B. Lippincott Co. p. 1486.

Spongiform appearance of Creutzfeld-Jakob disease degeneration in brain: based on slide provided by Ralph Rubin, The Johns Hopkins University School of Medicine.

Legionnaire's disease reference was from a personal communication from Donald Fredrickson.

The figures on recent cases of Creutzfeld-Jakob disease were kindly supplied by Paul Brown of NIH.

The New York Times, April 20, 1985. Harold M. Schmeck, Jr., on the pituitary hormone Creutzfeld-Jakob d isease story. This story may have been the only public announcement of the halt in the federally sponsored program of providing human growth hormone via harvested pituitary glands. The Department of Health, Education and Welfare notified parents of children who had taken the material, but that was apparently all.

"Doctors in the United States and Britain had halted the use of pituitary glands from cadavers in 1985. In France they continued to use pituitary glands, but subjected the material to an additional purification step." Source: "French scientists may face charges over Creutzfeld-Jakob disease outbreak." *Science*, Vol. 261, July 30, 1993. News and Comment by Michael Balter. p. 543.

Kuru Sorcery. Shirley Lindenbaum. 1979. Mayfield Publishing Company.

Slow Viruses. David H. Adams and Thomas M. Bell. 1976. Reading, MA: Addison-Wesley Publishing Company, Inc., Advanced Book Program.

The "brave new world" of infectious amyloidosis. Paul Brown. *Molecular Neurobiology*, Vol. 8, April–June, 1994.

The "Friendly fire" in medicine: hormones, homografts, and Creutzfeldt-Jakob disease. Review article by Paul Brown, Michael A. Preece, and Robert G. Will. *Lancet*. Vol. 340, July 4, 1992.

Iatrogenic Creutzfeldt-Jakob disease: an example of the interplay between ancient genes and modern medicine. Paul Brown, et al. 1994. *Neurology*. 44:291–293.

An example of the interplay between ancient genes and modern medicine. P. Brown, L. Cervenakova, L. G. Goldfarb, W. R. McCombie, R. Rubenstein, R. G. Wioll, M. Pocchiaria, J. F. Martinez-Lage, C. Scalici, C. Masulo, G. Graupera, J. Ligan, and D. C. Gajdusek. 1994. *Neurology*. 44:291–293.

Transmissible and non-transmissible amyloidoses: autocatalytic post-translational conversion of host precursor proteins to beta pleated sheet configurations. 1988. D. Carleton Gajdusek. *Journal of Neuroimmunology*. 20:95–110.

Neurological progress. The phenotypic expression of different mutations in transmissible human spongiform encephalopathy. Paul Brown. 1992. *Reviews of Neurology (Paris)*. 148:317–327.

Scrapie agent: prions or virinos? Richard H. Kimberlin. 1982. *Nature*. 297:107.

Gene knock-out technology: The "whys,'" "whats," and "hows" of gene targeting in neuroscience. A. J. Silva and K.P. Giese. Center for Learning and Memory. Cold Spring Harbor Laboratory, New York.

Mice devoid of PrP are resistant to scrapie. H. Bueler, A. Aguzzi, A. Sailer, R.-A. Greiner, P. Autenried, M. Aguet, and C. Weissmann. 1993. *Cell*. 73:1339–1347.

Slow, latent and temperate virus infections. D. Carleton Gajdusek, Clarence J. Gibbs, Jr., and Michael Alpers, editors. National Institute of Neurological Diseases and Blindness Monograph No. 2, NIH, 1965.

Studies on slow virus diseases. D. Carleton Gajdusek and C. J. Gibbs, Jr. In *NIH: An Account of Research in its Laboratories and Clinics*. DeWitt Stetten, Jr., editor, and W. T. Carrigan, associate editor. 1984. New York: Academic Press.

Human to human transmission of rabies virus by corneal transplant. S. A. Houff, J. L. Sever, et al. 1979. *New England Journal of Medicine*. 300:603–604.

Scrapie in sheep and goats. Alan G. Dickinson. In *Slow Virus Diseases of Animals and Man*. R. H. Kimberlin, editor. Amsterdam: North-Hollland Publishing Company.
    The specific references are: Cuille and Chelle. 1936. Contre Roundue Academy of Science, Paris. Vol. 203, p. 1552.
    W. S. Gordon, A. Brownlee, and B. R. Wilson. 1939. Proceedings of the Third International Congress of Microbiology, New York. p. 362.

Figure 13.1 represents results of positron emission tomography (PET) and is based on a diagram in *American Family Physician*, September, 1991, p. 979.

CHAPTER 14

Appearance of Alzheimer's brain tissue, based on *How Things Work: The Brain*. St. Remy Press, Time-Life Books, Inc.

Degeneration in vitro of neurons over-expressing the Alzheimer amyloid protein precursor. *Nature*, Sept. 3, 1992. p. 64.

Alzheimer's pathology begins to yield its secrets. Jean Marx. 1993. *Science*. 259:457–458.

New piece in Alzheimer's puzzle. John Travis. 1993. *Science*. 261:828–829.

The Early Story of Alzheimer's Disease. A. Alzheimer, O. Fischer, F. Bonfiglio, E. Kraepelin, and G. Perusini. Katherine Bick, Luigi Amaducci, and Giancarlo Pepeu, editors. Liviana Press.

Alzheimer's disease, Down's syndrome, and aging. 1982. *Annals of the New York Academy of Sciences*. Vol. 396.

Familial Alzheimer's disease linked to a defective gene on chromosome 14. Jean Marx. *Science*, Oct. 23, 1992, pp. 550 and 668.
Minireview: Identification of disease genes and somatic gene therapy; an overview and prospects for the aged. Pragna I. Patel. 1993. *Journal of Gerontology: Biological Sciences*. 48:B80–B85.

Observations in a preliminary open trial of estradiol therapy for senile dementia-Alzheimer's type. Howard Fillit, Herman Weinreb, Ina Cholst, Victoria Luine, Bruce McEwen, Roberto Amador, and John Zabriskie. 1986. *Psychoneuroendocrinology*. 11:337–345.

In vivo effects by estrone sulfate on the central nervous system-senile dementia (Alzheimer's type). Hideo Honjo, et al. 1989. *Journal of Steroid Biochemistry*. 34:521–525.

The prevalence of dementia and Alzheimer's disease in Shanghai, China: impact of age, gender and education. Mingyuan Zhang, et al. 1990. *Annals of Neurology*. 27:428–437.

Animal models of Alzheimer's disease: glutamatergic denervation as an alternative approach to cholinergic denervation. Trond Myhrer. 1993. *Neuroscience and Biobehavioral Reviews*. 17:195–202.

Hippocampal formation atrophy in the ageing and the prediction of Alzheimer's disease. Mony J. de Leon. In *Aging and Dementia: A Methodological Approach*. A. Burns, editor. 1993. London: Edward Arnold.

Differential rearing conditions in rats: effects on neurochemistry in neocortical areas and cognitive behaviors. Trond Myhrer, et al. 1992. *Brain Research Bulletin*. 28:427–434. He cites M. R. Rosenzweig, "Experience, memory and the brain." 1984. *American Psychologist*. 39:365–376, and M. R. Rosenzweig, et al., "Effects of environmental complexity and training on brain chemistry and anatomy: a replication and extension." 1962. *Journal of Comparative and Physiological Psychology*. 55:429–437. All this is pursuant to the statement in the introduction that "environmental factors can modify several aspects of the central nervous system. Rosenzweig and co-workers demonstrated some decades ago that rats housed in enriched environments displayed increased brain weight, higher levels of acetylcholinesterase in neocortex, and an increased number of dendritic spines compared to control rats reared in isolated social environments. The brain measures were found to correlate positively with learning and memory."

Brain aging and Alzheimer's disease, "wear and tear'" versus "use it or lose it." D. F. Swaab. 1991. *Neurobiology of Aging*. 12:317–324.
Commentaries on Swaab:
   James E. Black, Krystyna R. Isaacs, and William T. Greenough, *Usual vs Successful Aging: Some Notes on Experiential Factors*, pp. 325–328. Two interesting points in the abstract: "Exposure to complex expereince in old age can also generate new synapses in cerebral cortex and cerebellum." " ... use of environmental therapies should encompass the entire life span to produce succesful aging."
   Ian Davies, pp. 328–330, says, in conclusion, the Swaab concept is optimistic but doesn't "withstand critical examination."
   James W. Geddes and Carl W. Cotman, *Plasticity in Alzheimer's Disease: Too Much or Not Enough?* pp. 330–333.

Low body mass index in demented outpatients. W. G. Berlinger and J. F. Potter. 1991. *Journal of the American Gerontological Society*. 39:973-978.

Location of Alzheimer's disease degeneration in brain. *Pathology*. E. Rubin and J. L. Farber. Philadelphia: J. B. Lippincott Co. pp. 1481 and 1486.

CHAPTER 15

How the brain ages. Brain Concepts, by Joe Carey, Society for Neuroscience, 1992.

The impact of long-term exercise training on psychological function in older adults. Robert D. Hill, Martha Storandt, and Mary Malley. 1993. *Journal of Gerontology: Psychological Sciences*. 48:12–17.

Aging and mental health: primary care of the healthy older adult. A roundtable discussion: part 1. Panelists include Robert N. Butler, Sanford I. Finkel, Myrna I. Lewis, Fredrick T. Sherman, and Trey Sunderland. 1992. *Geriatrics*. 47:54–65.

Optimal time of day and the magnitude of age differences in memory. Cynthia P. May, Lynn Hasher, and Ellen R. Stoltzfus. 1993. *Psychological Science*. 4:326–330. Notes that it can be misleading to gauge memory loss in old people when they are tested, as is common, in late afternoon.

The molecular biology of aging. Jeffrey P. Cohn. 1987. *BioScience*. 37:99–102. (Used for the items from the Gerontology Research Center in Baltimore and for a reminder on Hayflick's cell research.)

The Neuro-Immune-Endocrine Connection. Carl W. Cotman, Roberta E. Brinton, Albert Galaburda, Bruce S. McEwen, and Diana M. Schneider, editors. 1987. New York: Raven Press.

Memory and Brain. Larry R. Squire. 1987. Oxford: Oxford University Press. Also interviews with him.

Steroid hormone interactions with the brain: cellular and molecular aspects. Bruce S. McEwen. 1979. *Reviews of Neuroscience.* 4:1–30.

Estrogen receptors colocalize with low affinity nerve growth factors receptors in cholinergic neurons of the basal forebrain. C. D. Toran-Allerand, R. C. Miranda, W. D. L. Bentham, et al. 1992. *Proceedings of the National Academy of Sciences USA.* 89:4668–4672.

The role of estrogen deficiency in the aging central nervous system. Stanley J. Birge. In *Treatment of the Postmenopausal Woman.* R. Lobo, editor. New York: Raven Press. pp. 153–161.

Diet restriction prevents aging-induced deficits in brain phosphoinositide metabolism. 1993. *Journal of Gerontology: Biological Science*s. 48:B62–B67. Cites Roy Walford, among others.

Exercise increases average longevity of female rats despite increased food intake and no growth retardation. John O. Holloszy. 1993. *Journal of Gerontology: Biological Sciences.* 48:B97–B100.

Review. Brain aging and Alzheimer's disease, "wear and tear" versus "use it or lose it." D. F Swaab. 1991. *Neurobiology of Aging.* 12:317–324. Commentaries on pp. 325–355, including one by Bruce McEwen.

The molecular biology of aging. Jeffrey P. Cohn. 1987. *Bioscience.* 37:99–102.

Environmentally-induced changes in the brains of elderly rats. R. A. Cummins, et al. *Nature*, June 29, 1973. pp. 516–518.

Diet restriction prevents aging-induced deficits in brain phosphoinositide metabolism. Ashiwel S. Undie and Eitan Friedman. 1993. *Journal of Gerontology: Biological Sciences.* 48:B62–B67.

The impact of long-term exercise training on psychological function in older adults. Robert D. Hill, et al. 1993. *Journal of Gerontology: Psychological Sciences.* 48:P12–P17.

Effects of estrogen replacement therapy on cerebral perfusion and cognition among postmenopausal women. Janice L. Funk, Karl F. Mortel, and John S. Meyer. 1991. *Dementia.* 2:268–272.

Effects of estrogen on memory function in surgically menopausal women. Susana M. Phillips and Barbara B. Sherwin. 1992. *Psychoneuroendocrinology.* 17:485–495.

An evaluation of psychological effects of sex hormone administration in aged women. II. Results of therapy after eighteen months. Betty McDonald Caldwell. 1954. *Journal of Gerontology.* 9:168–174.

Regionally specific loss of neurons in the aging human hippocampus. Mark J. West . 1993. *Neurobiology of Aging.* 14:287–293.

Age, gender, medical treatment, and medication effects on smell identification. Jonathan A. Ship and James M. Weiffenbach. 1993. *Journal of Gerontology: Medical Sciences.* 48:M26–M32.

Aging and mental health: primary care of the healthy older adult. A roundtable discussion: part 1. Panelists include Robert N. Butler, Trey Sunderland, Sanford Finkel, and Frederick Sherman. 1992. *Geriatrics.* 47:54–65.
Harvard Focus, Feb. 25, 1993. "While a significant effort has been made to understand the neural degeneration associated with diseases such as Alzheimer's, little is known about the varying degrees of memory loss seen in healthy individuals as they age."

The prevalence of dementia and Alzheimer's disease in Shanghai, China: impact of age, gender and education. Mingyuan Zhang, et al. 1990. *Annals of Neurology.* 27:428–437.

Steroid hormones are multifunctional messengers to the brain. Bruce S. McEwen. 1991. *Trends in Endocrinology and Metabolism.* 2:62–67. Among other things, the abstract says "Future research on the actions of steroids on the brain may advance the notion that the endocrine system has some responsibility for determining the individual traits of an animal in brain function and behavior."

Re-examination of the glucocorticoid hypothesis of stress and aging. Bruce S. McEwen. 1992. *Progress in*

Brain Research. 93:365–383.

Brain aging and Alzheimer's disease: "wear and tear" versus "use it or lose it." D. F. Swaab. 1991. *Neurobiology of Aging.* 12:317–324.
Commentaries on Swaab:

James E. Black, Krystyna R. Isaacs, and William T. Greenough. *Usual vs Successful Aging: Some Notes on Experiential Factors.* pp. 325–328. Two interesting points in the abstract: "Exposure to complex experience in old age can also generate new synapses in cerebral cortex and cerebellum." " ... use of environmental therapies should encompass the entire life span to produce successful aging."

Joan Davies. pp. 328–330. Says, in conclusion, that the Swaab concept is optimistic but doesn't "withstand critical examination."

James W. Geddes and Carl W. Cotman. Plasticity in Alzheimer's disease: too much or not enough? pp. 330–333.

J. Timothy Greenamyre. pp. 334–336.

Herbert Haug and Reinhard Eggers. pp. 336–338.

Michel A. Hofman. pp. 338–340.

David M.A. Mann. pp. 340–343.

Mark P. Mattson. pp. 343–346.

Bruce S. McEwen. When is stimulation too much of a good thing? pp. 346–348.

Robert M. Sapolsky. Energetics and neuron death: hibernating bears or starving refugees? pp. 348–349.

Stephen W. Scheff. Use or abuse. pp. 349–351.

Michael V. Sofroniew. Can activity modulate the susceptibility of neurons to degeneration? pp. 351-352.

D. F. Swaab. His final response to the comments. pp. 352–355.

Brain aging press conference at the Society for Neuroscience annual meeting, Nov. 9, 1993, in Washington, DC. Bruce McEwen, Michael Meaney, Sonia Lupien, James Golomb, and Mony deLeon. Based on the following abstracts:
Basal cortisol levels, neuropsychological performance and normal human aging. S. Lupien, S. Sharma, N. P. V. Nair, and M. J. Meaney. 1993. *Society for Neuroscience Abstracts.* 19: No. 247.2.
Hippocampal specific atrophy is associated with delayed secondary memory impairment in normal human aging. J. Golomb, A. Kluger, M. J. deLeon, A. Convit, H. Rusinek, A. E. George, S. de Santi, and S. H. Ferris. 1993. *Society for Neuroscience Abstracts.* 19: No. 447.12.

CHAPTER 16

Two articles presented as "A debate: is homosexuality biologically influenced?" On one side are Simon LeVay and Dean Hamer. On the other side is William Byne. *Scientific American*, May, 1994.

A linkage between DNA markers on the X chromosome and male sexual orientation. Dean H. Hamer, Stella Hu, Victoria L. Magnuson, Nan Hu, and Angela M. L. Pattatucci. *Science*, Vol. 261, July 16, 1993. pp. 321–327. There is also a Research News item by Robert Pool on page 291.

Minireview: Identification of disease genes and somatic gene therapy; an overview and prospects for the aged. Pragna I. Patel. 1993. *Journal of Gerontology: Biological Sciences.* 48:B80–B85. Abstract says " ... Once the success and reliability of ongoing gene therapy trials for various human diseases is established, it may then be considered in the prevention and treatment of chronic, disabling diseases such as Alzheimer's disease, Parkinson's disease, arthritis, and diabetes as well as intervention of immunosenescence, when the relevant genes have been cloned. Ethical considerations for gene therapy for aging are similar to those for gene therapy in general. In addition, the ethics of gene therapy for treating diseases versus intervention of the normal aging process must be considered."

Sounding Board: The Frankenstein factor. 1977. *New England Journal of Medicine.* 297:665. It is a commentary on the debates over psychosurgery and recombinant DNA work.

The New York Times, Nov. 15, 1992. Florida Court Rejects New Death Definition. Tallahassee, FL. The Florida Supreme Court has upheld a lower court's ruling that prevented a baby born with much of her brain missing from being declared dead so that her organs could be used for transplants.

The New York Times, Oct. 21, 1992. Court Says Killer Can't Be Forced to Be Sane Enough to Die. New Orleans. The Louisiana Supreme Court has decided that an incompetent prisoner cannot be forced to take drugs that might make him sane enough to be executed.

The New York Times, June 24, 1993. Geneticist Is Badly Hurt in Mail Bomb Explosion. San Francisco. A geneticist widely known for his research into Down's syndrome and other genetic defects was critically injured Tuesday when he opened a mail bomb sent to his home, the Federal Bureau of Investigation said today.

The New York Times, June 25, 1993. Yale Professor Is Injured by Blast: Mail Bomb Tied to Terror in 70's.

The Creative Loop. How the Brain Makes A Mind. Erich Harth. 1993. Reading, MA: Addison-Wesley Publishing Co. p. 196.

Behavioral Endocrinology. J. B. Becker, S. M. Breedlove, and D. Crews, editors. 1992. Cambridge, MA: MIT Press. *Nature*, Vol. 366, No. 6453, Nov. 25, 1993, p. 378. A review of behavioral endocrinology by Peter Marler.

Starting Points: Meeting the Needs of Our Youngest Children. Carnegie Corporation of New York. Published April 12, 1994.

The Limits of Science. Peter B. Medawar. 1984. New York: Harper & Row.

The Biology of Mental Disorders. Fourth in the series New Developments in Neuroscience. Sept. 1992. U. S. Congress. Office of Technology Assessment.

Science and Moral Priority. Merging Mind, Brain and Human Values. Roger Sperry. 1983. New York: Columbia University Press.

Summing up. The Ethical and Legal Problems in Medicine and Biomedical and Behavioral Research. President's Commission for the Study of Ethical Problems in Medicine and Biomedical and Behavioral Research.

314

Bruce S. McEwen is Professor and Head of the Harold and Margaret Milliken Hatch Laboratory of Neuroendocrinology at The Rockefeller University in New York City. Harold M. Schmeck, Jr., is former National Science Correspondent for *The New York Times*. He is the author of several books, including *The Semi-Artificial Man* (Walker) and *Immunology: The Many-Edged Sword* (Braziller), and scores of articles for such publications as Smithsonian, *The New York Times Magazine, Boys Life*, and *Science Digest*.

Lydia Kibiuk is a free-lance medical illustrator in Baltimore, MD, and a graduate of the Johns Hopkins Department of Art as Applied to Medicine.